AF323109

Neuromuscular Junction Disorders

Additional Volumes in Preparation

Drug-Induced Movement Disorders, *edited by Kapil D. Sethi*

Neuromuscular Junction Disorders

Diagnosis and Treatment

Matthew N. Meriggioli

Rush-Presbyterian–St. Luke's Medical Center
Chicago, Illinois, U.S.A.

James F. Howard, Jr.

University of North Carolina at Chapel Hill
Chapel Hill, North Carolina, U.S.A.

C. Michel Harper

Mayo Clinic Foundation
Rochester, Minnesota, U.S.A.

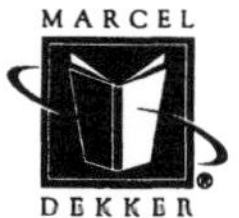

MARCEL DEKKER, INC.   NEW YORK · BASEL

Although great care has been taken to provide accurate and current information, neither the author(s) nor the publisher, nor anyone else associated with this publication, shall be liable for any loss, damage, or liability directly or indirectly caused or alleged to be caused by this book. The material contained herein is not intended to provide specific advice or recommendations for any specific situation.

Trademark notice: Product or corporate names may be trademarks or registered trademarks and are used only for identification and explanation without intent to infringe.

Library of Congress Cataloging-in-Publication Data
A catalog record for this book is available from the Library of Congress.

ISBN: 0-8247-4079-3

This book is printed on acid-free paper.

Headquarters
Marcel Dekker, Inc., 270 Madison Avenue, New York, NY 10016, U.S.A.
tel: 212-696-9000; fax: 212-685-4540

Distribution and Customer Service
Marcel Dekker, Inc., Cimarron Road, Monticello, New York 12701, U.S.A.
tel: 800-228-1160; fax: 845-796-1772

Eastern Hemisphere Distribution
Marcel Dekker AG, Hutgasse 4, Postfach 812, CH-4001 Basel, Switzerland
tel: 41-61-260-6300; fax: 41-61-260-6333

World Wide Web
http://www.dekker.com

The publisher offers discounts on this book when ordered in bulk quantities. For more information, write to Special Sales/Professional Marketing at the headquarters address above.

Current printing (last digit):

10 9 8 7 6 5 4 3 2 1

PRINTED IN THE UNITED STATES OF AMERICA

Foreword

Few practicing neurologists have the energy, commitment and expertise to complete a substantial monograph. With the publication of this text on neuromuscular junction disorders, Dr. Matthew Meriggioli has achieved this almost single-handed, aside from the valuable chapters contributed by Dr. Michel Harper on congenital myasthenia, and by Dr. James Howard on neurotoxicology as it relates to disorders of the neuromuscular junction. Monographs with a restricted authorship have practical advantages, ensuring a uniformity of style that readers will here find to be lucid and readily accessible.

Neurologists sometimes feel diffident in managing myasthenic disorders, not only because of the risks of respiratory or bulbar weakness that can sometimes be life-threatening but also because of the diverse and sometimes uncertain treatment options. This volume should serve to reassure them. It is intended as a clinician's guide, providing the scientific background with accompanying clear illustrations before turning to diagnosis and management. Readers can be confident that all three authors are themselves clinically active in the fields they cover, and are thus well qualified to provide an authoritative work. Indeed, the clinical chapters contain illustrative and informative case histories from the authors' own practice. Dr. Meriggioli stresses the relative lack of evidence-based criteria for many of the treatments used in myasthenia, but offers balanced recommendations where this is the case. I am confident that this text will be well received by practising neurologists, and I warmly commend it.

John Newsom-Davis, MD FRS
Professor Emeritus, University of Oxford
Department of Clinical Neurology
Radcliffe Infirmary
Oxford, England

Preface

Diseases of the neuromuscular junction (NMJ) include a large spectrum of acquired and inherited disorders mainly characterized by fluctuating muscle weakness and fatigability of ocular, bulbar or limb muscles. Remarkable progress has been made in our understanding of the pathogenesis of these disorders in recent years. Furthermore, our ability to diagnose these conditions has improved significantly due to the widespread availability of immunologic tests, the use of in vitro electrophysiologic and microstructural studies, and the refinement of sensitive clinical electrodiagnostic tests of neuromuscular transmission. Despite these advances, significant questions remain to be answered by the researcher and the clinician, and disagreement exists amongst specialists regarding therapy and management of patients. This lack of a "consensus opinion" makes it difficult for the physician as well as the physician–trainee to approach these disorders in a systematic fashion. Unfortunately, existing textbooks covering this topic do not present a detailed and concise resource for diagnosis and management of these patients.

This book is directed toward advanced students, residents and practitioners of neurology, and in particular those who are involved in the evaluation and care of patients with neuromuscular junction disorders. In response to the ever-increasing mass of neuroscience information, we have attempted to present a monograph offering a concise, comprehensive and up-to-date resource covering all aspects of the diagnosis and clinical management of patients with diseases of the neuromuscular junction with an emphasis on the clinical aspects of this very interesting group of conditions. The basic physiology, anatomy, pathophysiology and immunology pertaining to these diseases are covered in only sufficient depth to allow the clinician to better understand the mechanism of signs and symptoms, the physiologic basis for diagnostic tests, and the rationale for specific treatments.

It is important for the reader to realize that there are a number of approaches to the treatment of the common disorders of neuromuscular transmission. The reason for this disagreement is apparent when one considers the surprising paucity of randomized, controlled, prospective therapeutic studies addressing treatment issues in these diseases. This is particularly apparent in the most common disorder of neuromuscular transmission, myasthenia gravis. For this reason, we present the commonly prescribed treatments for these disorders, the apparent rationale for their use, and the strength of scientific evidence for efficacy of a certain intervention based on the existing international literature. We attempt to explain why all physicians do not use a particular intervention in the same way or in all clinical situations. The reader may develop his/her own approach based on this evidence. The art of providing optimal medical care to this group of patients often lies in deciding when to treat aggressively and when to proceed cautiously and conservatively. The information provided in this book will assist the clinician in making this important therapeutic decision by presenting data regarding the natural history of the disease in question and by detailing the adverse effects of specific treatment modalities. As in other areas of medicine, therapeutic decision-making in disorders of the NMJ is a risk/benefit assessment.

The book is formatted into two main parts. The first part (Chapters 1–3) covers the basic anatomy, physiology, pathophysiology, and diagnosis of the NMJ. The features of presynaptic, synaptic and postsynaptic disorders of the NMJ are discussed in general as an introduction to the more specific coverage of the individual disorders. A brief coverage of the immunology relevant to the immune-mediated disorders of the NMJ is also presented. Part I ends with a discussion of the diagnostic approach to NMJ disorders including immunologic, pharmacologic and electrophysiologic testing. The information presented in Part I provides a background for understanding concepts presented in Part II. Part II is comprised of the different individual disorders of neuromuscular transmission. Chapters examining myasthenia gravis, Lambert-Eaton syndrome, congenital myasthenic syndromes and human botulism, tetanus and venom poisoning are presented. The final chapter of the book covers the effects of pharmacologic agents on the NMJ. Tables and cross-referenced charts are used to facilitate understanding of the information and to allow for integration of the text.

It is our hope that this volume will aid students and clinicians to gain a better understanding of the clinical evaluation, investigation, diagnosis and treatment of diseases of the NMJ, and that investigators and more experienced clinicians will find it a valuable resource.

Matthew N. Meriggioli
James F. Howard, Jr.
C. Michel Harper

Contents

Contents

xi

Neuromuscular Junction Disorders

1

Anatomy and Physiology of the Neuromuscular Junction

I. INTRODUCTION

Clinicians who regularly care for patients with disorders of the neuromuscular junction (NMJ) realize the importance of understanding its anatomy and physiology. A working knowledge of the anatomy and physiology of the normal NMJ is obviously needed to fully understand the pathophysiology of disorders affecting this highly specialized structure. In addition, a full appreciation of its normal function also forms the basis for understanding the principles underlying diagnostic testing and the mechanisms of certain therapeutic interventions. A review of the clinically relevant aspects of the anatomy and physiology of normal neuromuscular transmission follows. A number of clinical examples are provided to illustrate the application of anatomic and physiologic concepts to the diagnosis and treatment of patients with NMJ disease.

II. THE NEUROMUSCULAR JUNCTION: A SPECIALIZED SYNAPSE

There are two main types of synapses: electrical and chemical. At an electrical synapse, two excitable cells communicate by direct passage of electrical current between them. At a chemical synapse, an action potential causes a transmitter substance to be released from the presynaptic neuron. The transmitter diffuses across the extracellular synaptic space and binds to receptors on the postsynaptic cell to change the electrical properties of the postsynaptic membrane.

The NMJ is a specialized chemical synapse between the axon of a motor neuron and a somatic muscle fiber. The unique structure and functional organization of this synapse allows for the process of transmitting an electrical impulse from a motor axon to the muscle fiber it innervates. The development of sophisticated techniques (including electron microscopy and in vitro neurophysiologic studies) has considerably enhanced our knowledge of the microanatomy (Fig. 1.1) and physiology of the NMJ. The NMJ has

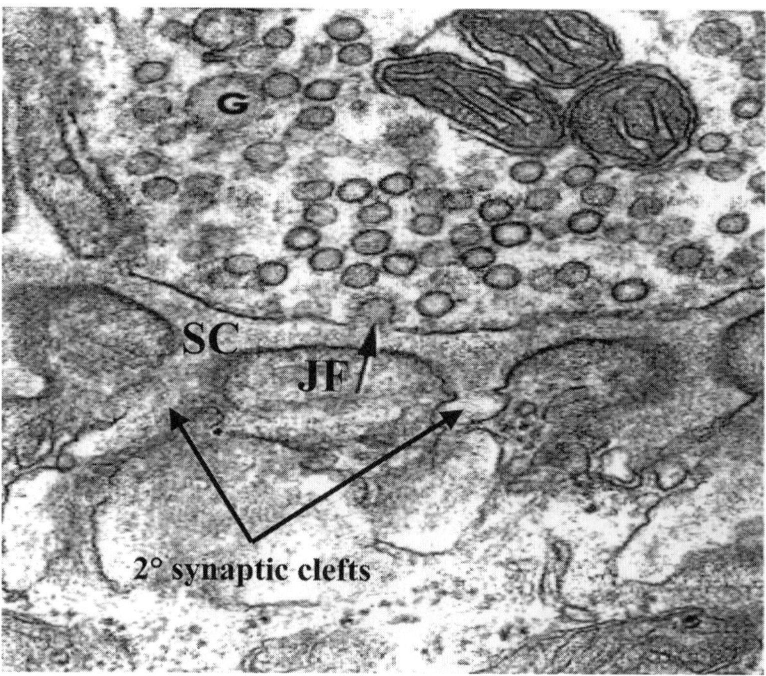

Figure 1.1 Electron micrograph of the normal neuromuscular junction. The presynaptic nerve terminal is on top with the postsynaptic muscle membrane on the bottom. The short arrow marks a synaptic vesicle that has fused with the presynaptic membrane and released its contents of acetylcholine molecules into the synaptic cleft (SC). The secondary synaptic clefts are the spaces between the junctional folds (JF). A giant synaptic vesicle (G) is seen within the presynaptic nerve terminal. (From Ref. 1.)

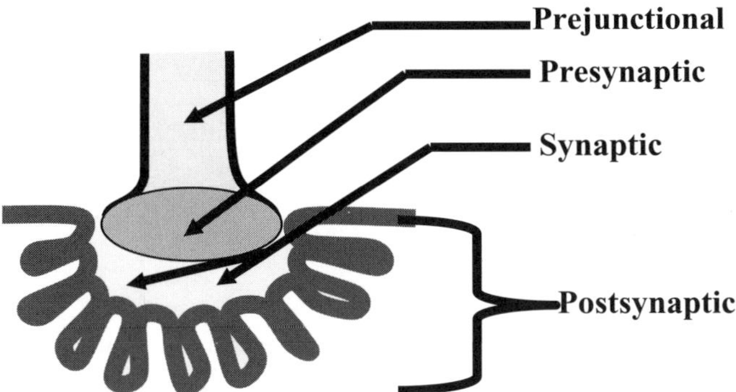

Figure 1.2 Diagrammatic representation of Fig. 1.1 illustrating the components of the neuromuscular junction: (1) the presynaptic nerve terminal, (2) the synaptic space, and (3) the postsynaptic muscle membrane.

three basic components (Figs. 1.1 and 1.2): (a) the presynaptic region, consisting of a terminal branch of a motor axon (the nerve terminal) in which the neurotransmitter is synthesized, stored, and released; (b) the synaptic space lined with a basement membrane; and (c) the postsynaptic membrane which contains the receptor for the neurotransmitter. In human voluntary muscle, the neurotransmitter is acetylcholine and the receptor is the nicotinic acetylcholine receptor.

III.　ANATOMY OF THE NEUROMUSCULAR JUNCTION

A.　The Presynaptic Region

Each motor neuron in the brainstem and spinal cord gives rise to an axon that branches distally to provide a single nerve terminal to each of the muscle fibers it innervates. (Fig. 1.3) (1). The motor neuron and the muscle fibers it innervates are collectively known as the *motor unit*. Each muscle fiber is innervated by only one motor neuron, but any single motor neuron may innervate multiple muscle fibers. In humans, an important exception to this rule is the extraocular muscles in which single muscle fibers may receive multiple innervation. This may play a role in the increased susceptibility of these muscles to certain disorders of neuromuscular transmission, such as myasthenia gravis (Chapter 4).

　　　Nerve terminals are highly specialized regions of the motor axon. An action potential originating in the brainstem or spinal cord propagates to the nerve terminal, where it sets into motion a complex chain of events resulting

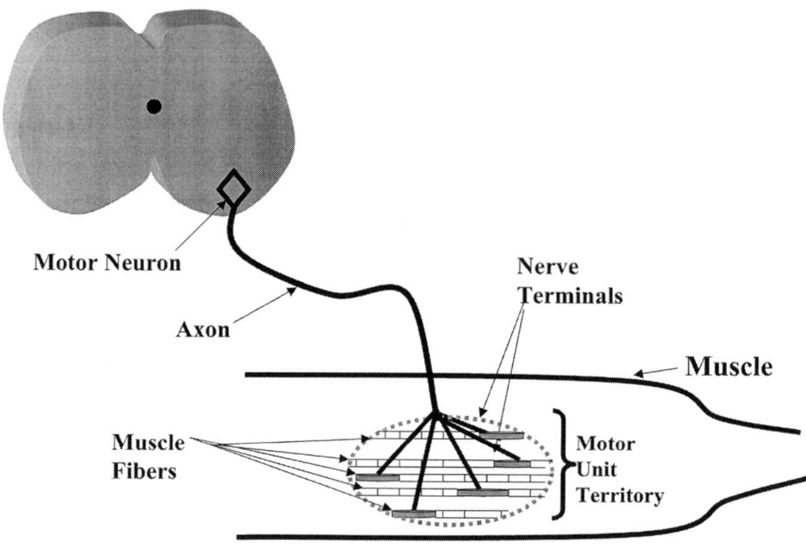

Figure 1.3 The motor unit consists of a motor neuron, its axon, and the muscle fibers innervated by that axon. A single anterior horn cell motor neuron gives rise to distal branches each supplying innervation to a single muscle fiber. Each muscle fiber receives innervation from one motor neuron (with rare exceptions; see text). The most distal aspect of the individual axonal branches is termed the nerve terminal and composes the presynaptic region of the neuromuscular junction.

in a 1000-fold increase in the rate of release of the neurotransmitter, acetylcholine (ACh). Near the NMJ, the motor nerve loses its myelin sheath and divides into fine terminal branches. As a terminal branch of an axon nears the muscle fiber, it expands into a presynaptic terminal bouton that lies in a depression in the muscle cell membrane. The terminal nerve fiber is surrounded by a sheath of epithelial cells (Henle's sheath), which also ends abruptly a short distance from the NMJ (2). The distal bulb of the nerve terminal is unmyelinated, but is "capped" by a Schwann cell (Fig. 1.4) which, in addition to its involvement in the formation of the nerve myelin sheath, may play an important role in synaptic maintenance and repair (3). A basement membrane overlies the Schwann cell laterally and becomes continuous with the basement membrane of the muscle fiber.

The nerve terminal contains a number of subcellular components. Since the primary function of the nerve terminal is to synthesize and release ACh, the enzymes and other machinery necessary for these functions are present within the nerve terminal. These include numerous mitochondria needed to meet the considerable metabolic demands of transmitter synthesis and

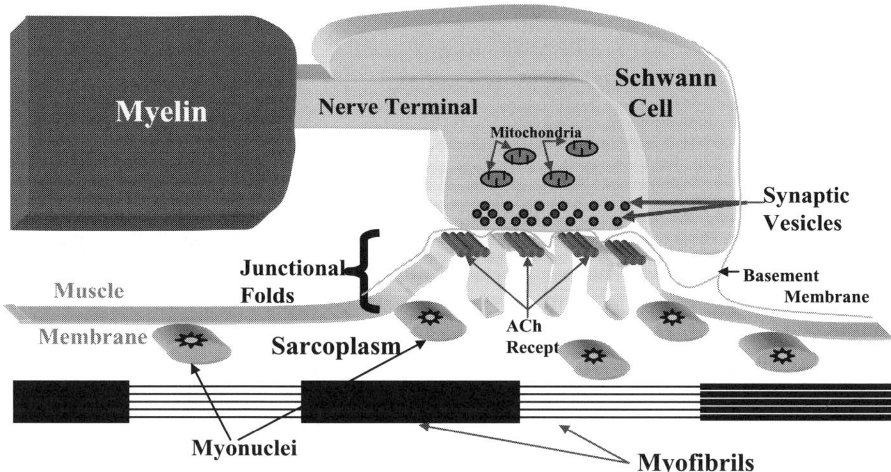

Figure 1.4 Diagrammatic representation of the major components of the mammalian neuromuscular junction. The nerve terminal is unmyelinated but is capped by a Schwann cell. It is directly aligned with the endplate region of a muscle fiber. A basement membrane overlies the Schwann cell laterally and becomes continuous with the basement membrane of the muscle fiber. The endplate region of the muscle fiber is thrown into a number of folds (junctional folds), with the acetylcholine receptors located on the crests of these folds.

release, as well as microtubules and microfilaments (4,5). The nerve terminal also contains the enzyme choline acetyltransferase, which is necessary for the synthesis of ACh (1).

The most important of the subcellular components of the nerve terminal are the synaptic vesicles, which are membrane-bound, smooth-surfaced structures containing the ACh molecules (1,6). The ACh molecules are synthesized in the nerve terminal, and packaged and stored in the synaptic vesicles. A single nerve terminal has approximately 200,000 synaptic vesicles (7). The amount of ACh in a vesicle constitutes a basic unit or *quantum* of neurotransmitter. One quantum of ACh is defined as the number of transmitter molecules contained in a single vesicle (about 6000–10,000 ACh molecules) (1).

The synaptic vesicles in the nerve terminal are arranged in at least two pools: the readily releasable pool and the reserve or storage pool. The synaptic vesicles comprising the readily releasable pool are aligned near release sites in the nerve terminal. These release sites are called the *active zones* and lie in direct opposition to the ACh receptors (AChRs) on the postsynaptic muscle membrane (Fig. 1.5) (8,9). When the vesicles fuse with the presynaptic nerve terminal membrane, they release their contents (ACh) into the synaptic cleft (7–9). As the pool of readily releasable vesicles is depleted, vesicles from the storage pool are mobilized to the release sites. The physiologic consequences of this process will be described in further detail below (see Section IV).

Voltage-gated calcium (Ca^{2+}) channels are also located in the active zones (9–11). They appear as double parallel rows of dense intramembrane particles (Fig. 1.6) by electron microscopy. Each row contains approximately five channels with 20-nm spacing between rows and 60-nm spacing between double rows (1,9). This high concentration of calcium channels at the active zones allows for the rapid increases in calcium concentration in regions where vesicle fusion occurs. The principal calcium channel type at human NMJs is the P/Q-type calcium channel (12). These calcium channels are believed to be the site of immunologic attack in Lambert-Eaton syndrome (Chapter 5).

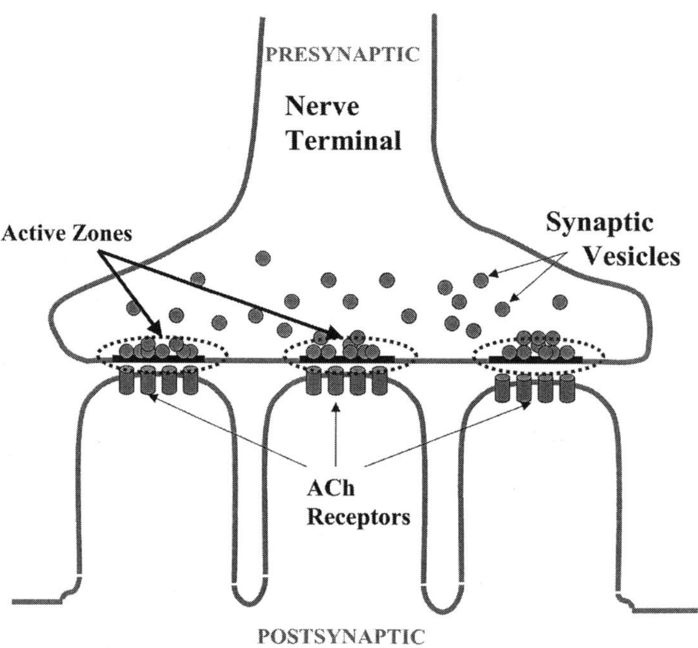

Figure 1.5 Organization of the motor endplate region. The sites of release of acetylcholine (active zones) are directly aligned with the cusps of the folds on the postsynaptic muscle membrane where the acetylcholine receptors are concentrated.

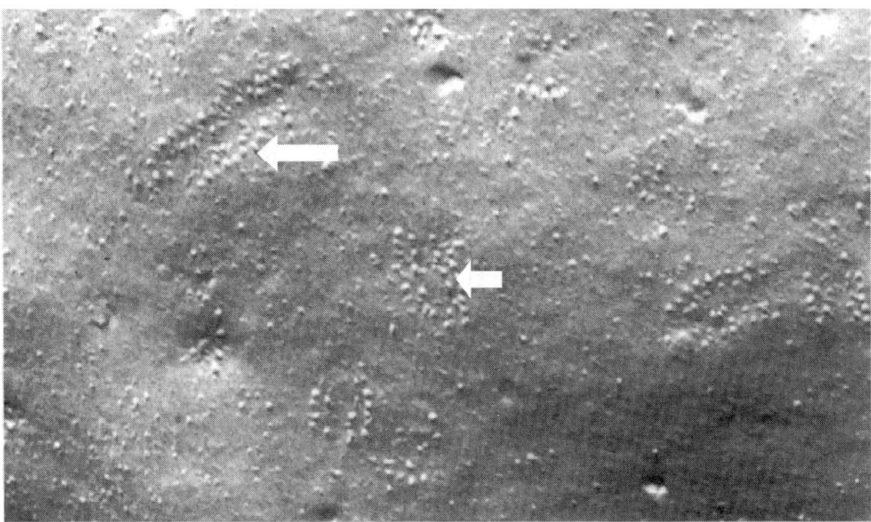

Figure 1.6 Freeze-fracture electron microscopy of the presynaptic membrane revealing scattered integral membrane particles arrayed in double parallel rows (arrows). These particles correspond to the voltage-gated calcium channels. (Reproduced from Engel AG, Myasthenia Gravis and Myasthenic Syndromes, New York: Oxford University Press, 1999.)

B. The Synaptic Space

The synaptic space is located between the presynaptic nerve terminal membrane and the postsynaptic muscle membrane. It consists of a primary cleft and a number of secondary clefts (1,13) (Figs. 1.1). The primary cleft is the space (about 50 nm wide) between the presynaptic membrane and the postsynaptic junctional folds. It is bounded laterally by basement membrane. The secondary clefts are the spaces between the junctional folds on the postsynaptic membrane. The synaptic cleft is essentially an extracellular compartment that is continuous with the external space around the NMJ. The short expanse of the primary synaptic cleft allows ACh receptors to reside very near the ACh release sites so that diffusion time across the cleft is short (see Section IV).

C. The Postsynaptic Region

The postsynaptic region is a highly specialized area of the muscle fiber membrane, which is also known as the endplate. In normal human muscle there is one endplate per muscle fiber, typically located about halfway along the length of the fiber. The muscle membrane comprising the endplate is thrown into numerous junctional folds, with the crest of each fold aligned with an active zone on the presynaptic terminal (1,5). These postsynaptic junctional folds produce a several-fold amplification of the postsynaptic surface area. Because the junctional folds are separated by the secondary synaptic clefts, this organization also increases the volume of the synaptic space. The density of the folding is much more extensive at the endplate compared to the extrajunctional membrane. The vast majority of AChRs are concentrated on the crests of the junctional folds (13,14) at a density of approximately 10^4 sites/μm^2 (1).

The muscle fiber membrane at the endplate is lined with a basal lamina containing the enzyme acetylcholinesterase (AChE) (15), which splits the ACh molecule into choline and acetate. AChE is located mainly in the troughs of the junctional folds (16). This location provides a "sink" for inactivation of ACh molecules (Fig. 1.7). Muscle activity is required for normal AChE expression in muscle and its accumulation at the NMJ (17). The concentration of AChE is approximately five- to eight-fold lower than the concentration of

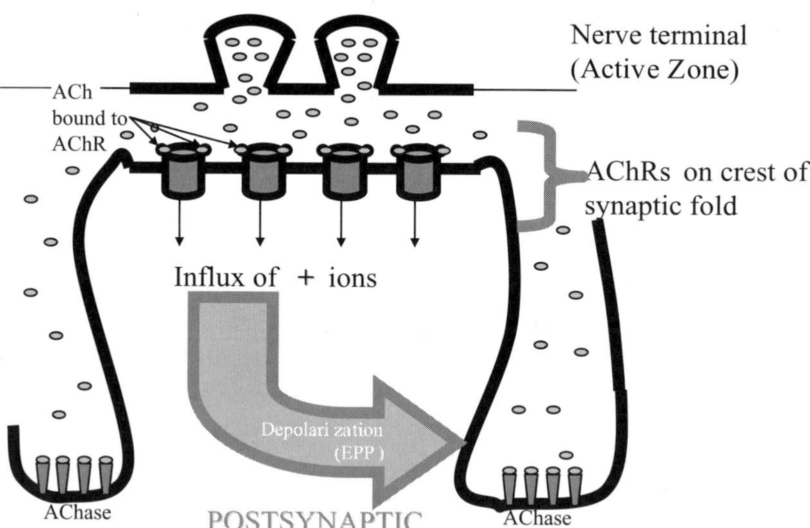

Figure 1.7   Location of acetylcholinesterase. The enzyme acetylcholinesterase is contained in the basal lamina lining the muscle endplate. It is mainly located in the troughs of the junctional folds, thereby providing a "sink" for inactivation of acetylcholine.

ACh receptors, but is adequate to hydrolyze most of the ACh released by the nerve terminal and to prevent repeated binding of ACh to the AChRs (18). Inactivation of AChE prolongs the duration of action of ACh and slows the decay of the ACh-induced ionic current.

Voltage-sensitive sodium channels are also present in large numbers on the postsynaptic membrane. These sodium channels are also concentrated in the depths of the secondary synaptic clefts (19,20). They are present in the endplate region at an increased concentration (three- to seven-fold) compared with the extrajunctional membrane (21). The density of sodium channels in the postsynaptic membrane varies according to fiber type with fast-twitch muscle fibers having a higher density of sodium channels than slow-twitch fibers (21).

1. The Acetylcholine Receptor

AChR is a transmembrane protein composed of five subunits and in humans exists in two isoforms (22). The mature or "innervated" isoform of the AChR is composed of two α subunits and one each of the β, δ, and ϵ subunits (Fig. 1.8A) (1). The fetal or "denervated" AChR has a γ subunit in place of the ϵ subunit (23). Interestingly, normal adult human extraocular muscle expresses a significant proportion of the fetal isoform of AChR in addition to the mature isoform, which may provide a unique target for immune-mediated damage of these muscles, as will be discussed in Chapter 4. After denervation, the γ subunit is expressed on AChRs of muscle fibers, both at and away from the endplate (24).

The AChR subunits are arranged in a ring, spanning the membrane and forming a water-filled transmembrane channel that is roughly funnel shaped with the narrow aspect oriented to the intracellular compartment (25). Each subunit is composed of four transmembrane domains (M1–M4), the M2 and M3 domains of each subunit contributing to the central pore of the channel (Fig. 1.8B). Clusters of negatively charged residues are located at either end of the channel to aid in excluding the passage of negative ions and encouraging the passage of positive ions. Ion binding sites are located within the channel and are critical to ion passage.

Each α subunit on the AChR has one binding site for ACh. Thus, there are two ACh binding sites on a single AChR. The binding site is located at the interface between the α subunit and the δ subunit and at the interface between the α subunit and either the ϵ or γ subunit (Fig. 1.8C). Because amino acids from both subunits contribute to each of the AChR binding sites, the properties of each of the binding sites on a single AChR are a little different. AChR channel opening requires that two ACh molecules bind to the AChR. A specific region of the α subunit has been found to be the binding site for

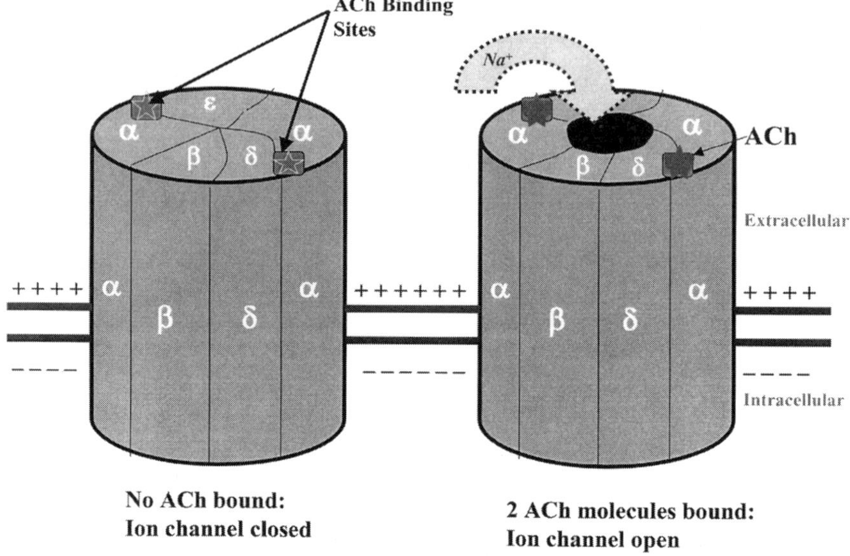

Figure 1.8A Structure of the adult acetylcholine receptor. The adult acetylcholine receptor is composed of five subunits (2α, β, δ, and ε). The acetylcholine binding sites are located on the two α subunits. The subunits are embedded in the post-synaptic membrane and are arranged in a ring surrounding a central pore that connects the extracellular and intracellular spaces. Binding of two acetylcholine molecules to the acetylcholine binding sites makes this pore permeable to the passage of positive ions.

most of the antibodies in myasthenia gravis, and has been designated as the *main immunogenic region* (MIR) (26). Although in close proximity, the MIR is separate and distinct from the AChR binding sites. There is one MIR on each of the two α subunits in an AChR. It is located on the extracellular surface of the AChR making it readily accessible to circulating antibodies.

CASE 1.1 A 53-year-old man develops fluctuating diplopia and right-sided eyelid ptosis. He has no complaints of bulbar or extremity weakness or fatigability. His examination reveals bilateral medial rectus weakness and fatigable right ptosis with normal facial, bulbar, and extremity muscle strength. AChR binding antibodies are negative, but electrodiagnostic studies confirm a defect in neuromuscular transmission.

His symptoms respond initially to treatment with AChE inhibitors but eventually recur despite dose escalation. Treatment with high-dose daily prednisone (50 mg/day) results in complete remission of all symptoms.

Discussion The patient has ocular myasthenia gravis (MG). As will be discussed in Chapter 4, MG is an autoimmune disease in which antibodies are directed against the AChRs on the muscle endplate. The reason for the selective vulnerability of the extraocular muscles in MG is not precisely known. However, there are at least three *anatomic features* that distinguish the neuromuscular junctions in extraocular muscles compared to other muscles:

1. Increased expression of fetal acetylcholine receptors.
2. Multiple innervation of extraocular muscles (i.e., an extraocular muscle may receive innervation from more than one motor neuron).
3. Decreased motor unit size (a motor neuron innervating an extraocular muscle supplies innervation to an average of 10–15 muscle fibers, compared to hundreds or even thousands in extremity muscles).

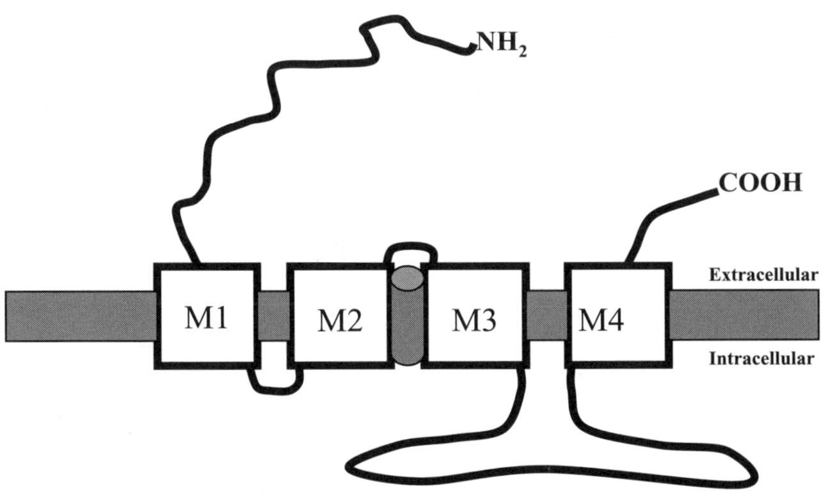

Figure 1.8B Basic structure of acetylcholine receptor subunits. Each acetylcholine receptor subunit is composed of four transmembrane domains (M1–M4). The M2 and M3 domains contribute to the central ion pore of the channel.

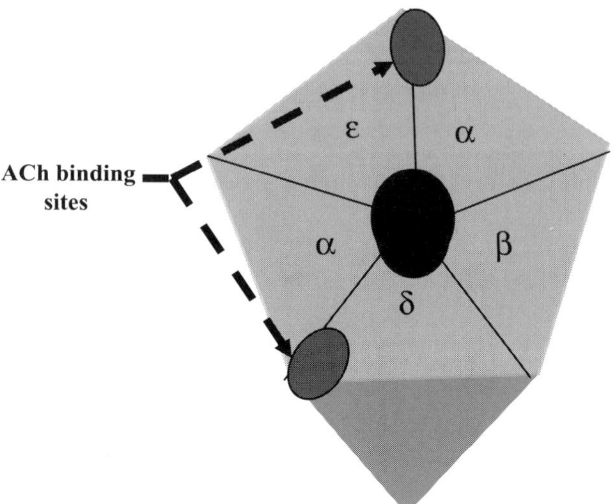

Figure 1.8C Acetylcholine receptor binding site. The acetylcholine receptor binding sites are located between the α_1 and δ subunits and between the α_2 and ε subunits. Binding of two molecules of acetylcholine is required for opening of the ion channel.

The AChRs are highly concentrated at the endplate region, their concentration being 1000-fold less outside the endplate (27). The half-life of mature AChRs is 8–11 days, while the half-life of fetal AChRs is less than 24 h (28). Mature AChRs are continuously turned over by internalization and degradation of "old" receptor molecules and replacement by new AChRs (29). They are not recycled. Thus, there must be some "signal" that accounts for the clustering of new AChRs in the postsynaptic region and specifically at the crests of the junctional folds. Nerve-derived factors, such as agrin (13,30–32), rapsyn, (33,34), and neuregulins (13,35,36), may provide this "signal" by affecting gene transcription of AChR subunits. Accordingly, there is a high concentration of AChR messenger RNA in these synaptic regions consistent with enhanced gene transcription (37). The clustering of AChRs and their alignment adjacent to areas of ACh release may also be regulated by a muscle-specific tyrosine kinase or MuSK (32). Complex interactions between agrin, rapsyn, and MuSK are involved in the development and maintenance of the normal nerve–muscle synapse. The process of AChR turnover and AChR clustering at the crests of postsynaptic junctional folds is of critical importance because a high density of these receptors on the crests of the postsynaptic junctional folds is absolutely required for normal neuromuscular transmission.

At the endplate, individual AChRs are connected to each other and anchored to the muscle fiber cytoskeleton. Rapsyn, a 43-kDa protein, connects AChRs to one another and also connects the clusters of AChRs to the muscle fiber cytoskeleton via the dystrophin–glycoprotein complex (DGC) (34,37). The DGC contains transmembrane (including α- and β-dystroglycan and the sarcoglycan complex) and submembrane proteins (dystrophin, utrophin, syntrophin, and the 87-kDa protein dystrobrevin); it connects to the cytoskeleton via F-actin and to the basal lamina via laminin (Fig. 1.9). In addition to anchoring the AChRs to the muscle cytoskeleton, any or all of the above-mentioned muscle cell membrane components may be involved in synaptic maintenance and development via a complex signaling pathway.

D. Overview

The NMJ is a specialized chemical synapse between a motor axon and a muscle fiber. The presynaptic region is the site of synthesis, storage, and release of the neurotransmitter ACh. The synaptic space consists of primary and secondary synaptic clefts and is the space that must be traversed by the neurotransmitter to interact with the receptor on the postsynaptic membrane.

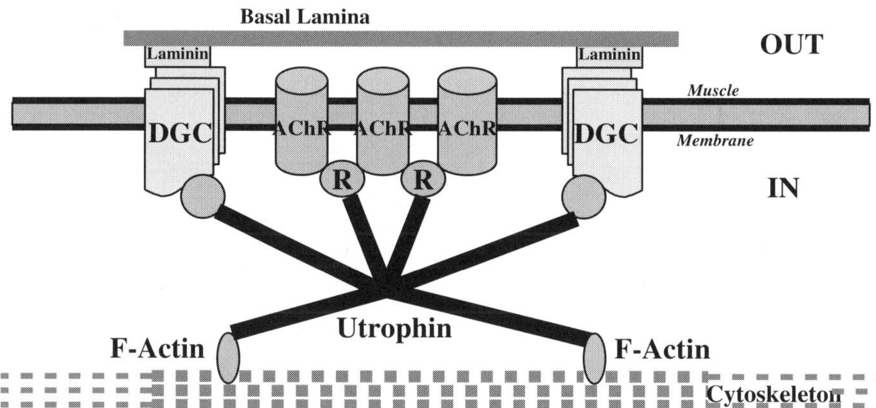

Figure 1.9 Diagrammatic representation of the microstructure of the muscle endplate region. Rapsyn (R) connects the acetylcholine receptors (AChR) to one another and also connects the clusters of AChRs to the muscle fiber cytoskeleton via the dystrophin–glycoprotein complex (DGC). The DGC contains a number of proteins and connects to the cytoskeleton via F-actin and to the basal lamina via laminin.

The postsynaptic membrane or motor endplate contains numerous AChRs, each of which consists of two ACh binding domains as well as the ionic channel. When the AChR is activated by binding of two ACh molecules to the binding domains, the ion channel opens allowing cations to flow across the membrane and causing a depolarizing current. AChE is located in the basal lamina of the postsynaptic membrane and speeds the decline in ACh concentration in the synaptic space. The anatomic configuration of the NMJ places AChRs at the site of ACh release, and allows for rapid diffusion and metabolism of ACh after detachment from the AChR.

The above discussion of the anatomy of the NMJ forms the basis for a review of the physiology of neuromuscular transmission. As will become apparent, important structure–function correlations exist, providing effective interaction of ACh molecules with their receptors on the postsynaptic membrane.

IV. PHYSIOLOGY OF NEUROMUSCULAR TRANSMISSION

The time that elapses between the arrival of a nerve action potential at the nerve terminal and the subsequent depolarization of the postjunctional membrane is only a few milliseconds. However, a number of different and complex processes occur during this brief period of time. The steps involved in neuromuscular transmission are summarized in Table 1.1 and Fig. 1.10, and are discussed in further detail below.

Table 1.1 The Physiologic Events of Neuromuscular Transmission

1. Depolarization of presynaptic nerve terminal.
2. Opening of voltage-gated calcium channels in response to depolarization.
3. Movement of calcium into the nerve terminal.
4. Synaptic vesicles fuse with the presynaptic membrane, releasing ACh into the synaptic space.
5. Diffusion of ACh to the postsynaptic membrane.
6. ACh molecules bind AChR (2 ACh molecules/AChR) or are hydrolyzed by AChase.
7. AChRs with bound ACh undergo conformational change, opening ion channel.
8. Net influx of positive charge (Na^+ in, K^+ out) resulting in depolarization of endplate region $\Rightarrow$ endplate potential (EPP).
9. If the EPP is of sufficient magnitude to depolarize the muscle fiber membrane to threshold, an action potential is generated in the muscle fiber membrane that propagates in both directions away from the endplate.
10. Muscle fiber contraction.

ACh, acetylcholine; AChR, acetylcholine receptor; Na^+, sodium ions; K^+, potassium ions.

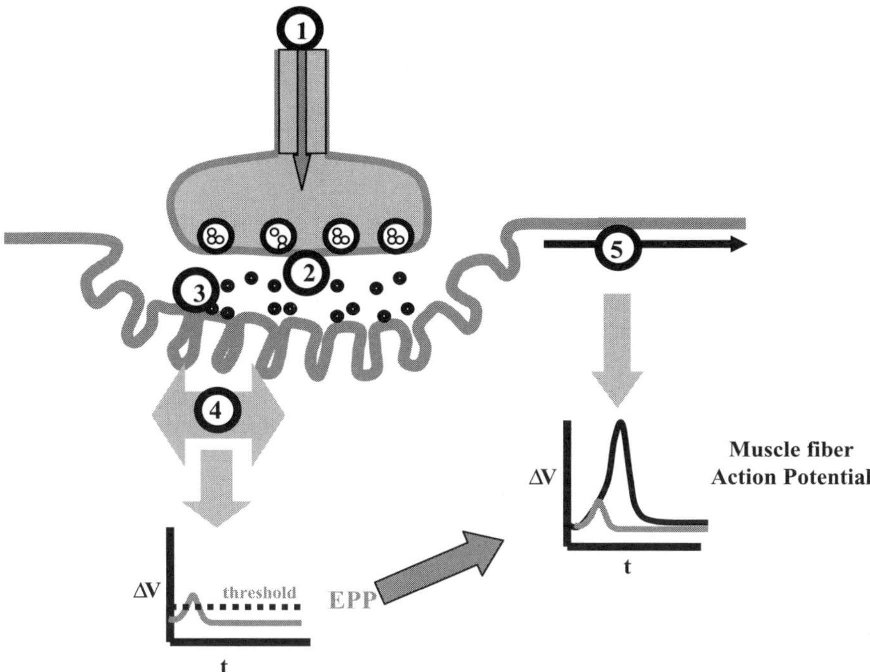

Figure 1.10 The main events of neuromuscular transmission. (1) Nerve action potential propagates down the axon and depolarizes the nerve terminal resulting in opening of voltage-gated calcium channels. (2) Synaptic vesicles fuse with the presynaptic membrane releasing their contents of acetylcholine (ACh) into the synaptic cleft. (3) ACh molecules bind to the ACh receptors (AChR) on the postsynaptic membrane opening the AChR ion pore (4) Membrane conductance to positive ions increases, producing a depolarization of the endplate region (endplate potential, EPP). (5) The endplate is electrically coupled to the adjacent muscle membrane such that it may be brought to the threshold of firing by spread of current from the endplate resulting in a muscle fiber action potential. The EPP *must* be of sufficient magnitude to depolarize the adjacent muscle membrane to threshold or a muscle fiber action potential will not occur.

A. Presynaptic Events

The initial event in neuromuscular transmission is the propagation of a nerve action potential down the motor axon resulting in depolarization of the presynaptic nerve terminal. As a result of this depolarization, voltage-gated calcium channels are opened and calcium enters the nerve terminal. It is this influx of calcium that mediates transmitter release, promoting synaptic vesicle exocytosis (1,16,39,40). The quantity of calcium that enters the nerve terminal determines the number of quanta released in response to a nerve action potential. Reducing the concentration of calcium in the extracellular fluid reduces the number of quanta released by any given presynaptic membrane depolarization.

CASE 1.2 A 66-year-old man with myasthenia gravis ("in remission") receives an aminoglycoside antibiotic for management of a gram-negative bacteremia. Shortly after initiation of treatment, he develops severe ptosis, diplopia, dysphagia, and shortness of breath. His physicians realize that aminoglycoside antibiotics may exacerbate weakness in patients with NMJ disease. They immediately stop the infusion and treat him symptomatically with AChE inhibitors.

Discussion Aminoglycoside antibiotics inhibit ACh release from the nerve terminal through competition with Ca^{2+}. Administration of calcium salts overcomes this effect and is the preferred treatment for this toxicity (see Chapter 8).

The calcium-regulated exocytosis of the synaptic vesicles is a complicated process involving the coordinated actions of a number of proteins located on the synaptic vesicles themselves, in the cytosol, and on the presynaptic membrane (41–43) (Fig. 1.11). Calcium entry is proposed to lead to phosphorylation of synapsin I (a vesicle-associated protein), which then dissociates from the synaptic vesicles, allowing them to detach from the cytoskeleton and making them available for release (44). This is followed by a number of calcium-dependent protein interactions that result in (a) the movement of the synaptic vesicles toward the proximity of the active zone; (b) the docking of the vesicles at the active zones; and (c) the fusion of the vesicles with the presynaptic membrane (45). Table 1.2 summarizes the main calcium-dependent proteins involved in these processes. The importance of these proteins is emphasized by the effects of specific clostridial neurotoxins, each of which cleaves a particular protein involved in vesicle movement, docking, and fusion. The result in each case is a failure of exocytosis. Other factors may be relevant in the calcium-dependent process of synaptic vesicle exocytosis. The approximation of the synaptic vesicles and the presynaptic membrane may be inhibited by electrostatic forces caused by the like polarity of surface charges on the vesicle membrane and the nerve terminal membrane. Calcium may play an additional role by binding to the vesicle

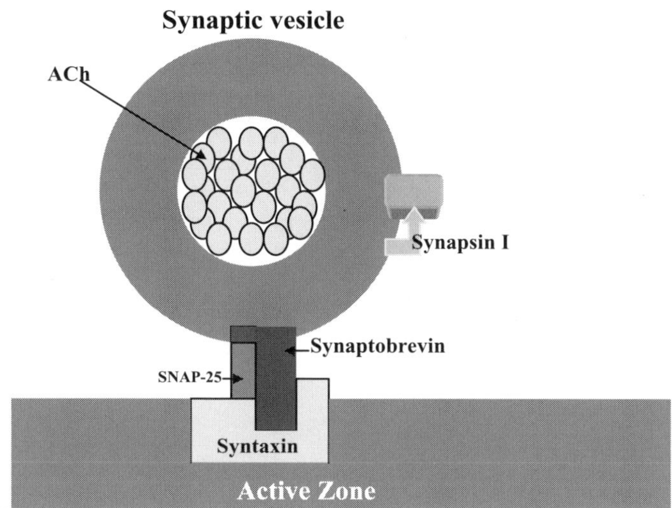

Figure 1.11 Calcium-regulated exocytosis of the synaptic vesicles. Synapsin I links synaptic vesicles to the cytoskeleton. Calcium-dependent phosphorylation of synapsin I releases the synaptic vesicles. Once freed from their cytoskeletal attachments, the synaptic vesicles are transported from deeper regions of the nerve terminal to the proximity of the active zone. Docking of vesicles at the active zone likely occurs through the interaction of vesicle-associated synaptotagmin with the voltage-gated calcium channels on the presynaptic membrane. The calcium-regulated exocytosis of the synaptic vesicles involves the coordinated actions of a number of proteins depicted in the figure. Synaptobrevin on the synaptic vesicle and syntaxin on the presynaptic membrane serve as the "anchors" that pull the respective membranes together. The precise exocytotic mechanism is complex, but it is believed that SNAP-25 (SNAP=soluble NSF attachment protein), a protein anchored to the presynaptic membrane, binds two molecules of syntaxin, forming a complex. Synaptobrevin then binds to this complex, displacing one of the syntaxin molecules and bringing the membrane of the synaptic vesicle and the presynaptic membrane into close proximity. The precise driving force behind actual membrane fusion is not clear.

membrane surface and neutralizing the negative charges, allowing for fusion with the presynaptic membrane (46).

One of the earliest observations resulting from intracellular recordings from neuromuscular junctions was the presence of spontaneous, low-amplitude depolarizations of the endplate region (47). These potentials apparently resulted from the nearly simultaneous release of many molecules of ACh from the nerve terminal. The frequency of these *miniature endplate*

Table 1.2 Proteins Involved in Synaptic Vesicle Transport, Docking, and Fusion

Protein	Location	Function	Neurotoxin
Synapsin I	Synaptic vesicle	Links vesicles to cytoplasm	
Synaptobrevin	Synaptic vesicle	Docking/fusion	Botulinum B, D, F, and G; tetanus
Synaptotagmin	Synaptic vesicle	Docking	
SNAP-25	Presynaptic membrane	Docking/fusion	Botulinum A, E
Syntaxin	Presynaptic membrane	Docking/fusion	Botulinum C

potentials (MEPPs) varied with time, but their amplitudes were within a very narrow range. These observations led to the quantal hypothesis of transmitter release; namely, the depolarization that occurs a the endplate after nerve stimulation results from release of a large number of "packets" of ACh from the nerve terminal with each packet containing the amount of ACh that would in itself produce an MEPP (48). According to this hypothesis, an MEPP represents the depolarization induced at the endplate by the *spontaneous* release of a single quanta (contents of a single synaptic vesicle) of ACh, and an *endplate potential* (EPP) represents the depolarization produced by all of the vesicles released after a nerve action potential. Interestingly, the precise function of MEPPs is not presently known.

Depolarization of the nerve terminal by a nerve impulse results in the nearly synchronous release of 50–300 synaptic vesicles (49). The number of quanta released in response to a nerve impulse is called the *quantal content* and depends on a number of factors. Synaptic vesicles in the nerve terminal are sequestered in at least two well-defined pools: one is composed of the vesicles ready for immediate release and the other is the reserve pool. At each nerve terminal, a number of synaptic vesicles are positioned at the active zones prepared for release (*readily releasable stores*). These vesicles have a certain probability of release dependent on nerve terminal calcium concentration, which is very low in the absence of nerve terminal stimulation and increases significantly after depolarization. This relationship may be expressed using the formula $m = np$ (1,48), where m represents the quantal content, p the probability of release, and n the number of readily available quanta positioned at the release sites. In the resting state, p is very low and consequently m is minimal. During a nerve action potential, p is increased dramatically due to the influx of calcium into the nerve terminal and subsequently m is quite large. As one might predict, the quantal content *normally* varies from one nerve action potential to another depending on the size of the releasable store of synaptic vesicles and the (calcium-dependent) probability of release. The releasable store is in equilibrium with the reserve store of vesicles (N) in the nerve terminal. Immediately following a nerve action potential and the subsequent quantal release of synaptic vesicles, the releasable store is diminished.

With repetitive nerve stimulation, two competing forces act at the nerve terminal (Fig. 1.12). First, repeated stimulation depletes the pool of readily releasable synaptic vesicles (n), resulting in a reduction in the quantal content. However, this effect is countered by the effects of changing nerve terminal calcium concentrations. Release of ACh by the presynaptic terminal is terminated by removal of calcium from the region of the active zones, which

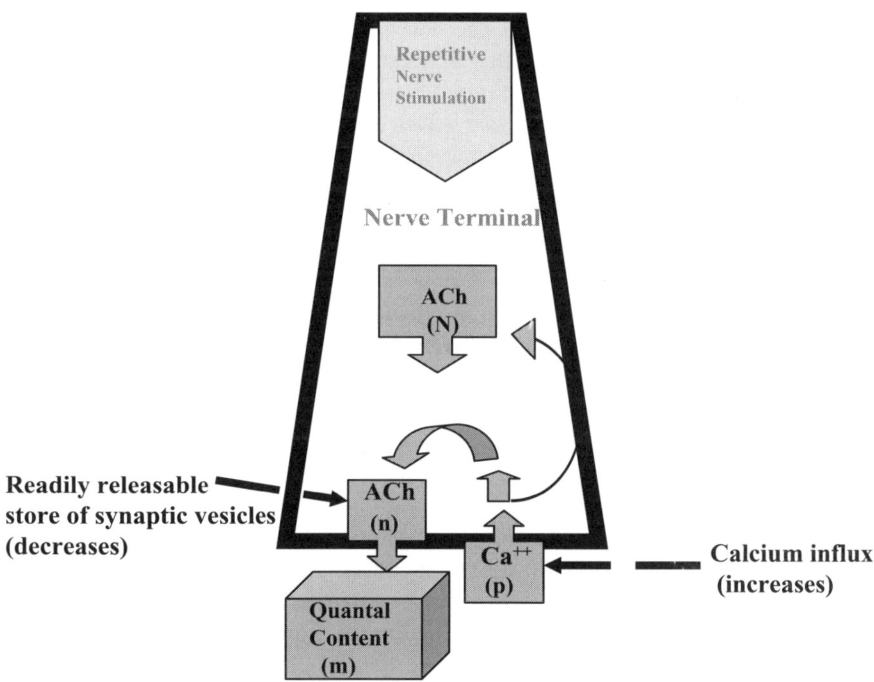

Figure 1.12 Competing forces at the presynaptic nerve terminal. Repetitive nerve stimulation causes depletion of the readily releasable stores of synaptic vesicles, but also causes accumulation of intracellular calcium, which enhances release and mobilization of synaptic vesicles. The rate of stimulation is critical in determining which of these competing forces is predominant. At high rates of stimulation (>5 Hz), there is saturation of the normal calcium buffering processes in the nerve terminal and the effect of increased intracellular calcium predominates over vesicle depletion. At slow rates of stimulation the effects of vesicle depletion are dominant. These principles are directly applied to the clinical electrodiagnostic testing of patients with suspected disorders of neuromuscular transmission (Chapter 3).

is accomplished by sequestration into organelles (smooth endoplasmic reticulum and mitochondria) in the terminal, diffusion away from the release sites, and extrusion into the extracellular space (50,51). Most of the calcium is removed from the nerve terminal within 100–200 ms of release of a quantal content (52). If the nerve terminal is stimulated at rapid rates (faster than every 100–200 ms), there is a saturation of this calcium-buffering system and the calcium concentration builds up in the nerve terminal increasing the probability (p) of synaptic vesicle release.

The excess calcium allows more synaptic vesicles to be freed from their cytoskeletal restraints and to be mobilized to the active zones, resulting in enhanced release of ACh. This phenomenon is known as *posttetanic facilitation* (53,54) (Fig. 1.13). Thus, at high rates of stimulation (>5–10 Hz), the effect of calcium build-up within the nerve terminal predominates over the rundown of synaptic vesicles. This effect lasts for approximately 30–60 s; the enhanced quantal content that persists for a brief period of time is referred to as *posttetanic potentiation*. After a period of rest of approximately 60 s, the quantal content declines. This is called *posttetanic exhaustion* (54) and lasts until synaptic vesicles from the reserve pool are mobilized, thus replenishing the readily releasable store.

CASE 1.3 A 25-year-old woman with myasthenia gravis is examined by her physician. The physician observes mild right ptosis at rest. The patient is asked to sustain upward gaze for 2 min. After 90 s, the right ptosis has worsened, completely covering the right eye.
What is the physiologic explanation for this phenomenon?
Why didn't the ptosis improve as a result of posttetanic facilitation?

Discussion The clinical description is an example of fatigable muscle weakness, in this case affecting the levator palpebrae muscle. At rest, there are a number of dysfunctional endplates causing muscle weakness and partial right ptosis. With sustained activation, there is depletion of the readily releasable stores of synaptic vesicles and the quantal content decreases resulting in dysfunction (failure) at additional endplates and worsening weakness (complete ptosis). It is important to realize that with repetitive or sustained activation there are two competing forces acting on the nerve terminal: (1) depletion of readily releasable vesicles and (2) accumulation of calcium. The quantal content is either decreased or increased depending on which force predominates. In this case, the quantal content decreased because the effect of vesicle depletion outweighed the effect of calcium build-up in the nerve terminal.

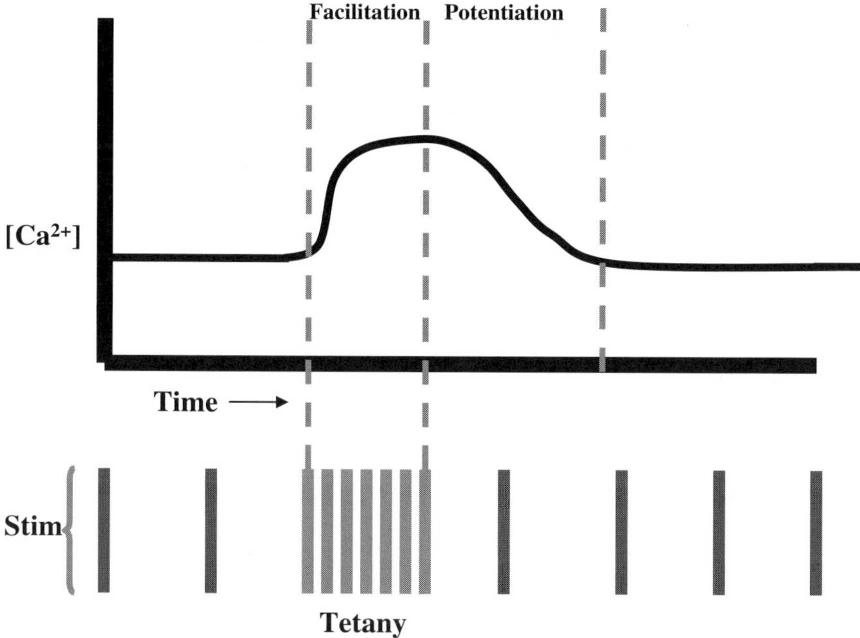

Figure 1.13 Posttetanic facilitation. With high rates of nerve stimulation (>5 Hz), the calcium concentration (Ca^{2+}) increases in the nerve terminal resulting in fusion of increased numbers of synaptic vesicles with the presynaptic membrane (increased quantal content). Facilitation is a normal phenomenon occurring at high rates of nerve stimulation. This effect persists for 30–60 s after cessation of the stimulus (potentiation). In normal muscle the added amount of calcium in the nerve terminal resulting from a brief interstimulus interval (facilitation) is not significant since the amount of ACh released is always more than sufficient to depolarize the muscle fiber to threshold. (See discussion of the safety factor of neuromuscular transmission.)

Stimulation of the nerve terminal at slow rates (1–4 Hz) results in a progressive decrease in the quantal content due to a depletion in the readily releasable stores of synaptic vesicles. Decreasing numbers of quanta are released by the first several nerve discharges in a train of stimuli, until the fourth, fifth, or sixth stimulus, after which the mean amount of ACh released per impulse becomes relatively constant. The initial decrease in quantal content is known as *posttetanic depression* (54) and (as noted) is probably due to depletion of readily available synaptic vesicles. By the fourth, fifth, or sixth consecutive stimulus, the number of quanta released no longer declines but remains stable and may even increase (55). This may be explained in the following way: repetitive nerve stimulation causes depletion of the readily releasable pool of synaptic vesicles and forces mobilization of vesicles from the reserve pool and local recycling of vesicles. When the replenishment of vesicles equals the release, no further decrease in quantal content occurs (Fig. 1.14). The decrease in quantal content persists as long as low-frequency stimulation is continued. After cessation of stimuli, a short period of time (20–30 s) is required for the mobilization process to restore the readily releasable pool of vesicles to the resting level.

It is helpful to keep in mind that the above processes occur in normal muscle. Thus, under normal circumstances, the additional calcium in the nerve terminal caused by high-frequency stimulation (posttetanic facilitation) is clinically inconsequential since the quantal content is always more than sufficient to result in a single muscle action potential. Similarly, with low rates of stimulation, the reduced quantal content (posttetanic depression) never falls below that required for threshold firing of the muscle fiber. However,

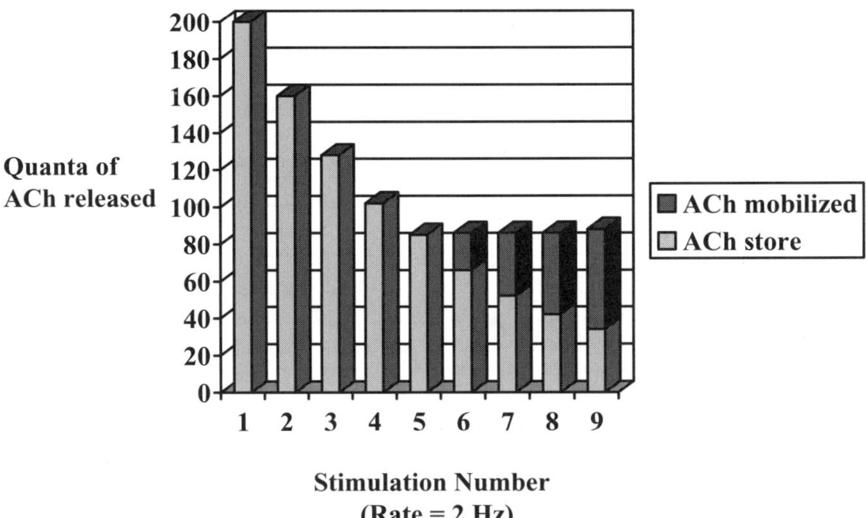

Figure 1.14 Posttetanic depression. At slow rates of stimulation, there is a progressive decrease in the amount of acetylcholine released from the nerve terminal with each stimulus. This is due to depletion of the readily releasable stores of synaptic vesicles. However, after the fourth or fifth stimulus the amount of ACh released stabilizes due to mobilization of synaptic vesicles from various storage compartments in the nerve terminal so that the amount of ACh mobilized keeps up with the amount released.

these processes become critical in diseased muscle, and the basic principles discussed above are applied to the electrodiagnostic evaluation of patients with disorders of the neuromuscular junction (Chapter 3).

1. Synthesis of Acetylcholine and Recycling of Synaptic Vesicles

Nerve terminal ACh concentrations are maintained at relatively constant levels at physiological stimulation rates (55). The rate of ACh synthesis can be markedly increased by stimulation in a calcium-dependent manner. The molecular events believed to be involved in ACh synthesis and vesicle recycling are depicted in Fig. 1.15. ACh is synthesized within the nerve terminal from choline and acetyl coenzyme A (acetyl-CoA). AChE hydrolyzes ACh released from the nerve terminal to choline and acetate. Choline is returned

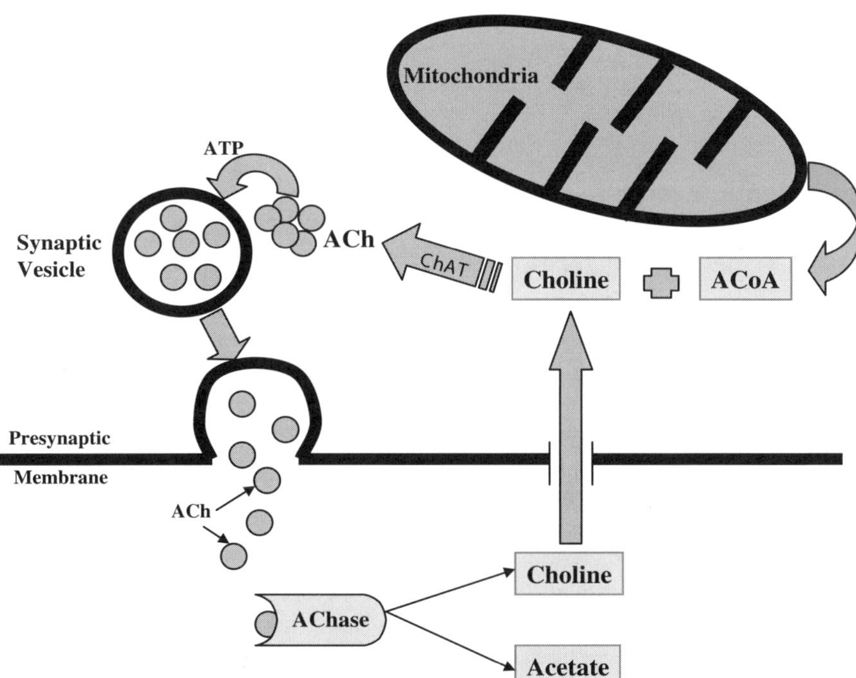

Figure 1.15 Synthesis of acetylcholine. Acetylcholine is synthesized within the nerve terminal from choline and acetyl-CoA (ACoA) through the action of choline acetyltransferase (ChAT). Acetyl-CoA is made in the mitochondria and transported to the cytosol. Uptake of choline from the synaptic space occurs via a high-affinity uptake system.

to the nerve terminal via a high-affinity, sodium-dependent uptake system (56). Acetyl-CoA is normally made in the mitochondria and transported into the cytoplasm in a calcium-dependent manner (1). Choline acetyltransferase present in the nerve terminal cytoplasm synthesizes ACh from choline and acetyl-CoA.

When ACh is released from the synaptic vesicles by exocytosis, the membrane of the vesicle fuses with the membrane of the nerve terminal. If no process compensated for this, the membrane of the nerve terminal would enlarge as a result of neuromuscular transmission. This does not occur because the membrane of the vesicle is retrieved and recycled rapidly. How this recycling occurs in nerve terminals is complicated and not completely understood (57). After fusion of the vesicle membrane with the nerve terminal membrane, the vesicle membrane collapses and coalesces into the nerve terminal membrane. Retrieval of vesicle membrane occurs by endocytosis, which is also calcium dependent. Paradoxically, the rate of endocytosis is reduced by increased cytosolic calcium concentration (58). Under normal circumstances, endocytosis keeps up with exocytosis, so that there is no appreciable difference between the stimulated nerve terminal membrane and the terminal at rest.

B. Synaptic Events

The fusion of the synaptic vesicles with the presynaptic membrane results in the release of approximately 10,000 ACh molecules into the synaptic space. The diffusion of ACh across the synaptic cleft is very rapid due to the small distance to be traversed and the relatively high diffusion constant for ACh (54). Most ACh molecules are not initially hydrolyzed by AChE because of saturation of AChE by the very high concentration of ACh (16). A high proportion of ACh molecules reach the postsynaptic membrane and collide with the AChR. Some of these collisions result in the binding of ACh to specific binding sites on the AChR. Binding of two ACh molecules to an AChR induces a conformational change in the AChR that opens the ion channel (see Section C below). After a brief period, the ACh molecules dissociate from the AChR and the ion channel closes. After ACh dissociates from the AChR, it is either rapidly hydrolyzed by AChE to choline and acetate or diffuses out of the synaptic cleft (16).

With AChE fully active, ACh molecules in a single quantum exert their effect within a very limited area (within a radius of 0.8 μm from the site of release) (67). This effectively "saturates" the AChRs in a very small region of the postsynaptic membrane directly adjacent to the ACh release sites, ensuring efficient binding of ACh to AChRs in a 2:1 ratio. This is known as the *saturating disc model* of ACh–AChR interaction (16). Since the ACh release sites are discreet and vary from impulse to impulse, different sets of "discs" become saturated on repetitive stimulation. This prevents desensitization of the AChR from extended exposure to ACh. AChE limits the number of collisions of ACh with the AChRs in addition to limiting the radius of ACh spread. Inactivation or absence of AChE increases the number of collisions of ACh with AChR and increases the radius of diffusion of ACh. This allows for sequential binding of ACh to multiple AChRs and opening of multiple ion channels before diffusion of ACh from the synaptic space (59,60).

C. Postsynaptic Events

The large number of AChRs on the muscle endplate membrane makes it very sensitive to ACh released from the nerve terminal. The AChR forms a cation-selective channel that is relatively nonselective for individual cations (i.e., sodium, potassium, calcium) (61). This is due to the fact that the size of the channel at its narrowest point (*ion pore*) is significantly larger than voltage-sensitive channels, which are very ion selective (62). Thus, the relative contributions of the different cations to the current through the channel depend primarily on their concentrations and the electrochemical driving forces. Ions do not pass through the channel in a bulk flow fashion, but instead bind to specific sites within the pore and move from one site to the next. The structure of the binding site within the channel is critical to ion passage (61,62). If the interaction between the ion and the binding site is too weak, it will not pass through the channel. If it is too strong, the ion may remain fixed to the binding site, effectively blocking the channel. This is the proposed mechanism of action of several noncompetitive AChR antagonists used clinically as neuromuscular blocking agent (see Chapter 8). The binding of ACh to the AChR likely allows the passage of ions across the channel by leading to a change in pore structure or by altering the properties of the ion binding sites.

In addition to the AChRs, the endplate membrane also has a high density of voltage-sensitive sodium channels (63–65). As noted, these channels are concentrated in the depths of the secondary synaptic folds; their density is approximately three-to sevenfold greater at the endplate membrane than the extrajunctional membrane, and fast-twitch muscle fibers have a higher density of sodium channels than slow-twitch fibers. The depolarization of the endplate region due to opening of the AChR ion channels in turn causes rapid opening of the voltage-sensitive sodium channels. This results in further depolarization of the muscle membrane (Fig. 1.16). The amplitude of the sodium current for a region of membrane depends on the density of sodium channels in the membrane, the conductance of these channel, and the fraction of channels that open in response to membrane depolarization. The

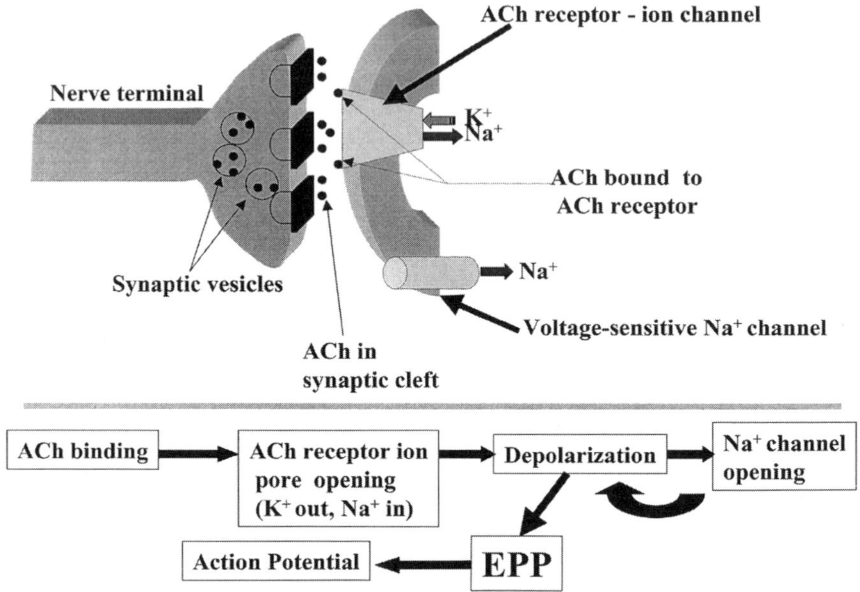

Figure 1.16 Voltage-sensitive sodium channels. Voltage-sensitive sodium channels are found in high concentrations in the troughs of the junctional folds of the postsynaptic membrane. Depolarization of the postsynaptic membrane opens these sodium channels, resulting in further depolarization of the endplate region.

high concentration of voltage-sensitive sodium channels at the endplate lowers the threshold of depolarization needed to generate a muscle fiber action potential.

Opening of the AChR ion channels allows cations to flow across the muscle membrane producing a depolarizing generator potential known as the *endplate potential* (EPP). The AChR ion channel has an effective open time of approximately 1 ms (66). While two ACh molecules are bound to the AChR, the ion pore may repeatedly open and close, producing bursts of channel openings. Normal adult AChRs have channel open times and "burst" durations within a certain range. Adult (mature) and fetal AChRs may be distinguished on the basis of their single-channel conductance and channel open times. Adult AChRs have shorter mean open times and larger single-channel conductances.

By the time the muscle action potential has occurred, the majority of the activated AChRs have closed their ion channel, so that any current in the few remaining open AChR ion channels is not sufficient to generate a second action potential. As discussed, AChE in the basal lamina of the postsynaptic membrane speeds the decline in concentration of ACh in the synaptic cleft, effectively preventing sequential binding of ACh with multiple AChRs. Thus, each nerve terminal action potential generates a single action potential in the muscle cell. This action potential propagates in both directions along the muscle fiber from the endplate region, and invades and depolarizes the T-tubule system of muscle which results in release of calcium from the adjacent sarcoplasmic reticulum stores leading to muscle contraction. Any process that affects either the function of AChE or channel open time may result in prolonged depolarization at the endplate and the generation of multiple muscle action potentials by a single nerve impulse.

D. The Safety Factor of Neuromuscular Transmission

Neuromuscular transmission is successful when the muscle fiber contracts. In order for this to occur, the EPP must exceed the threshold required for initiation of a muscle fiber action potential. As we have seen, the EPP is a *graded* potential varying in magnitude from one to another depending a number of factors. The muscle fiber action potential is *all-or-none*: the EPP either produces depolarization sufficient for generation of an action potential in the muscle fiber, or it does not occur (Fig. 1.17). The ratio between the EPP amplitude and the amount of endplate depolarization required for a muscle fiber action potential to occur is termed the *safety factor (SF) of neuromuscular transmission*, and may be expressed by the formula:

$$SF = EPP/E_{AP} - E_{M}$$

where EPP represents the endplate potential amplitude, E_{AP} the muscle fiber action potential threshold, and E_{M} the muscle resting membrane potential (54). Normally, the safety factor of neuromuscular transmission is quite large, preventing failure of neuromuscular transmission even during maximal, sustained voluntary muscle contraction. During repetitive stimulation in normal muscle, the amount of transmitter released by each nerve impulse is decreased, the EPP is smaller, and consequently the safety factor is reduced. This does not result in failure of neuromuscular transmission because of the magnitude of the safety factor (Fig. 1.18). This large margin of error is primarily due to the fact that (a) the nerve terminal releases more quantal packets of ACh than needed, and (b) there are more AChRs on the postsynaptic membrane than are necessary to depolarize the muscle fiber to threshold. As we shall see in the next chapter, the major physiologic consequence of all disorders of the neuromuscular junction is a critical reduction in the safety factor of neuromuscular transmission.

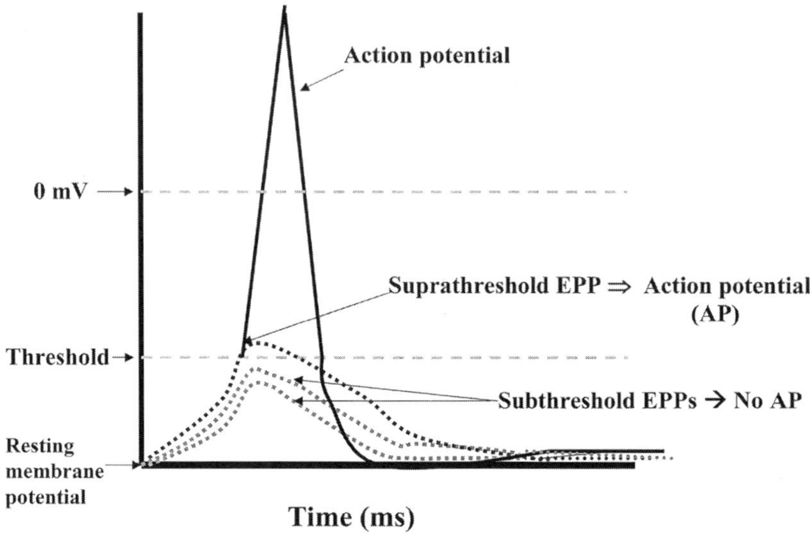

Figure 1.17 The endplate potential. The depolarization of the postsynaptic membrane (endplate) in response to a nerve impulse is called the endplate potential (EPP). If the EPP is of sufficient magnitude (i.e., greater than the threshold for firing of the muscle fiber action potential), an action potential is generated in the muscle fiber. The EPP normally varies slightly from one nerve impulse to another but must reach a threshold depolarization in order for a muscle fiber action potential to occur.

E. Overview

Neuromuscular transmission begins when a nerve action potential reaches the nerve terminal and depolarizes its membrane. The resulting depolarization opens voltage-gated Ca^{2+} channels and Ca^{2+} from the interstitial fluid flows down its electrochemical gradient into the nerve terminal. The influx of Ca^{2+} causes synaptic vesicles to fuse with the plasma membrane and empty their ACh into the synaptic space by exocytosis. ACh diffuses across the synaptic space and interacts with a specific AChR protein on the external surface of the muscle plasma membrane of the motor endplate. The combination of ACh with its receptor transiently increases the conductance of the postjunctional membrane to cations (Na^+ and K^+), resulting in a transient depolarization of the endplate region. This transient depolarization is called the endplate potential (EPP). If the EPP is of sufficient magnitude, a muscle fiber action potential is generated. The difference between the EPP amplitude and the amount of depolarization

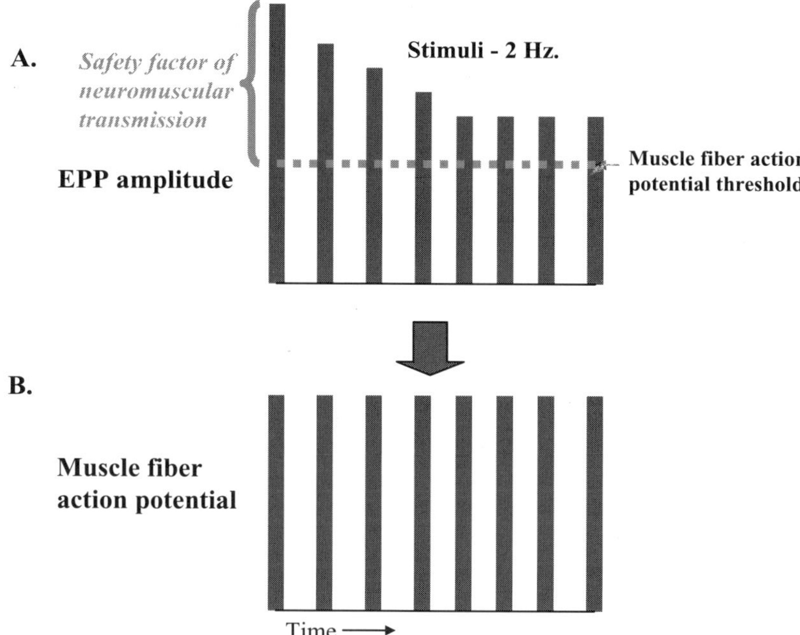

Figure 1.18 The safety factor of neuromuscular transmission. The safety factor of neuromuscular transmission may be defined as the ratio of the endplate potential (EPP) amplitude and the depolarization needed to generate a muscle fiber action potential. In normal muscle, this ratio is quite large. Repetitive stimulation of a nerve at a rate of 2–3 Hz results in a progressive decrease in the EPP. This is a *normal* phenomenon. This decrease in the EPP does not result in failure of neuromuscular transmission in normal muscle because of the magnitude of the safety factor (A). Thus, all EPPs will result in propagated muscle fiber action potentials (B).

required for generation of a muscle action potential is referred to as the safety factor of neuromuscular transmission.

The endplate potential is transient because the action of ACh is ended by the hydrolysis of ACh to choline and acetate by the enzyme AChE, which is present in high concentrations in the postsynaptic membrane. After the endplate region is depolarized, adjacent regions of the muscle cell membrane are depolarized by electrotonic conduction. When those regions reach threshold, action potentials are generated that are propagated along the muscle fiber at high velocities initiating the chain of events that lead to muscle contraction.

The next chapter will examine the consequences of functional abnormalities at many of the steps in the process of neuromuscular transmission discussed above. How these physiologic abnormalities result in clinical symptoms of muscle weakness and fatigability will also be considered.

REFERENCES

1. Engel AG. The neuromuscular junction. In: Engel AG, Franzini-Armstrong C, eds. Myology, 2d ed. New York: McGraw-Hill, 1994:261–302.
2. Saito A, Zacks SI. Ultrastructure of Schwann and perineural sheaths at the mouse neuromuscular junction. Anat Rec 1969; 164:379.
3. Balice-Gordon RJ. Dynamic roles at the neuromuscular junction. Curr Biol 1996; 6:1054–1056.
4. Engel AG, Santa T. Histometric analysis of the ultrastructure of the neuromuscular junction in myasthenia gravis and the myasthenic syndrome. Ann NY Acad Sci 1971; 183:46–63.
5. Engel AG, Tsujihata M, Lindstrom JM, et al. The motor end-plate in myasthenia gravis and experimental autoimmune myasthenia gravis: a quantitative ultrastructural study. Ann NY Acad Sci 1976; 274:60–79.
6. Birks R, Huxley HE, Katz B. The fine structure of the neuromuscular junction in the frog. J Physiol (Lond) 1960; 150:134–144.
7. Pascuzzi RM. Introduction to the neuromuscular junction and neuromuscular transmission. Semin Neurol 1990; 10:1–5.
8. Augustine GJ, Adler EM, Charlton MP. The calcium signal for transmitter secretion from presynaptic nerve terminals. Ann NY Acad Sci 1991; 635:365–381.
9. Smith SJ, Augustine GJ. Calcium ions, active zones and synaptic transmitter release. Trends Neurosci 1988; 10:458–464.
10. Engel AG. Review of evidence for loss of motor nerve terminal calcium channels in Lambert-Eaton myasthenic syndrome. Ann NY Acad Sci 1991; 635:246–258.
11. Pumplin DW, Reese TS, Llinas R. Are the presynaptic membrane particles calcium channels? Proc Natl Acad Sci USA 1981; 78:7210–7213.
12. Protti DA, Sanchez VA, Cherksey BD, Sugimori M, Llinas RR, Uchitel OD. Mammalian neuromuscular transmission blocked by funnel web toxin. Ann NY Acad Sci 1993; 681:405–407.
13. Hall ZW, Sanes JR. Synaptic structure and development: the neuromuscular junction. Cell 1993; 72:99–121.
14. Witzemann V, Barg B, Criado M, Stein E, Sakmann B. Developmental regulation of five subunit specific mRNAs encoding acetylcholine receptor subtypes in rat muscle. FEBS Lett 1989; 242:419–424.
15. McMahan UJ, Sanes JR, Marshall LM. Cholinesterase is associated with the basal lamina at the neuromuscular junction. Nature 1978; 271:172–174.
16. Salpeter MM. Vertebrate neuromuscular junctions: general morphology, molec-

ular organization, and functional consequences. In: Salpeter MM, ed. The Vertebrate Neuromuscular Junction. New York: Alan Liss, 1987:1–54.

17. Gaspersic R, Koritnik B, Crne-Finderle N, Sketelj J. Acetylcholinesterase in the neuromuscular junction. Chem Biol Interact 1999; 119–120:301–308.

18. Land BR, Salpeter EE, Salpeter MM. Kinetic parameters for acetylcholine interaction in intact neuromuscular junction. Proc Natl Acad Sci USA 1981; 78:7200–7204.

19. Ruff RL, Whittlesey D. Na$^+$ current densities and voltage dependence in human intercostals muscle fibres. J Physiol (Lond) 1992; 458:85–97.

20. Flucher BE, Daniels MP. Distribution of Na$^+$ channels and ankyrin in neuromuscular junctions is complementary to that of acetylcholine receptors and the 43 kD protein. Neuron 1989; 3:163–175.

21. Ruff RL, Whittlesey D. Na$^+$ currents near and away from endplates on human fast and slow twitch muscle fibers. Muscle Nerve 1993; 16:922–929.

22. Lindstrom JM. Acetylcholine receptors and myasthenia. Muscle Nerve 2000; 23:453–477.

23. Mishina M, Taki T, Imoto K, Noda M, Takahashi T, Numa S, Methfessl C, Sakmann B. Molecular distinction between fetal and adult forms of muscle acetylcholine receptor. Nature 1986; 321:406–411.

24. Schuetze SM, Role LW. Developmental regulation of nicotinic acetylcholine receptors. Annu Rev Neurosci 1987; 10:403–407.

25. Guy HR, Hucho F. The ion channel of the nicotinic acetylcholine receptor. Trends Neurosci 1987; 10:318–322.

26. Lindstrom JM, Seybold MD, Lennon VA, Whitingham S, Duane DD. Antibody to acetylcholine receptor in myasthenia gravis: prevalence, clinical correlates and diagnostic value. Neurology 1976; 26:1054–1059.

27. Kuffler SW, Yoshikami D. The distribution of acetylcholine sensitivity at the post-synaptic membrane of vertebrate skeletal twitch muscles: iontophoretic mapping in the micron range. J Physiol (Lond) 1975; 244:703–730.

28. Salpeter MM, Loring RH. Nicotinic acetylcholine receptors in vertebrate muscle: properties, distribution and neural control. Prog Neurobiol 1985; 25: 297–325.

29. Kaminski HJ, Suarez JL, Ruff RL. Neuromuscular junction physiology in myasthenia gravis: isoforms of the acetylcholine receptor in extraocular muscle and the contribution of sodium channels to the safety factor. Neurology 1997; 48(suppl 5):8–17.

30. Reist NE, Werle MJ, McMahan UJ. Agrin released by motor neurons induces the aggregation of acetylcholine receptors at neuromuscular junctions. Neuron 1992; 8:865–868.

31. Duclert A, Changeux JP. Acetylcholine gene expression at the developing neuromuscular junction. Physiol Rev 1995; 75:339–368.

32. Sanes JR, Apel ED, Gautam M, Glass D, Grady RM, Martin PT, Nichol MC, Yancopoulos GD. Agrin receptors at the neuromuscular junction. Ann NY Acad Sci 1998; 841:1–13.

33. Flucher BE, Daniels MP. Distribution of Na$^+$ channels and ankyrin in

neuromuscular junctions is complementary to that of the acetylcholine receptors and the 43 kD protein. Neuron 1989; 3:163–175.

34. Apel ED, Roberds SL, Campbell KP, Merlie JP. Rapsyn may function as a link between the acetylcholine receptor and the agrin binding dystrophin-associated glycoprotein complex. Neuron 1995; 15:115–126.

35. Jo SA, Zhu X, Marchionni MA, et al. Neuregulins are concentrated at nerve–muscle synapses and activate ACh-receptor gene expression. Nature 1995; 373:158–161.

36. Fischbach GD, Rosen KM. ARIA: a neuromuscular junction neuregulin. Annu Rev Neurosci 1997; 20:429–458.

37. Merlie JP, Sanes JR. Concentration of acetylcholine receptor mRNA in synaptic regions of adult muscle fibers. Nature 1985; 317:66–68.

38. Froehner SC. The submembrane machinery for nicotinic acetylcholine receptor clustering. J Cell Biol 1991; 114:1–7.

39. Barrett EF, Magleby KL. Physiology of cholinergic transmission. In: Goldberg AM, Hanin I, eds. Biology of Cholinergic Function. New York: Raven Press, 1976:29–100.

40. Hubbard JI, Jones SF, Landau EM. On the mechanism by which calcium and magnesium affect the release of transmitter by nerve impulses. J Physiol (Lond) 1968; 196:75–87.

41. Sudhof TC. The synaptic vesicle cycle: a cascade of protein–protein interactions. Nature 1995; 375:645–653.

42. Sudhof TC, Jahn R. Proteins of synaptic vesicles involved in exocytosis and membrane recycling. Neuron 1991; 6:665–677.

43. Whittaker VP. The structure and function of cholinergic synaptic vesicles. Biochem Soc Trans 1984; 12:561–576.

44. Perin MS, Fried VA, Mignery G, Jahn R, Sudhof TC. Phospholipid binding by a specific synaptic vesicle protein homologous to the regulatory region of protein kinase C. Nature 1990; 345:260–263.

45. Sheng Z-H, Westenbroek RE, Catterall WA. Physical link and functional coupling of presynaptic calcium channels and the synaptic docking/fusion machinery. J Bioenerg Biomembr 1998; 30:335–345.

46. Niles WD, Cohen FS. Video-microscopy studies of vesicle-planar membrane adhesion and fusion. Ann NY Acad Sci 1991; 635:273–306.

47. Fatt P, Katz B. Spontaneous subthreshold activity at motor nerve endings. J Physiol (Lond) 1952; 117:109–128.

48. del Castillo J, Katz B. Quantal components of the endplate potential. J Physiol (Lond) 1956; 124:560–573.

49. Katz B, Miledi R. Estimates of quantal content during chemical potentiation of transmitter release. Proc R Soc Lond 1979; 205:369–378.

50. Blaustein MP. Calcium transport and buffering in neurons. Trends Neurosci 1988; 11:438–443.

51. Brinley JF, Tiffert T, Scarpa A. Mitochondria and other calcium buffers of squid axon studied in situ. J Physiol 1978; 72:101–127.

52. Katz B, Miledi R. The role of calcium in neuromuscular facilitation. J Physiol 1968; 195:481–492.

53. Magleby KL. The effect of repetitive stimulation on facilitation of transmitter release at the frog neuromuscular junction. J Physiol 1976; 257:449–470.
54. Magleby KL. Neuromuscular transmission. In: Engel AG, Franzini-Armstrong C, eds. Myology, 2d ed. New York: McGraw-Hill, 1994:442–463.
55. Ali HH, Savarese JJ. Monitoring of neuromuscular function. Anesthesiology 1976; 45:216–249.
56. Beach RL, Vaca K, Pilar G. Ionic and metabolic requirements for high-affinity choline uptake and acetylcholine synthesis in nerve terminals at a neuromuscular junction. J Neurochem 1980; 34:1387–1398.
57. Heuser JE, Reese TS. Evidence for recycling of synaptic vesicle membrane during transmitter release at the frog neuromuscular junction. J Cell Biol 1973; 57:315–344.
58. Matthews G. Neurotransmitter release. Annu Rev Neurosci 1996; 19:219–233.
59. Heuser JE, Reese TS. Structural changes after transmitter release at the frog neuromuscular junction. J Cell Biol 1981; 88:564–580.
60. Heuser JE, Reese TS, Dennis MJ, Jan Y, Jan L, Evans L. Synaptic vesicle exocytosis captured by quick freezing and correlated with quantal transmitter release. J Cell Biol 1979; 81:275–300.
61. Dwyer TM, Adams DJ, Hille B. The permeability of the end plate channel to organic cations in frog muscle. J Gen Physiol 1980; 75:469–492.
62. Ruff RL. Ionic channels: I. The biophysical basis for ion passage and channel gating. Muscle Nerve 1986; 9:675–699.
63. Engel AG, Lambert EH, Howard FM. Immune complexes (IgG and C3) at the motor end-plate in myasthenia gravis. Ultrastructure and light microscopic localization and electrophysiological correlations. Mayo Clin Proc 1977; 52:267–280.
64. Haimovich B, Schotland DL, Fieles WE, Barchi RL. Localization of sodium channel subtypes in rat skeletal muscle using channel-specific monoclonal antibodies. J Neurosci 1987; 7:2957–2966.
65. Ruff RL. Sodium channel current density at and away from end plates on rat fast- and slow-twitch skeletal muscle fibers. Am J Physiol 1992; 262:C229–C234.
66. Lindstrom J. Acetylcholine receptors: Structure, function, synthesis destruction and antigenicity. In: Engel AG, Franzini-Armstrong C, eds. Myology, 2d ed. New York: McGraw-Hill, 1994:586–606.

2

Pathophysiology of Neuromuscular Junction Disorders

I. INTRODUCTION

The basic defect that all disorders of the neuromuscular junction (NMJ) have in common is a reduced *safety factor of neuromuscular transmission*. The complex electrical and molecular interactions that underlie the process of neuromuscular transmission may fail at any point from the nerve terminal to the muscle fiber endplate. The end result is the same: the difference between the endplate potential (EPP) and the threshold potential for firing of the muscle fiber is lessened. If the EPP fails to reach the threshold of the muscle fiber, an action potential is not generated and muscle fiber contraction does not occur. This is called *neuromuscular transmission failure*, and if this occurs at a critical number of endplates, clinical weakness results.

From a purely pathophysiologic point of view, disorders of the NMJ may be classified according to the location of failure. Thus, we will consider four sites of dysfunction: (a) the prejunctional level, (b) the presynaptic region, (c) the synaptic space, and (d) the postsynaptic region (see Fig. 1.2). The precise etiology of dysfunction in diseases affecting the NMJ may be autoimmune, congenital, pharmacologic, or toxic and will be discussed in subsequent chapters. It is important to keep in mind that disorders of the NMJ are very complex, and "pure" levels of failure probably do not exist in vivo where multiple mechanisms may be operative.

We will, nevertheless, examine the effect of each primary site of dysfunction on the following physiologic variables introduced in the previous chapter: (a) quantal content (m), probability of quantal release (p), and miniature endplate potential (MEPP) amplitude, duration, and frequency. These parameters are defined in Table 2.1, and their relative contributions in determining the amplitude of the EPP and consequently the *safety factor of neuromuscular transmission* are depicted in Fig. 2.1.

The quantal content (m) is a measure of presynaptic integrity and is determined by the probability (p) of quantal release (which is dependent on nerve terminal calcium concentration) multiplied by the number (n) of readily releasable synaptic vesicles ($m = np$) (1). The quantal store (N) also has a role in ensuring the effectiveness of normal neuromuscular transmission particularly during periods of sustained activation (Fig. 2.2). With rundown of the supply of readily releasable synaptic vesicles, the quantal stores must be effectively mobilized to ensure adequate quantal content during repetitive or prolonged neural stimulation (2).

The *MEPP frequency* is primarily a measure of presynaptic function. Recall that the MEPP refers to the spontaneous release of a single quanta

Table 2.1 Microphysiologic Parameters Relevant to NMJ Function

Parameter	Definition	NMJ localization
Quantal content (m)	Number of synaptic vesicles released after a nerve AP	Presynaptic
Probabilty of quantal release (p)	Likelihood of synaptic vesicle release (increases with $\uparrow$ [Ca^{2+}])	Presynaptic
Readily releasable vesicles (n)	Number of synaptic vesicles positioned at the active zones ready to fuse with the presynaptic membrane	Presynaptic
Miniature endplate potential (MEPP)	Depolarization caused by release of the contents of a single synaptic vesicle	Presynaptic (frequency) Presynaptic, synaptic, and postsynaptic (amplitude) Synaptic and postsynaptic (duration)

AP, action potential; [Ca^{2+}], intracellular calcium concentration.

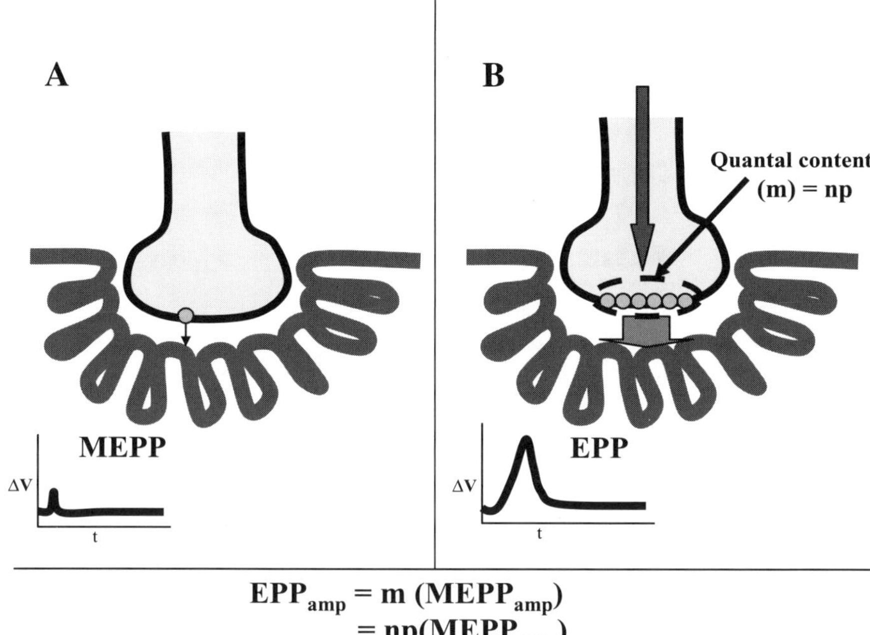

$$EPP_{amp} = m \, (MEPP_{amp})$$
$$= np(MEPP_{amp})$$

Figure 2.1 Depolarization at the endplate. (A) The miniature endplate potential (MEPP) refers to the depolarization produced at the endplate by the liberation of the acetylcholine molecules contained in a single synaptic vesicle. (B) The endplate potential (EPP) is the depolarization produced by the sum total of all the synaptic vesicles released from the nerve terminal in response to a nerve action potential. Thus, the EPP represents the product of the MEPP amplitude and the number of synaptic vesicles released after a nerve action potential (quantal content = *m*).

from the presynaptic nerve terminal. The complex presynaptic machinery discussed in Chapter 1 that ensures normal production and packaging of acetylcholine (ACh) as well as normal cycling, docking, and fusion of the synaptic vesicles may have an effect on MEPP frequency. On the other hand, the *MEPP amplitude* depends on the number of ACh molecules per quanta, the geometry of the endplate (accessibility of the ACh receptors), and the number and functional state of the ACh receptors (AChRs). Thus, presynaptic, synaptic, and postsynaptic factors determine the amplitude of the MEPP. Finally, the *MEPP duration* is a reflection of the open time of the AChR ion channel (postsynaptic) and the functional status of the endplate

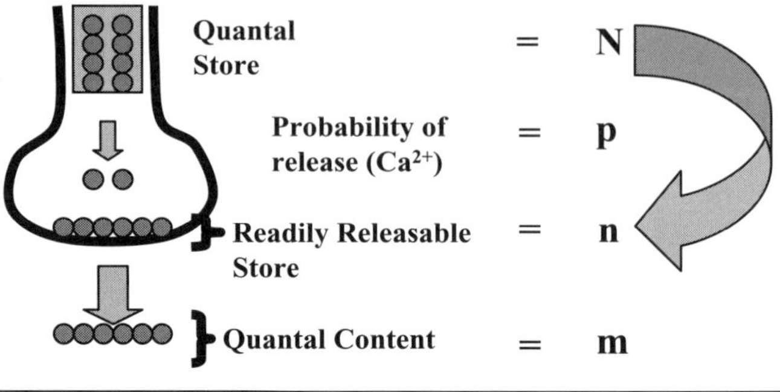

Figure 2.2 Presynaptic function. The quantal content (*m*) is dependent on the probability (*p*) of synaptic vesicle release (which increases with increased intracellular calcium concentration) and the store of synaptic vesicles (*n*) which are positioned appropriately for ready release. With sustained or repetitive neural stimulation, the store of readily releasable synaptic vesicles (*n*) is depleted and must be replaced by synaptic vesicles comprising the quantal store (*N*).

acetylcholinesterase (AChE, synaptic). The microphysiologic consequences of dysfunction at specific levels of the NMJ along with clinical examples of each level of dysfunction are shown in Table 2.2.

II. PREJUNCTIONAL (NEUROGENIC) NEUROMUSCULAR TRANSMISSION FAILURE

Diseases primarily affecting the motor axon proximal to the nerve terminal may cause abnormal neuromuscular transmission. This is most commonly observed in rapidly progressing neurogenic disorders characterized by prominent ongoing reinnervation and denervation. A classic example is amyotrophic lateral sclerosis (ALS) in which there is partial axonal degeneration due to anterior horn cell disease and subsequent collateral reinnervation of denervated muscle fibers by surviving axons. This reinnervation takes place by subterminal sprouting of nerve twigs from healthy motor axons to "orphaned" muscle fibers (3,4). The stimulus for collateral sprouting is not known but may involve the loss of an inhibitory factor provided by normal muscle.

Table 2.2 Neuromuscular Junction Disorders: General Classification

Level of dysfunction	Nature of disturbance	Electrophysiologic consequence	Examples
Prejunctional	↓ Synaptic vesicles (readily releasable and storage supply)	↓n ↓N	ALS
Presynaptic	↓ ACh molecules/ quanta	↓m ↓ MEPP amplitude	CMS—defect in ACh synthesis
	Derangement in quantal release mechanisms	↓ m ↓ p ↓MEPP frequency	LES, botulism
Synaptic	Dysfunction of endplate acetylcholinesterase	↑ MEPP duration (? Compensatory changes)	CMS—endplate cholinesterase deficiency
Postsynaptic	Impaired ACh–AChR interaction	↓ MEPP amplitude	MG
	Deranged AChR ion channel kinetics	↑ or ↓ MEPP duration	CMS—slow channel CMS—fast channel

m, quantal content; n, quantity of readily releasable synaptic vesicles; p, probability of synaptic vesicle release; N, quantal store; MEPP, miniature endplate potential; CMS, congenital myasthenic syndrome; ACh, acetylcholine; LES, Lambert-Eaton syndrome; MG, myasthenia gravis.

CASE 2.1 A 75-year-old woman presented to her neurologist with an 8-month history of progressive weakness, dysarthria, and fatigue. Her neurologist made the diagnosis of myasthenia gravis on the basis of a "positive tensilon test" and an 18% decrement in compound muscle action potential amplitude with repetitive stimulation of the ulnar nerve at 3 Hz. She failed to improve significantly when treated with AChE inhibitors. She was referred for a second opinion. A repeat electrodiagnostic study revealed the presence of a diffuse motor neuronopathy consistent with the clinical diagnosis of ALS.

Discussion This woman's complaints of fatigue and the results of pharmacologic and electrophysiologic tests of the NMJ were indicative of a disorder of neuromuscular transmission. However, her physicians failed to realize that a primary neurogenic disorder (prejunctional) may have a very prominent effect on neuromuscular transmission. As

> we will see in Chapter 3, many of the diagnostic tests used to confirm a neuromuscular transmission defect are not 100% specific for a *primary* NMJ (presynaptic, synaptic, postsynaptic) disorder, and may be "falsely positive" in other diseases of the motor unit, particularly those causing subacute denervation/reinnervation.

Experimental studies have demonstrated that immature nerve terminals release smaller amounts of ACh (5–7). In rapidly progressive processes, such as ALS, there is no time for maturation of these newly formed neuromuscular junctions due to continuous denervation and reinnervation. In addition, the surviving motor neurons may be marginally functional and incapable of supporting new axonal sprouts. In ALS the reinnervating motor unit may die before effective sprouting has developed. Single-fiber electromyography (EMG) studies (see Chapter 3) confirm a defect in neuromuscular transmission in patients with motor neuron disease (8). In the early stages of reinnervation, neuromuscular transmission is very uncertain, with frequent neuromuscular transmission failure often showing a dependence on firing rate (see below). This effect is largely due to a decreased release of ACh at immature, reinnervating sprouts, and is most pronounced in rapidly progressive denervating disorders like ALS.

A number of reports have demonstrated evidence for abnormal neuromuscular transmission in motor neuron disease (9–12). In one study, in vitro microelectrode recordings were reported in 10 patients with ALS (11). MEPP amplitudes and the mean quantal content were decreased. The mean probability of quantal release was normal or low, and the mean MEPP frequency was not significantly different compared to controls. However, the *quantal store* was decreased, and the mean probability of *quantal store mobilization* was high. Histologic evidence of denervation and small or absent nerve terminals were observed in all patients. Only a few of these endplates were innervated by regenerating nerve fibers. Failure of electrical stimulation to generate EPPs was observed and was frequency dependent, *increasing* with higher rates of stimulation.

These microphysiologic data suggest that the neuromuscular transmission defect in ALS is primarily due to a decreased number of synaptic vesicles at the release sites (n) and in storage sites (N) in the nerve terminal. The probability of quantal release is normal, but the probability of mobilizing vesicle stores is increased. Thus, with high-frequency stimulation, the nerve terminals are rapidly depleted of available ACh stores, likely underlying the frequent clinical complaint of muscle fatigue in these patients.

As we have seen, high-frequency nerve stimulation enhances release of ACh due to build-up of calcium in the nerve terminal. This effectively counters the effect of stimulation-induced vesicle depletion in normal nerve terminals. However, an increase in nerve terminal calcium concentrations also increases mobilization of vesicles and their exocytosis. This effect predominates when quantal stores are reduced since increased mobilization rapidly depletes these stores, particularly at high rates of stimulation. This results in decreasing quantal release and subsequently decreased EPP amplitudes with fast frequency stimulation. In motor neuron disease, this reduction in quantal stores is likely explained by the diminished size of the atrophic nerve terminals (11).

From the clinical point of view, the above discussion yields two critical points. First, it is important to realize that finding evidence of an abnormality in neuromuscular transmission in a subacutely evolving primary neurogenic disorder usually does not necessarily imply a separate pathologic process at the neuromuscular junction. Second, a prejunctional level of failure can potentially be distinguished from a presynaptic NMJ disorder by their responses to high rates of stimulation. Neuromuscular transmission in prejunctional disorders may be worsened with higher rates of stimulation, whereas higher stimulus rates transiently improve neuromuscular transmission in presynaptic disorders (see below).

III.　PRESYNAPTIC DISORDERS

Diseases primarily affecting the normal function of the nerve terminal, and in particular the release of ACh, are classified as presynaptic disorders. There are three main categories of dysfunction in the presynaptic region that may lead to clinical symptoms: (a) reduced calcium ion entry into the nerve terminal, (b) impaired acetylcholine release *not* due to diminished calcium entry, and (c) defective ACh synthesis or packaging (Table 2.3). Sophisticated micro-physiologic techniques have enhanced our understanding of the nature of these disorders.

Table 2.3　Presynaptic Disorders

1. Reduced calcium ion entry into the nerve terminal 　　Example: LES
2. Impaired acetylcholine release not due to diminished calcium entry 　　Example: Botulism 　　Example: CMS—reduced quantal release
3. Defective acetylcholine synthesis or packaging 　　Example: CMS—defective ACh synthesis or packaging, paucity 　　　or reduced size of synaptic vesicles

LES, Lambert-Eaton syndrome; CMS, congenital myasthenic syndrome.

A.   Reduced Calcium Ion Entry into the Nerve Terminal

As we have seen, calcium enters the nerve terminal via voltage-gated calcium channels located in the region of the active zones of the presynaptic membrane and increases the probability (p) of synaptic vesicle release. Calcium is believed to be involved in vesicular docking, mobilization of synaptic vesicles from storage compartments in the nerve terminal, and fusion of the synaptic vesicles with the presynaptic membrane (13,14). Impairment of calcium entry results in a decreased probability of synaptic vesicle release, a low quantal content, but a normal MEPP amplitude. The classic example is Lambert-Eaton myasthenic syndrome in which antibodies are directed against the voltage-gated calcium channels (see Chapter 5). Experimentally, the effects of reduced calcium entry can be produced by magnesium, which decreases the probability of synaptic vesicle release by antagonizing the effect of calcium. This has important clinical ramifications in patients with diseases of the NMJ given the frequency of magnesium supplementation in general medical practice (15,16).

Repetitive stimulation at high rates or sustained muscle contraction improve the neuromuscular transmission defect in these disorders by causing a build-up of calcium in the nerve terminal. The initially low intracellular calcium concentration increases as calcium ions move into the nerve terminal before the calcium-buffering mechanisms can clear the calcium from the previous nerve impulses. Repetitive stimulation at slow rates will worsen the problem by causing depletion of readily releasable stores of synaptic vesicles. However, very few vesicles are released in the first place, so that the depletion of vesicles may not have as prominent an effect. Neuromuscular transmission failure often occurs after a *single* stimulus in nerve terminals with severely impaired calcium ion entry. Clinically this situation would cause muscle weakness at baseline (fixed weakness) in addition to muscle fatigability.

CASE 2.2 A 63-year-old man with Lambert-Eaton syndrome is examined by his neurologist. The man has mild weakness in the hip girdle muscles but otherwise appears to be quite strong in other muscle groups despite his complaints of "severe fatigue." He has no elicitable muscle stretch reflexes at rest. However, after resisted extension of the right knee for 10 s, a knee-jerk reflex is obtained. What is the physiologic explanation for this patient's examination findings?

Discussion Lambert-Eaton syndrome (Chapter 5) is a presynaptic disorder of neuromuscular transmission in which antibodies are directed against the voltage-gated calcium channels on the presynaptic nerve terminal. Calcium influx in response to nerve terminal depolarization is impaired resulting in a decreased quantal content. Frequently neuromuscular transmission fails at a number of endplates prior to exercise causing muscle weakness at baseline and hypoactive muscle stretch reflexes. A short period of sustained exercise of the affected muscles will increase quantal content due to build-up of calcium in the nerve terminal. The result is enhanced release of ACh producing an endplate potential of sufficient amplitude for muscle fiber action potential generation. This is the explanation for the "facilitated" knee-jerk reflex in this case. However, more prolonged exercise will eventually exhaust the supply of readily releasable synaptic vesicles and the quantal content will decrease despite the increased intracellular calcium. This underlies the patient's complaints of severe muscle fatigue. Because the facilatory response is very brief, it is rarely clinically demonstrable with the exception of facilitation of reflexes.

B. Decreased Probability of ACh Release with Normal Calcium Entry

Decreased probability of ACh release with normal calcium entry arises from an inability to facilitate synaptic vesicle fusion with the nerve terminal membrane. An example of this is botulism in which there is blockade of vesicle docking to the presynaptic membrane (17). Thus, with depolarization of the nerve terminal, calcium channels open normally allowing calcium to enter and increasing the intracellular calcium concentration. However, the calcium-mediated fusion of the synaptic vesicle membrane with the presynaptic membrane is impaired, resulting in a decreased quantal content. The mean probability of quantal release is also reduced. The MEPP amplitude is normal since the amount of ACh per vesicle is normal, but the MEPP frequency is reduced.

As would be expected, rapid repetitive stimulation or sustained contraction results in accumulation of calcium in the nerve terminal, facilitating the release of more vesicles. This facilitation may be rather modest depending on the severity of the impairment in vesicular docking and/or fusion, which diminishes the release of ACh no matter how much calcium accumulates in the nerve terminal. Slow repetitive stimulation worsens the problem by adding transient vesicular depletion to the abnormality preventing normal fusion of the synaptic vesicles.

The decreased probability of release of the synaptic vesicles reduces the quantal content (m), and may lead to failure of the EPP to reach threshold in a significant number of muscle fibers leading to clinical weakness. The level of weakness would be expected to worsen with activity because the readily releasable stores of vesicles that are capable of undergoing exocytosis and releasing their content of ACh are used up. Brief, sustained maximal voluntary contraction of affected muscles would be expected to transiently improve clinical strength.

C. Defective ACh Synthesis or Synaptic Vesicle Packaging, Paucity or Reduced Size of Synaptic Vesicles, Impaired Quantal Release (Presynaptic Congenital Myasthenic Syndromes)

The nerve terminal takes up choline from the synaptic space and converts it to ACh which then must be packaged into the synaptic vesicles, which subsequently must be positioned appropriately for fusion with the presynaptic membrane and release of ACh into the synaptic cleft. Failure or decreased function may occur at the following levels in this process: (a) uptake of choline by the nerve terminal, (b) enzymatic synthesis of ACh from choline and acetyl-CoA, (c) ACh packaging into the synaptic vesicles, (d) synaptic vesicle number or size, and (e) synaptic vesicle release.

In defects of ACh synthesis or packaging, the longer the synaptic vesicles remain in the nerve terminal, the more likely they are to release a quantity of ACh that approaches normal (18,19). Accordingly, MEPPs that arise from these vesicles would be normal or near-normal in amplitude. However, with repeated depolarizations of the nerve terminal and subsequent rundown of readily releasable stores of vesicles, new vesicles must be mobilized from the reserve pool. These vesicles contain more recently synthesized and packaged ACh molecules and, consequently, lower quantities. It is only when these more recently synthesized vesicles comprise a major portion of the quantal content that an abnormally low quantal content and resultant subthreshold EPP are likely to occur. As might be predicted from the above discussion, electrophysiologic confirmation of a disorder causing diminished ACh synthesis or impaired packaging is often difficult and may require prolonged nerve stimulation at physiologic rates (18,19).

In the rare defects causing a reduced number of synaptic vesicles (20,21), the EPP is reduced due to the decreased number of readily releasable quanta (n). The probability of quantal release (p) is normal. The postsynaptic region is normal so that, as one would expect, the MEPP amplitudes are normal. These defects may superficially resemble Lambert-Eaton syndrome, except that the reduced quantal content (m) is due to a decrease in n rather than p. Congenital defects causing reduced synaptic vesicle size and abnormalities of synaptic vesicle release have also been described and will be discussed in Chapter 6.

IV. SYNAPTIC DISORDERS

The principal pathologic process associated with the synaptic space is a deficiency or impaired function of the enzyme acetylcholinesterase (AChE). In this situation, a nerve impulse will result in release of a normal quantity of ACh from the nerve terminal. However, with an absence or deficiency of AChE, the ACh molecules will be allowed to diffuse more widely along the postsynaptic membrane and bind sequentially to more than one AChR or repeatedly to the same AChR. This will result in an EPP of higher amplitude and prolonged duration. The duration of the EPP may exceed the refractory period of the muscle membrane, potentially resulting in multiple depolarizations of the muscle in response to a single nerve stimulus.

If the nerve terminal is depolarized excessively, desensitization of the AChRs may occur because of the accumulation of large quantities of ACh which leads to repeated binding to the same AChR (22,23) (see Section V). The survival of the patient depends on compensatory mechanisms that prevent eventual complete desensitization of the AChRs in these disorders. This compensation may occur presynaptically by a decrease in the number of vesicles released per nerve impulse or postsynaptically by a decrease in the number of AChRs capable of responding to a nerve terminal depolarization. Microelectrode recordings in congenital endplate AChE deficiency reveal that there is a diminished reserve pool of synaptic vesicles (N) structurally associated with small-diameter but mature nerve terminals (24), similar to the findings described in prejunctional disorders. The subsequent reduction in the quantal content restores the EPP to a more "normal" level.

From the above discussion, one would predict that in isolated AChE deficiency or absence, MEPPs would be increased in amplitude and duration and likely normal in frequency. The quantal content and probability of quantal release should be normal. However, with time, compensatory mechanisms may lead to changes in presynaptic and/or postsynaptic function. For example, the primary clinical, naturally occurring illustration of this phenomenon is congenital endplate AChE deficiency (Chapter 6), in which microelectrode studies show MEPP amplitudes to be normal with a prolonged duration, and quantal content is actually reduced due to a diminished n (24). The explanation for this lies in the NMJ morphology where decreased nerve terminal size and degeneration of postsynaptic junctional folds indicate significant pre- and postsynaptic compensatory changes. Cholinesterase inhibitor toxicity and neuromuscular agonist drugs have similar effects on the NMJ, although pre- and postsynaptic compensatory mechanisms are not common unless the effects of these agents is excessively prolonged.

V. POSTSYNAPTIC DISORDERS

Disorders of neuromuscular transmission primarily affecting the postsynaptic region may be divided into two main categories as proposed by Engel (25). His classification divides the postsynaptic disorders into those with or without associated kinetic abnormalities of the AChR ion channel. Disorders *without* associated kinetic abnormalities of the ion channel result from a decreased number of functional AChRs. This may be due to a decrease in their total numbers, a malfunction with normal total numbers, or a combination of the two. The relevant clinical example is myasthenia gravis (Chapter 4) in which pathogenic antibodies are directed against the AChRs of skeletal muscle.

If the number of functional AChRs is reduced for whatever reason, the EPP is obviously reduced in amplitude. MEPPs occur with normal frequency but are of reduced amplitude. Quantal content and probability of quantal release are unaffected. Assuming AChE is functioning normally, a larger proportion of ACh is hydrolyzed than normal because of fewer available AChRs. Depending on the severity of the problem, the EPP produced may be barely suprathreshold or even subthreshold. Sustained voluntary activity will produce the normal relative reduction in quantal content due to depletion of vesicles. However, the already reduced EPP will decrease even further until it is insufficient to trigger threshold firing of the muscle fiber. The muscle fiber fails to contract, and fatigable muscle weakness is the clinical result. Continued activity results in a progressive decline in strength as more muscle fibers fail to contract.

Brief maximal activation of the involved muscle may enhance vesicle release due to build-up of residual calcium in the nerve terminal. This effect is short lived as the depletion of the readily releasable store of vesicles eventually results in a reduced quantal content, often below pre-exercise levels. This phenomenon is known as *postexercise exhaustion* and is employed in the diagnostic testing of disorders of the neuromuscular junction (see Chapter 3).

The postsynaptic disorders causing abnormalities in the kinetics of the AChR ion channel may be categorized as those resulting in a prolonged EPP (slow channel) and those resulting in a shortened (fast-decaying) EPP (fast channel). The prolonged EPPs and endplate currents in the slow-channel syndrome are the result of prolonged activation of the AChR. The best characterized clinical example is congenital slow-channel syndrome (26). As in congenital absence of endplate AChE, the prolonged EPP in slow-channel syndrome may exceed the refractory period of the muscle fiber and result in multiple muscle fiber action potentials in response to a single nerve stimulus. One might expect MEPP amplitude to be increased in these disorders, but the opposite is true (27). The prolonged and repeated depolarizations of the muscle membrane lead to cationic overloading of the postsynaptic membrane and consequently an endplate myopathy with degeneration of the junctional folds and loss of AChRs (22,23). Treatment with agents that enhance ACh release (3,4-diaminopyridine) or inhibit the action of AChE (pyridostigmine) may actually worsen the endplate myopathy in these patients.

In fast-channel syndromes, the EPPs rapidly decay. This brief AChR ion channel openings and a reduced probability of channel opening by ACh. Quantal content and probability of quantal release are normal as expected. MEPP amplitude is reduced due to reduced probability of channel opening. This markedly reduces the probability of effective channel openings (i.e., leading to subthreshold EPPs) and decreases the duration of channel opening events. Three congenital fast-channel myasthenic syndromes have been reported (28–30). Each is caused by mutations in different domains of the AChR subunit. Treatment with agents that enhance release of ACh or inhibit AChE may improve the defect by effectively saturating more AChRs and increasing the likelihood of a more sustained channel opening.

A. Sodium Channels

A reduced number of functioning voltage-sensitive sodium channels on the postsynaptic muscle membrane (see Fig. 1.17) may also adversely affect neuromuscular transmission by increasing the threshold for muscle fiber action potential generation, thus decreasing the safety factor of neuromuscular transmission. This is likely to occur in any synaptic or postsynaptic process that results in significant alteration of endplate or peri-endplate morphology, i.e., myasthenia gravis (31) and congenital absence of endplate AChE (32).

CASE 2.3 A 26-year-old woman is evaluated for complaints of ptosis, diplopia, fatigue with chewing, and lower extremity weakness. Her physician decides to perform a tensilon test and administers the recommended dose of edrophonium as a single intravenous infusion. The woman's ptosis worsens and she develops slurred speech. These effects last for approximately 10 min and she returns to her baseline level. What happened?

Discussion Inhibitors of ACh will not produce weakness in patients with normal neuromuscular junctions. In most patients with postsynaptic disorders of neuromuscular transmission like myasthenia gravis,

ACh inhibitors will prolong the action of ACh at the postsynaptic membrane resulting in a longer and larger EPP and subsequent symptomatic improvement. There are two possible explanations for the symptomatic worsening in this patient. First, it is possible that this patient's disease caused a profound reduction in the number of functioning AChRs, and that the inhibition of AChE effectively "overloaded" the remaining functional AChRs and caused *desensitization*. Second, it is possible that the prolonged action of the ACh molecules induced by blocking the activity of acetylcholinesterase may have caused an abnormally sustained depolarization at the endplate, resulting in a *depolarization block* (see Chapter 8) of the AChRs. In either case, the significant depletion of functioning AChRs (likely due to myasthenia gravis in this patient) made her especially sensitive to the effects of inhibition of AChE.

B. Postsynaptic Desensitization

In the previous discussion of the synaptic level of neuromuscular transmission failure, the consequences of failure of rapid termination of the action of ACh were considered. We saw that compensatory mechanisms were critical to prevent "overstimulation" of the postsynaptic membrane. If the AChR is exposed to the actions of ACh for prolonged periods of time, the receptors become inactive or *desensitized* and no longer open their channels in response to ACh (33). In addition to congenital defects resulting in a deficiency of endplate AChE, agents that mimic the agonist action of ACh (see Chapter 8), or the excessive use of AChE inhibitors may induce *desensitization*. Desensitization likely contributes to the "cholinergic crisis" that sometimes occurs in myasthenia gravis patients treated with AChE inhibitors.

VI. CLINICAL CORRELATION

All of the concepts discussed above can be applied to the clinical diagnosis and management of NMJ disorders. The discussion below provides clinical illustrations of the principal pathophysiologic alterations at each level of the NMJ (prejunctional, presynaptic, synaptic, and postsynaptic).

A. Prejunctional Failure

It is known that fatigability very similar to that experienced by patients with "primary" neuromuscular transmission disorders is a common complaint in a subset of patients with ALS (34) and in patients with a remote history of poliomyelitis (35,36). Electromyographic evidence of failure of neuromuscular transmission in patients with these disorders has also been reported (8,37). Furthermore, electrophysiologic evidence of neuromuscular transmission abnormalities has been observed in other primary neurogenic conditions. The common denominator in these disorders is the presence of ongoing denervation and reinnervation; the mechanisms of impaired neuromuscular transmission is a reduced release of neurotransmitter at immature, reinnervating axonal sprouts, and reduced release of transmitter at atrophic nerve terminals with decreased quantal stores.

Clinically, these patients will have baseline weakness prior to exercise, but will also complain of significant fatigable muscle weakness with prolonged use of the affected muscle group. Treatment with cholinesterase inhibitors may result in a mild symptomatic benefit in some patients. Although this "neurogenic neuromuscular transmission defect" is encountered most frequently in ALS patients, it may seen in any patient with a subacute to chronic axonopathy/neuronopathy. Recognition of this phenomenon will prevent unnecessary concern regarding a superimposed primary disorder of the NMJ.

B. Presynaptic Failure

In patients with presynaptic dysfunction, such as Lambert-Eaton syndrome, the safety margin of neuromuscular transmission is reduced due to a deficiency in the nerve-evoked quantal release of ACh (reduced probability of quantal release, reduced quantal content). These patients often have baseline (prior to exercise) weakness because the amount of ACh released after a nerve impulse is often insufficient to lead to threshold firing of the muscle fiber at a significant number of endplates. Thus, there may be a marked decrease in the EPP amplitude in the resting state (Fig. 2.3). With maximal voluntary contraction or high-frequency nerve stimulation, there is a rapid development of increased strength associated with an increase in the EPP amplitude. This effect is due to build-up of calcium in the nerve terminal facilitating the release of synaptic vesicles. The improvement in strength is very short lived, usually not appreciated by patients, and difficult to demonstrate clinically (see Chapter 5). After approximately 30–50 s the EPPs return to the pre-exercise baseline.

With low-frequency stimulation (or sustained exercise), the already reduced quantal content decreases even further due to the normal physiologic depletion of readily releasable vesicles, causing neuromuscular transmission failure at an increasing number of endplates and fatigable muscle weakness (see Case 2). Treatment with cholinesterase inhibitors usually has minimal if any effect. This is not surprising since prolonging the action of ACh at

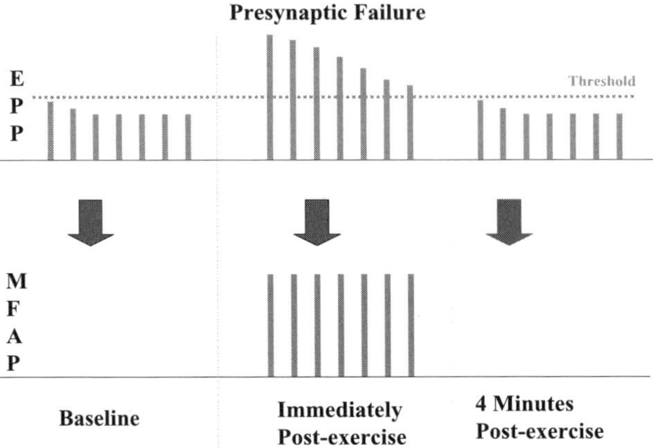

Figure 2.3 Presynaptic failure. In this example, the endplate potential (EPP) is reduced at this particular endplate such that none of the EPPs generated by repetitive stimulation at 2 Hz reach threshold. This suggests that the amount of acetylcholine released by the nerve terminal is severely decreased at rest (prior to exercise). Thus, no muscle fiber action potentials (MFAP) occur (neuromuscular transmission failure). With sustained exercise for approximately 10 s, calcium accumulates in the nerve terminal and facilitates the release of more synaptic vesicles resulting in EPPs of increased amplitude which are adequate for the generation of MFAPs. After 60–90 s of rest, the EPPs return to baseline due to sequestration/diffusion of calcium.

the endplate cannot completely compensate for the critical reduction in the number of ACh molecules released into the synaptic cleft.

C. Synaptic Dysfunction

As noted, the main defect involving the synaptic space is a dysfunction/deficiency of the enzyme acetylcholinesterase. In the absence of a normal amount of functioning AChE at the endplate, ACh can bind to more than one AChR prolonging the duration of the endplate potential. The prolonged endplate potential can trigger one or more additional muscle fiber action potentials if its amplitude remains above threshold longer than the relative refractory period of the preceding action potential. This accounts for the electrophysiologic finding (Chapter 3) of a repetitive compound muscle action potential (CMAP) after a single nerve stimulus. Accordingly, the disorders in which a repetitive CMAP have been reported are those that result in an EPP of increased duration (i.e., congenital endplate cholinesterase deficiency, slow-channel syndrome, and excessive use of cholinesterase inhibitors).

The compensatory response to prolonged endplate exposure to ACh may involve both the presynaptic and postsynaptic regions of the NMJ. A number of the nerve terminals may become reduced in size and release fewer vesicles. As a result of overstimulation by ACh, the endplate region degenerates with loss of AChRs and simplification of junctional folds. This can lead to severe fixed clinical weakness and muscle atrophy in addition to abnormal fatigability in affected patients. As one would expect, all symptoms are refractory to treatment with anticholinesterase drugs.

D. Postsynaptic Failure

In postsynaptic disorders of the neuromuscular junction, like myasthenia gravis, the EPP amplitudes may be sufficient to generate muscle fiber action potentials after single or a few nerve stimulations (Fig. 2.4). However, with repeated or sustained muscular effort, they fall below threshold and muscle fiber action potentials do not occur. Since the force of muscle contraction is dependent on the number of muscle fibers firing, repeated stimulations in these patients result in activation of fewer and fewer muscle fibers, leading to the clinical complaint of fatigable muscle weakness.

Brief, sustained, maximal muscle contraction may improve the safety margin by increasing the residual calcium concentration in the nerve terminal, thereby increasing the number of synaptic vesicles released. This effect is short lived but can be demonstrated on electrodiagnostic testing (see Chapter 3, Section III.B.1.). Unfortunately, this transient benefit has its price as the depletion of synaptic vesicles becomes critical approximately 3–5 min after completion of exercise leading to further lowering of the EPP. This phenomenon is termed *post activation exhaustion* (Fig. 2.4).

Treatment with cholinesterase inhibitors improves the defect in neuromuscular transmission by creating a more favorable ACh to AChR ratio, thereby increasing the number of neuromuscular junctions achieving suprathreshold EPPs.

E. Overview

The basic defect common to all disorders of the NMJ is a reduced safety margin of neuromuscular transmission. When an EPP fails to reach the magnitude of depolarization required for threshold firing of the muscle fiber, an action potential does not occur and the muscle fiber does not contract. This is called neuromuscular transmission failure or block. The different disorders

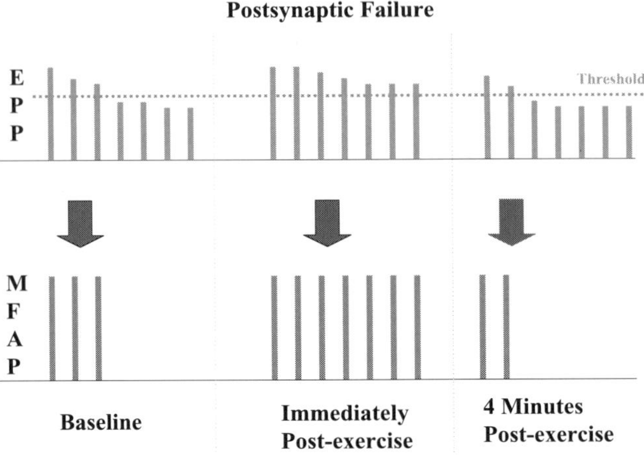

Figure 2.4 Postsynaptic failure. Initially the EPP at this endplate is sufficient for generation of a MFAP. However, after the third of seven stimuli delivered at 2 Hz, the EPP drops below threshold and neuromuscular transmission fails. After sustained exercise for 20 s, the accumulation of calcium in the nerve terminal results in enhanced acetylcholine release and a larger EPP amplitude that does not drop below threshold with repetitive stimulation. However, approximately 4 min after exercise, the baseline EPP amplitude is reduced even further and neuromuscular transmission failure occurs after the second stimulus (postexercise exhaustion).

affecting the NMJ may be classified according to the primary location of failure: prejunctional, presynaptic, synaptic, and postsynaptic. This classification may be an oversimplification as failure may occur at multiple levels simultaneously and dysfunction at a particular level may lead to compensatory changes involving other levels of the NMJ. Nevertheless, the discussion above forms a basis for a thorough understanding of the electrodiagnostic evaluation of disorders of the NMJ, which will be covered in the next chapter. The precise disease mechanisms causing these physiologic disturbances will be covered in subsequent chapters dealing with specific NMJ disorders.

VII. BASIC IMMUNE MECHANISMS IN DISORDERS OF THE NEUROMUSCULAR JUNCTION

The two classic clinical examples of NMJ disorders are myasthenia gravis (MG) and Lambert-Eaton syndrome (LES). The defect in neuromuscular transmission in both diseases is due to an autoimmune attack directed against the skeletal muscle AChRs for MG and the voltage-gated calcium channels for LES. To understand the principles underlying management and serologic diagnosis of these disorders, it is very helpful to have a basic knowledge of the immune system and autoimmunity. A simplified summary of the immune mechanisms that are believed to underlie the development of autoimmunity is presented below. The reader is referred to other sources for a more detailed discussion (38,39).

The immune system is designed to protect the host against pathogens. It is composed of lymphocytes, monocytes, and macrophages. It is crucial to the survival of the host that the immune system have the ability to recognize a diverse range of potential pathogens. These potential pathogens (antigens) are recognized by their molecular conformation by specific receptors on cells of the immune system. Only T and B lymphocytes have receptors that are specific for particular antigens. The population of T and B lymphocytes has a broad repertoire of antigenic specificities, some of which are potentially re-active against host tissues. Prevention of self-reactivity or "immune toler-ance" is believed to be accomplished by three main mechanisms (40,41):

1. Selection of autoreactive lymphocytes for apoptosis (*clonal deletion*)
2. Lack of encounter with self-antigen (*clonal ignorance*).
3. The production of inactivating signals which render lymphocytes nonfunctional (*clonal anergy*).

These mechanisms are not fail-safe, and it is the breakdown of self-tolerance that underlies the development of autoimmune disease. The precise cause of this breakdown is not known, but infections (42), malignancy (43), expo-sure to toxins (44), and disruption of cell or tissue barriers are some of the "triggers" that may play a role. Age, genetics, and hormonal factors may pre-dispose to the breakdown of tolerance explaining why certain individuals develop more than one autoimmune illness.

The induction of an antigen-specific autoimmune response requires the presence of antigen-specific lymphocytes and the presentation of the specific antigen in a manner that activates these lymphocytes. B lympho-cytes recognize the three-dimensional conformation of antigens through their B-cell receptors. T lymphocytes also recognize antigens via a T-cell receptor (TCR), but the antigen must be processed by specialized antigen-presenting cells, which present small antigenic peptide determinants in the context of major histocompatibility complex (MHC) molecules (38). The MHC molecules, which differ in their ability to bind antigenic peptides, con-trol what will be presented to the TCR. Thus, the TCR recognizes a specific antigen/MHC combination that is required for its activation. Costimulatory signals called cytokines are required for activation of T and B lymphocytes. Under certain conditions (i.e., infection, malignancy, toxin exposure, injury), MHC and costimulatory molecules may be up-regulated potentially resulting in activation of previously dormant or anergic self-reactive lymphocytes.

Once the immune response is initiated, there are complex interactions between T and B lymphocytes that may lead to lymphocyte proliferation, cytokine release, and production of antibodies (Fig. 2.5). In MG, it is antibody binding to self-antigen (i.e., the AChR) with activation of complement,

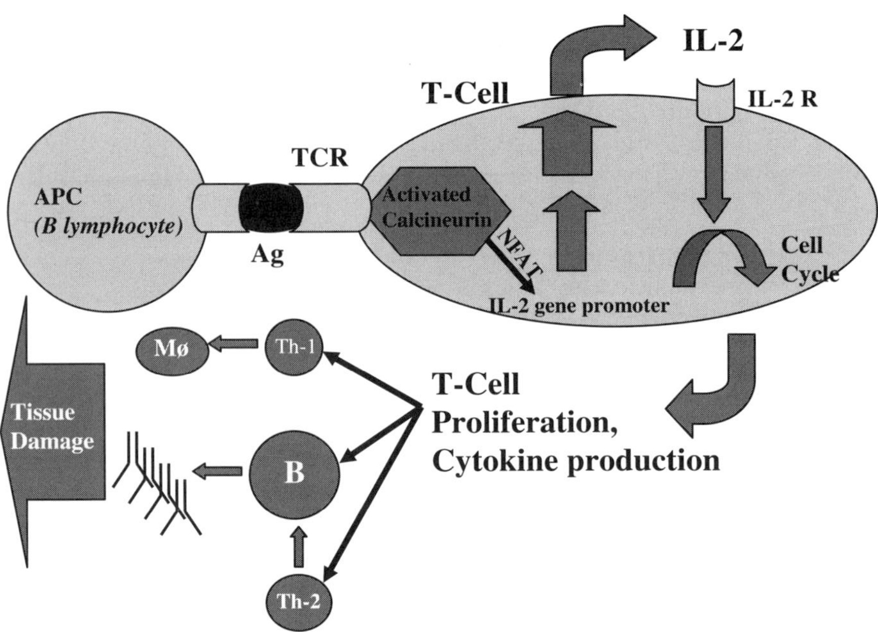

Figure 2.5 Cellular interactions leading to the immune response. T lymphocytes recognize antigen presented in the context of major histocompatibility complex (MHC) molecules by the antigen-presenting cell (APC). The APC may be a B lymphocyte which has bound antigen via its B-cell receptor (BCR). T-cell stimulation results in calcineurin activation, which dephosphorylates a nuclear factor of activated T cells (NFAT) enabling it to enter the nucleus and bind to interleukin-2 (IL-2) promoter. Stimulation of the IL-2 receptor induces the cell to enter the cell cycle and proliferate. Proliferating and activated T lymphocytes produce costimulatory molecules (cytokines) that activate B lymphocytes (to produce antibodies), cytotoxic T lymphocytes (Th-1), and macrophages (Mø) leading to tissue (NMJ) injury.

and macrophage activation that are believed to result in tissue injury and subsequent NMJ dysfunction.

VIII. OVERVIEW

Normal individuals may have lymphocytes that react against self-antigens, including the skeletal muscle AChR and the nerve terminal voltage-gated calcium channels. However, their presence does not result in a clinically significant autoimmune response in these individuals, a phenomenon called self-tolerance. The cause or causes of breakdown of self-tolerance leading to the development of autoimmune diseases is unknown. Systemic infections, malignancy (i.e., thymoma, small cell lung cancer), toxic exposure (i.e., penicillamine), or other tissue injury may play a role.

REFERENCES

1. Del Castillo J, Katz B. Quantal components of the end-plate potential. J Physiol 1954; 124:560–573.
2. Ceccarelli B, Hurlbut WP. Vesicle hypothesis of the release of quanta of acetylcholine. Physiol Rev 1980; 60:396–441.
3. Edds MV. Collateral reinnervation of residual motor axons in partially denervated muscles. J Exp Zool 1950; 113:517–552.
4. Hoffman H. Local reinnervation in partially denervated muscle. Aust J Exp Biol Med Sci 1950; 28:383–397.
5. Bennett MR, McLachlan EM, Taylor RS. The formation of synapses in reinnervated mammalian striated muscle. J Physiol (Lond) 1973; 233:481–500.
6. Bennett MR, Raftos J. The formation and regression of synapses during reinnervation of axolotl striated muscle. J Physiol (Lond) 1977; 265:261–295.
7. Grubb BD, Harris JB, Scofield IS. Neuromuscular transmission at newly formed neuromuscular junctions in the regenerating soleus muscle of the rat. J Physiol (Lond) 1991; 441:405–421.
8. Stalberg E, Schwartz MS, Trontelj JV. Single fiber electromyography in various processes affecting the anterior horn cell. J Neurol Sci 1975; 24:403–415.
9. Bernstein LP, Antel JP. Motor neuron disease: decremental responses to repetitive nerve stimulation. Neurology 1981; 31:204–207.
10. Denys EH, Norris FH. Amyotrophic lateral sclerosis: impairment of neuromuscular transmission. Arch Neurol 1979; 36:202–205.
11. Maselli RA, Wollman RL, Leung C, Distad B, Palombi S, Richman DP, Salazar-Grueso EF, Roos RP. Neuromuscular transmission in amyotrophic lateral sclerosis. Muscle Nerve 1993; 16:1193–1203.
12. Mulder DW, Lambert EH, Eaton LM. Myasthenic syndrome in patients with amyotrophic lateral sclerosis. Neurology 1959; 9:627–631.
13. Van der Kloot W, Molgo J. Quantal acetylcholine release at the vertebrate neuromuscular junction. Physiol Rev 1994; 74:899–991.

14. Augustine GJ. How does calcium trigger neurotransmitter release? Curr Opin Neurobiol 2001; 11(3):320–326.
15. Bashuk RG, Krendel DA. Myasthenia gravis presenting as weakness after magnesium administration. Muscle Nerve 1990; 13:708–712.
16. Fuchs-Buder T, Tassonyi E. Magnesium sulphate enhances residual neuromuscular block induced by vecuronium. Br J Anaesth 1996; 76:565–566.
17. Maselli RA. Pathogenesis of human botulism. Ann NY Acad Sci 1998; 841: 122–139.
18. Mora M, Lambert EH, Engel AG. Synaptic vesicle abnormality in familial infantile myasthenia. Neurology 1987; 37:206–214.
19. Engel AG, Lambert EH. Congenital myasthenic syndromes. Electroencephalogr Clin Neurophysiol Suppl 1987; 39:91–102.
20. Engel AG, Walls TJ, Nagel A, Uchitel O. Newly recognized congenital myasthenic syndromes: I Congenital paucity of synaptic vesicles and reduced quantal release. II. High conductance fast-channel syndrome. III. Abnormal acetylcholine receptor (AChR) interaction with acetylcholine. IV. AChR deficiency and short channel-open time. Prog Brain Res 1990; 84:125–137.
21. Walls TJ, Engel AG, Nagel AS, Harper CM, Trastek VF. Congenital myasthenic syndrome associated with paucity of synaptic vesicles and reduced quantal release. Ann NY Acad Sci 1993; 681:461–468.
22. Engel AG, Lambert EH, Santa T. Study of long-term anticholinesterase therapy. Effects on neuromuscular transmission and on motor endplate fine structure. Neurology 1973; 23:1273–1281.
23. Salpeter MM, Kasprzak H, Feng H, Fertuck H. End-plates after esterase inactivation in vivo: correlation between esterase concentration, functional response and fine structure. J Neurocytol 1979; 8:95–115.
24. Engel AG. Myasthenic syndromes. In: Engel AG, Franzini-Armstrong C, eds. Myology. 2nd ed. New York: McGraw-Hill, 1994:1798–1835.
25. Engel AG. Congenital myasthenic syndromes. Neurol Clin 1994; 12:401–437.
26. Engel AG, Lambert EH, Mulder DM, Torres CF, Sahashi K, Bertorini TE, Whitaker JN. A newly recognized congenital myasthenic syndrome attributed to a prolonged open time of the acetylcholine-induced ion channel. Ann Neurol 1982; 11:553–569.
27. Milone M, Wang H-L, Ohno K, Fukudome T, Pruitt JN, Bren N, Sine SM, Engel AG. Slow-channel syndrome caused by enhanced activation, desensitization, and agonist binding affinity due to mutation in the M2 domain of the acetylcholine receptor alpha subunit. J Neurosci 1997; 17:5651–5665.
28. Milone M, Ohno K, Brengman JM, Batocchi AP, Tonali P, Engel AG. Low-affinity fast-channel congenital myasthenic syndrome caused by new missense mutations in the acetylcholine receptor α subunit. Neurology 1998; 50:432–433.
29. Wang H-L, Milone M, Ohno K, Shen X-M, Tsujino A, Batocchi AP, Tonali P, Brengman JM, Engel AG, Sine SM. Naturally occurring mutation in the acetylcholine receptor α subunit reveals stereochemical and volume contributions of the M3 domain to channel gating. Nature Neurosci 1999; 2:226–233.

30. Ohno K, Wang H-L, Milone M. Congenital myasthenic syndrome caused by decreased agonist binding affinity due to a mutation in the acetylcholine receptor epsilon subunit. Neuron 1996; 17:157–170.
31. Ruff RL, Lennon VA. End-plate voltage-gated sodium channels are lost in clinical and experimental myasthenia gravis. Ann Neurol 1998; 43:370–379.
32. Engel AG, Lambert EH, Gomez MR. A new myasthenic syndrome with end-plate acetylcholinesterase deficiency, small nerve terminals, and reduced acetylcholine release. Ann Neurol 1977; 1:315–330.
33. Maselli RA, Leung C. Analysis of anticholinesterase-induced neuromuscular transmission failure. Muscle Nerve 1993; 16:548–553.
34. Sharma KR, Kent-Braun JA, Majumdar S, Huang Y, Mynhier M, Weiner MW, Miller RG. Physiology of fatigue in amyotrophic lateral sclerosis. Neurology 1995; 45:733–740.
35. Ravits J, Hallett M, Baker M, Nilsson J, Dalakas M. Clinical and electromyographic studies of postpoliomyelitis muscular atrophy. Muscle Nerve 1990; 13:667–674.
36. Trojan DA, Gendron G, Cashman NR. Anticholinesterase-responsive neuromuscular junction transmission defects in post-poliomyelitis fatigue. J Neurol Sci 1993; 114:170–177.
37. Stalberg E, Trontelj JV. Single Fiber Electromyography. 2nd ed. New York: Raven Press, 1994:156–158.
38. Janeway C, Travers P, Walport M, Capra J. Immunobiology: The Immune System in Health and Disease. New York: Garland, 1999.
39. Ragheb S, Lisak RP. Immune regulation and myasthenia gravis. Ann NY Acad Sci 1998; 841:210–224.
40. Miller J, Morahan G. Peripheral T cell tolerance. Annu Rev Immunol 1992; 10: 51–69.
41. MacLennan I. Deletion of autoreactive B cells. Curr Biol 1995; 5:103–106.
42. Rose NR. The role of infection in the pathogenesis of autoimmune disease. Semin Immunol 1998; 10:5–13.
43. Dropcho E. Autoimmune CNS paraneoplastic disorders: mechanisms, diagnosis and therapeutic options. Ann Neurol 1995; 37(suppl 1):S102–S133.
44. Penn AS, Low BW, Jaffe IA, Luo L, Jacques JJ. Drug-induced autoimmune myasthenia gravis. Ann NY Acad Sci 1998; 841:433–449.

3

Diagnostic Tests for Neuromuscular Junction Disorders

I. INTRODUCTION

Disorders of neuromuscular transmission produce symptomatic weakness that predominates in certain muscle groups and typically fluctuates in response to effort and rest. The diagnosis of myasthenia gravis and other disorders of neuromuscular transmission is primarily based on the clinical history and examination findings demonstrating this distinctive pattern of weakness. Laboratory confirmation of the clinical diagnosis may be obtained using pharmacologic, electrophysiologic, and (for certain neuromuscular junction disorders) serologic tests. The diagnostic examinations used to evaluate patients with suspected disorders of neuromuscular transmission are reviewed in this chapter.

II. PHYSIOLOGY OF NEUROMUSCULAR TRANSMISSION REVISITED

As discussed in Chapter 1, the summated action of a large number of acetylcholine (ACh) molecules (released after a nerve action potential reaches the nerve terminal) on the postsynaptic receptors produces the endplate potential (EPP). If the magnitude of the EPP is greater than or equal to the excitation threshold for depolarization of the surrounding sarcolemma, a muscle fiber action potential is produced. The concept of the *safety factor of neuromuscular transmission* was stressed in Chapters 1 and 2 as the difference between the magnitude of the EPP and the depolarization required for threshold firing of the muscle fiber.

Under normal circumstances, the safety factor of neuromuscular transmission is quite large (several times larger than the threshold potential required for generation of a muscle fiber action potential). With repetitive stimulation of the nerve (2–5 Hz.), there is a sequential decrease in the number of available ACh quanta, the number of ACh molecules released, and subsequently the magnitude of the EPP. In normal muscle, this is not a problem since the safety factor of neuromuscular transmission is so large (see Fig. 1.19). Patients with defects of neuromuscular transmission, such as myasthenia gravis (MG) and Lambert-Eaton syndrome (LES), have a reduced safety factor so that with repetitive nerve stimulation, the EPP may not allow for generation of a muscle fiber action potential (neuromuscular transmission failure) (see Chapter 2). As will become apparent, the tests used to diagnose disorders of the neuromuscular junction (NMJ) utilize the above principles to expose the reduced safety factor of neuromuscular transmission in these patients.

III. DIAGNOSTIC TESTING

The major tools used to confirm the clinical suspicion of a disorder of the NMJ may be divided into two main groups: pharmacologic tests and electrophysiologic tests (Table 3.1). At times these two types of examinations are used in combination to improve the objectivity or sensitivity of these tests in isolation. Although not all NMJ disorders have an autoimmune etiology, use of serologic (immunologic) tests has become standard in the diagnosis of MG and LES, and has the advantage of being more disease specific. The applications of these different categories of tests in the diagnosis of disorders of the NMJ will be summarized in this chapter.

A. Pharmacologic Testing

Clinical observation of the response to administration of pharmacologic agents that affect neuromuscular transmission forms the basis for a number of diagnostic tests. These include tests that demonstrate improved strength induced by agents that enhance neuromuscular transmission (i.e., edrophonium, pyridostigmine), or an exaggerated response to agents that block the NMJ (i.e., curare). The utility of these tests has diminished in recent years with the development of more sensitive electrophysiologic techniques.

Table 3.1 Diagnosis of Neuromuscular Junction Disorders

Pharmacologic tests
  Edrophonium
  Neostigmine
  Pyridostigmine
Electrophysiologic tests
  Repetitive nerve stimulation
  Conventional electromyography
  Single-fiber electromyography
Serologic tests
Myasthenia gravis
  Acetylcholine receptor antibodies
  Antistriational antibodies
  Antititin, antiryanodine antibodies
  Antibodies to muscle-specific tyrosine kinase (MuSK)
Lambert-Eaton syndrome
  Antibodies to the voltage-gated calcium channel

1. Edrophonium Chloride (Tensilon) Test

The use of edrophonium chloride (tensilon) as a diagnostic test for MG was described in 1952 (1). Its rapid onset (30 s) and short duration of effect (about 5 min) make it an ideal agent for this purpose. By inhibiting the normal action of acetylcholinesterase (AChE), edrophonium chloride and other cholinesterase inhibitors allow acetylcholine molecules to diffuse more widely throughout the synaptic cleft and to interact with acetylcholine receptors AChRs sequentially (2). This increases the amplitude and duration of the EPP and subsequently increases the safety factor of neuromuscular transmission.

The dose of edrophonium that will produce improvement varies among patients and cannot be predicted in advance. A dose that is too high may exacerbate weakness in patients with abnormal neuromuscular transmission (Case 2.2). Because of this, it is recommended that edrophonium be administered in incremental doses. Most clinicians start by administering a dose of 2 mg and observing the response for 45–60 s. This is followed by doses of 3 and 5 mg and observation for a clinical response for 1–2 min following each dose. The dose for newborns and infants is 0.15 mg/ kg subcutaneously. The response to the injection should be carefully monitored in a clinically weak muscle. Clinical improvement should be seen in 30 s and should last approximately 3–5 min. During the injection, patients often experience 1–3 min of increased salivation, mild sweating, perioral fasciculations, and mild nausea. Hypotension and bradycardia are extremely rare but precautions should be taken. Atropine sulfate (0.6 mg intramuscular or intravenously) should be available in case of an emergency. Some advocate continuous monitoring of heart rate and blood pressure. Bronchial asthma and cardiac dysrhythmias are relative contraindications for tensilon testing.

A tensilon test is considered positive when there is unequivocal improvement in an objectively weak muscle (3). The test is limited by the dependence on patient effort to give maximal exertion both before and after the drug is administered. For this reason, sentinel muscles should be chosen that are definitely weak and are most likely to demonstrate a clear-cut change (Fig. 3.1). Eyelid elevation and extraocular muscle functions are best for these purposes.

Interpretation of the results of a tensilon test is often difficult because the test is subjective. A dramatic response in any muscle group is usually sufficient to constitute a positive test. Conversely, exacerbation of weakness following administration of edrophonium, as previously noted, is strong evidence of abnormal neuromuscular transmission (4). Apparent slight to moderate improvement in muscle strength must be interpreted with extreme caution. Mild to moderate clinical improvement after administration of tensilon has been reported in a number of other conditions, including, brainstem lesions (5,6), oculomotor palsy due to cerebral artery aneurysm (7), diabetic abducens paresis (3), and even in normal control subjects (8).

While an improvement after administering edrophonium is evidence in favor of a defect in neuromuscular transmission, it is neither absolutely sensitive nor specific. Diagnostic sensitivity and specificity is acceptable only

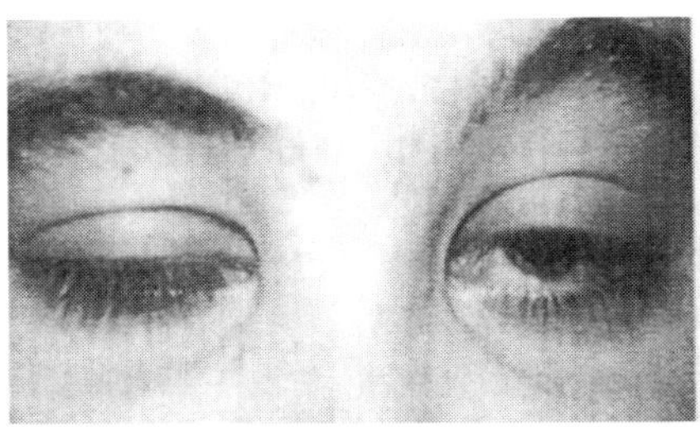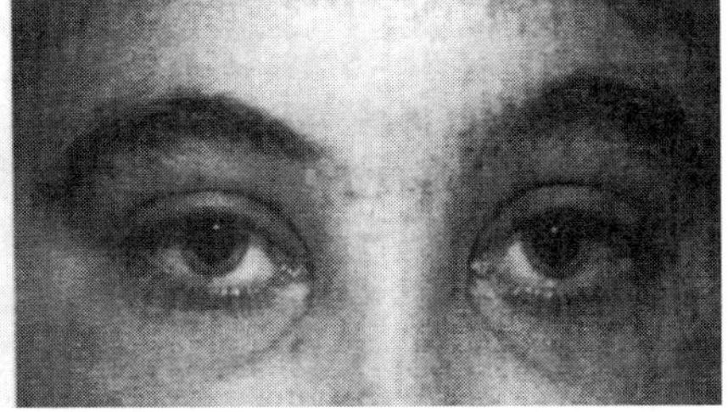

Figure 3.1 Edrophonium test. Patient with severe bilateral ptosis prior to administration of edrophonium (left). Marked improvement after administration of edrophonium (right) is apparent. (Reproduced from Grob D, Natural History of Myasthenia Gravis. In: Engel AG, ed. Myasthenia Gravis and Myasthenic Disorders. New York: Oxford University Press, 1999, p 133).

in patients with clear-cut weakness in muscles that can be assessed in a serial and objective manner, i.e., eyelid elevators and extraocular muscles. Thus, in the absence of ptosis or clinically obvious ophthalmoparesis, the edrophonium test should probably not be performed and other methods should be used to establish the diagnosis. The effect of cholinesterase inhibitors can also be assessed by monitoring electrophysiologic tests (see below), which may give a more objective measure of a positive response.

CASE 3.1 A 58-year-old woman with generalized MG of greater than 20 years duration is referred for a second opinion regarding her diagnosis. Her examination reveals severe bilateral ptosis and oph-thalmoparesis, and severe upper and lower limb weakness which is fatigable. She indicates that she has been on pyridostigmine (an AChE inhibitor) as her only treatment for the past 20 years. She states that "the medicine used to work like a charm, but doesn't do much for me now." The reason for her referral was that a local neurologist had performed a tensilon test and noted "absolutely no improvement in her severe ptosis." Did this patient have MG? What is the likelihood of a negative tensilon test in a patient with MG?

Discussion This patient indeed had MG. It is important to be cognizant of the potential false-negative as well as the false-positive results of the edrophonium test. Not all patients with MG will respond to edrophonium. The likelihood of a positive response depends on the clinical status of the patient and the muscle chosen for observation; as discussed above. In this case, despite selecting an obviously weak muscle, there was no observable clinical response. One reason for this may be the clinical status of this patient. She had long-standing, essentially untreated MG and very likely had developed an "endplate myopathy" (see Chapter 4) causing permanent changes in endplate morphology (i.e., loss of junctional folds, decreased numbers of ACh receptors), explaining her lack of response to inhibition of AChE. In general, false-negative examinations occur in 3–21% of MG patients, being more common in patients with purely ocular weakness (9,10).

---

2. Other Cholinesterase Inhibitors

Some patients with MG do not improve after administration of edrophonium but do respond to neostigmine methyl sulfate or prostigmine (11,12). The onset of action after the intravenous (IV) administration of neostigmine is 1–2 min; the onset of action after an intramuscular (IM) dose is approximately 5–15 min. The drug has maximal effect approximately 2–3 min after IV administration and 20 min after IM administration. The clinical effects of neostigmine last from 2.5 to 4 h after IM injection. This longer duration of action compared to edrophonium is especially useful in the evaluation of children. It also allows for functional testing of muscle groups for more prolonged periods of time (i.e., sustained arm elevation, stair climbing, and pulmonary function testing). The same precautions regarding potential false-positive tests are applicable as with edrophonium. However, patients are less likely to have a false-positive test due to brief, effort-related increases in strength because of the more prolonged duration of drug effect.

Finally, administration of oral pyridostigmine (Mestinon) as a therapeutic trial may demonstrate a beneficial effect on muscle strength and fatigability that is not apparent after a single dose of edrophonium. Once again, caution is advised in interpretation of such trials since the patient's subjective reports are the main measure of a positive response, and it is often difficult to objectively document the improvement. Nevertheless, a beneficial response to pyridostigmine may be quite helpful in certain patients when other diagnostic tests are negative or borderline.

3. Neuromuscular Blocking Agents

Drugs that block the AChRs on the postsynaptic muscle membrane have an exaggerated effect in patients with NMJ disease. On this basis, both curare (13) and quinine (14,15) have been used as diagnostic tests in patients with suspected disorders of neuromuscular transmission. Currently, neither agent is routinely used for this purpose. Curare is sometimes used as a provocative agent in electrophysiologic testing (see below). The enhanced effect of neuromuscular blocking drugs on patients with NMJ disease is probably most frequently encountered clinically when patients with previously undiagnosed MG or LES undergo a surgical procedure in which neuromuscular blocking drugs are used. These patients often develop prolonged paralysis with respiratory failure and ventilator dependence "unmasking" the NMJ disorder.

B. Electrophysiologic Testing

Electrophysiologic studies are performed in patients with suspected NMJ disease to confirm a defect in neuromuscular transmission, as well as to exclude other diseases of the motor unit that may confound or contribute to the clinical findings. Furthermore, these studies are useful in assessing the severity of involvement and in providing a quantitative baseline for comparison and documentation of disease evolution and response to treatment. It is important to understand that the electrophysiologic findings in patients with NMJ disease are not disease specific but, when interpreted in light of the clinical presentation and examination, lead the physician to the appropriate diagnosis.

The two principal electrophysiologic tests used to confirm a defect in neuromuscular transmission are repetitive nerve stimulation studies and single-fiber electromyography. Conventional needle electromyography may also aid in discovering a defect in neuromuscular transmission. These electrophysiologic techniques are described below and the typical findings in specific disorders of neuromuscular transmission are illustrated.

1.   Repetitive Nerve Stimulation

Repetitive nerve stimulation (RNS) is the most commonly used electrophysiologic test of neuromuscular transmission. In 1895, Jolly (16) first described the technique in which an electric current was applied to excite a motor nerve while the force of muscle contraction was recorded. Harvey and Masland (17) refined the technique in 1941 by recording the response to RNS to detect disorders of neuromuscular transmission. In this technique, a motor nerve is stimulated repetitively while recording compound muscle action potentials (CMAPs) from an appropriate muscle. A CMAP represents the electrophysiologic composite of the muscle fibers belonging to all the motor units in a supramaximally stimulated nerve. Failure of neuromuscular transmission in a number of motor endplates will result in fewer muscle fibers contributing to the amplitude of the CMAP (Fig. 3.2). This is the physiologic basis for the *decremental response* (see below) that is observed in patients with NMJ disease.

RNS serves to "stress" motor endplates with marginal safety factors by depleting the store of readily releasable synaptic vesicles. In clinical practice, a train of 8–10 stimuli are delivered at a rate of 2–3 Hz. This rate is effective for this purpose because it normally results in a sequential decrease in the amount of acetylcholine released from the nerve terminal up to the fifth or sixth stimulus at which point mobilization of storage ACh vesicles keeps pace with ACh release (see Chapter 1). The normal physiologic decrease in the magnitude of the safety factor of neuromuscular transmission due to this phenomenon becomes crucial in myasthenic endplates and the EPP drops below threshold. As this occurs in a larger number of endplates, the resulting CMAP is reduced in amplitude and area (decremental response).

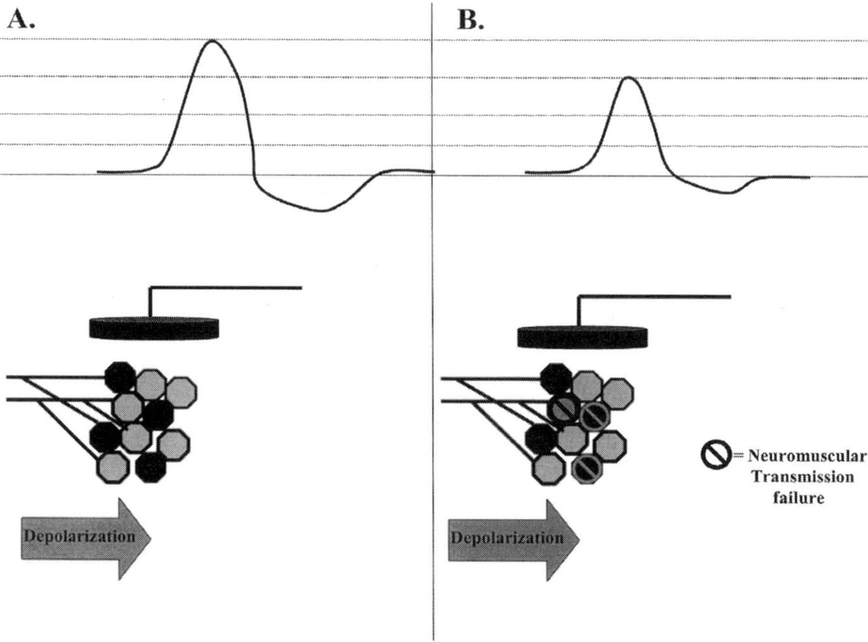

Figure 3.2 Cause of a decremental response. (A) The compound muscle action potential (CMAP) represents the sum of the electrical activity of all muscle fibers belonging to the motor units in a supramaximally stimulated nerve. (B) If neuromuscular transmission fails at a critical number of endplates, the amplitude of the recorded CMAP is reduced. This is the physiologic basis for the *decremental response* to repetitive nerve stimulation observed in patients with disorders of the NMJ.

The diagnostic yield of RNS may be improved by a number of activation techniques. The most commonly employed involves maximal exercise of the tested muscle for a prescribed period of time. Similar to the effect of rapid-rate (20–50 Hz) neural stimulation, this results in accumulation of calcium in the nerve terminal, enhancing the release of ACh. Recall from Chapter 2 that in LES and other presynaptic disorders, there is a marked increase in the CMAP amplitude following brief (~10–15 s) maximal exercise or rapid-rate nerve stimulation, a phenomenon referred to as *postactivation facilitation* (PAF). Following more sustained (i.e., 30–60 s or longer) maximal exercise, there is a depletion of readily releasable synaptic vesicles which in MG (and other postsynaptic disorders) results in a worsening of the decremental response compared to pre-exercise values. This is referred to as *postactivation exhaustion* (PAE), and is maximal 2–4 min following exercise. The test procedures described below are designed to elicit these phenomena, facilitating the diagnosis of an NMJ disorder.

Recording Technique The technique of RNS is similar to that used for the recording of routine motor nerve conduction studies (18). A peripheral nerve is stimulated supramaximally and the CMAP is recorded. Stimulation is performed with surface electrodes. The CMAP is recorded with a surface electrode placed over the motor point of the muscle; a reference recording electrode is placed on a distal point where minimal electrical activity is recorded, usually a tendon or bony prominence. The appropriate joints should be stabilized to minimize movement artifact.

Test Procedure

1. Determine supramaximal CMAP response.
2. Stimulate at 20–50% greater than stimulus intensity required for the above.
3. Test muscle at rest with a train of five to nine supramaximal stimuli at a frequency of 2–3 Hz.
4. After several minutes rest, repeat step 3 to ensure reproducibility.
5. Voluntarily activate muscle:

    a. If postsynaptic defect suspected and > 10% decrement at rest, exercise for 20 s, looking for *"repair of decrement"* (see below), facilitation of baseline amplitude, and PAE.
    b. If postsynaptic defect suspected and no significant decrement at rest, exercise for at least 60 s looking for PAE.
    c. If presynaptic defect suspected, note baseline CMAP amplitude and look for decrement at rest (this may be difficult to quantitate if baseline CMAP amplitude is very low). Exercise for 10–15 s looking for PAF.

6. Repeat train of five to nine supramaximal stimuli immediately after activation. Postactivation facilitation is usually maximal *immediately* after exercise.
7. Repeat the train of stimuli every minute for 5 min. PAE will usually be maximal 2–4 min post exercise.

A diagrammatic representation of some of the possible results of RNS testing is shown in Fig. 3.3. Stimulation rates of 1, 2, 3, or 5 Hz has been used in the diagnosis of NMJ disorders. Desmedt (19) found that stimulation rates between 3 and 5 Hz are most likely to produce a decremental response in MG.

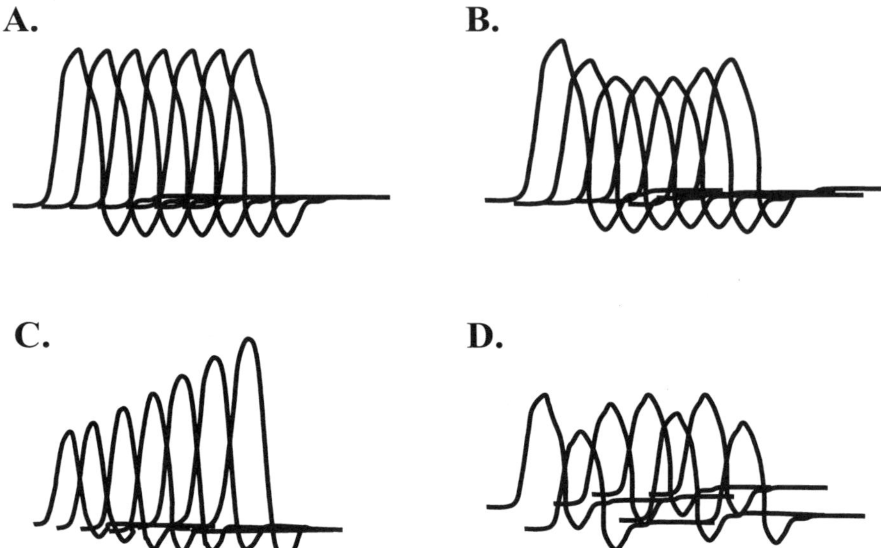

Figure 3.3 Diagrammatic representation of possible results of repetitive nerve stimulation. (A) Normal response. (B) Typical decremental response as may be seen in a patient with NMJ disease. (C) Incremental response or neuromuscular facilitation. (D) Artifact.

Excessively fast rates of stimulation in patients with NMJ disease may produce an increase in CMAP amplitude due to build-up of calcium in the nerve terminal and the resulting facilitated release of ACh (true facilitation). This occurs only in diseased endplates since in normal NMJs *all* endplate potentials result in muscle fiber action potential generation.

In normal as well as abnormal individuals, a rapid rate of stimulation may result in an increased CMAP amplitude by a different mechanism. Rapid rate stimulation causes increased synchronization of the action potential velocities in the tested muscle fibers (20). This produces a CMAP of increased amplitude but decreased duration (the negative peak area is essentially unchanged). This phenomenon is called *pseudofacilitation*. Diagrammatic representations of pseudofacilitation vs. true facilitation are shown in Fig. 3.4. It is obviously important to distinguish pseudofacilitation from true neuromuscular facilitation in which *both* the amplitude *and* area are increased.

The negative peak amplitude or negative peak area are the critical meausurements when performing RNS (20). The area is a more accurate measure of the number of muscle fibers contributing to the CMAP and as

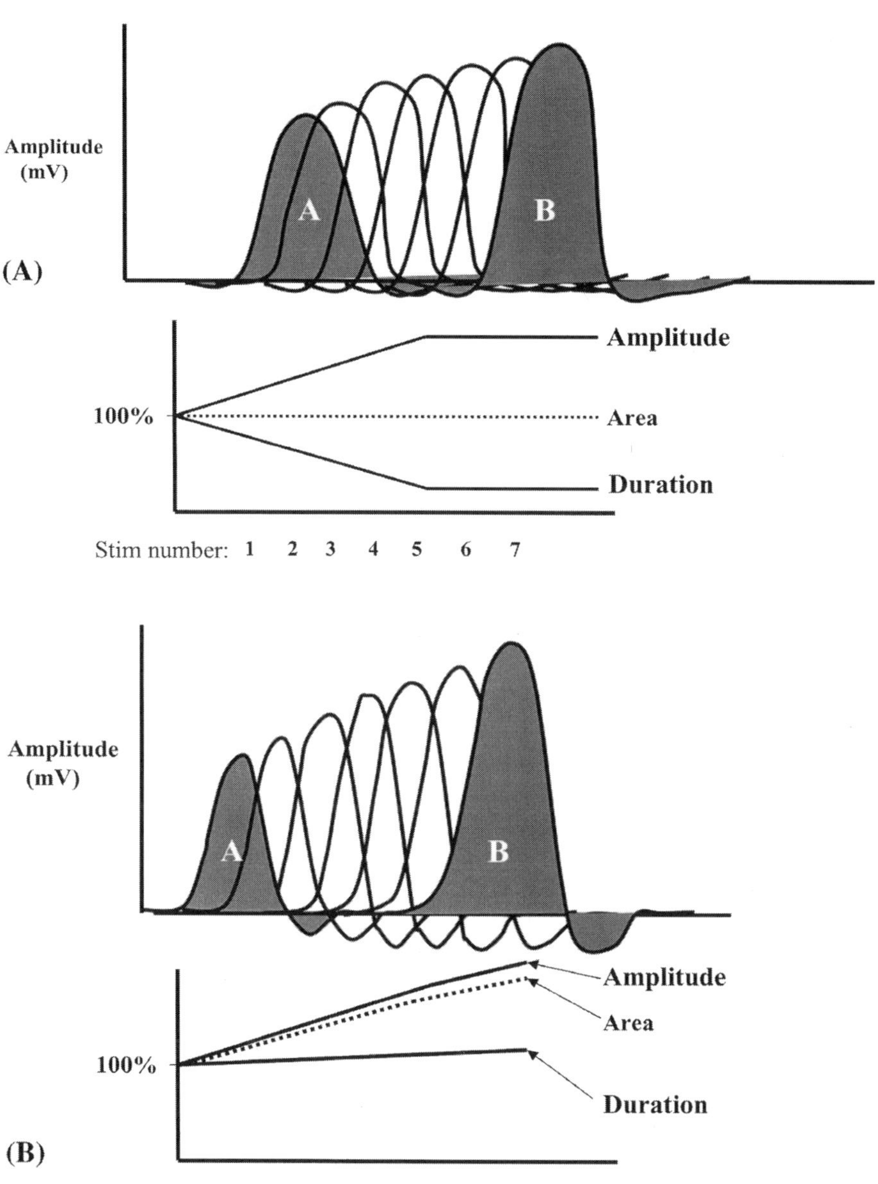

Figure 3.4 True neuromuscular facilitation vs. pseudofacilitation. The CMAP amplitude (A) is increased in both diagrammatic examples, in true facilitation (B), *both* the amplitude and negative peak area are increased.

noted above is not affected by pseudofacilitation. The decrement is defined as the percentage of change between the amplitude or area of the fourth, fifth, or lowest potential (usually the fourth) compared to the first potential, and is given by the formula:

$$\% \text{ Decrement} = (1 - (\text{potential}_n/\text{potential}_1)) \times 100\%$$

PAF can be calculated by the formula:

$$\% \text{ Facilitation} = [(\text{potential}_n/\text{potential}_1) - 1)] \times 100\%$$

where n is the amplitude or area of the potential to which the first potential is compared.

Criteria for Abnormality At 3–5 Hz stimulation frequency, decrements in CMAP amplitude up to 8% may be seen in normal subjects (21). A decrement greater than 10% is considered abnormal. However, the criteria for abnormality will vary to some degree between laboratories.

Any degree of PAF that is not due to pseudofacilitation is evidence of abnormal neuromuscular transmission. PAF of greater than 100% usually indicates a presynaptic disorder of neuromuscular transmission. However, PAF of up to 100% has been observed in patients with MG. The mechanism underlying these findings in a presumed purely postsynaptic disorder is not clear. Thus, a profound PAF is clear, objective evidence of abnormal neuromuscular transmission, and if greater than 100%, is consistent with a presynaptic localization.

Technical Considerations The following considerations are useful to maximize diagnostic sensitivity and prevent artifactual changes:

1. *Reproducibility.* The same decrement should be seen on repeat testing after a period of rest. The muscle should be rested for at least 30 s between trials. The average decrement after three trials may be reported and is often more accurate than the measurement after a single trial. Widely varying measurements from one trial to another are an indication of poor technique, or may be caused by incomplete muscle relaxation (see below).
2. *The stimulating and recording electrodes must be adequately immobilized.* Movement of the stimulating or recording electrodes, or the muscle itself, may produce irregular patterns of change in CMAP size and configuration during repetitive stimulation. It is important to recognize these patterns as not conforming to those expected in disease of the NMJ (Fig. 3.3D).
3. *Muscle temperature.* The decremental response in endplate diseases is less when the muscle is cool (22). Hand or foot muscles should be

warmed to at least 36°C to ensure the maximal diagnostic sensitivity.

4. Anticholinesterase medications can mask a decrement and should be stopped at least 12 hours prior to the study.

Muscle Selection The distribution of muscle weakness varies in patients with NMJ disease. In MG, proximal muscles are more likely to be clinically involved, although distal muscles may occasionally be preferentially affected (see Chapter 4). Thus, RNS is more likely to be abnormal in a proximal or facial muscle in patients with MG (20). To obtain the maximal diagnostic yield, multiple muscles should be tested, particularly clinically weak muscles. However, since hand muscles are the most convenient to test and are well tolerated by patients, most investigators begin with RNS studies in a distal hand muscle. A list of commonly tested muscles given in order of preference by the author follows:

1. Ulnar nerve, recording hypothenar muscle
2. Median nerve, recording thenar muscle
3. Spinal accessory nerve, recording trapezius muscle
4. Facial nerve, recording nasalis muscle
5. Musculocutaneous nerve, recording biceps brachii muscle

The technique for RNS of an intrinsic hand muscle (i.e., ulnar or median nerves) involves placing a recording electrode over the belly of the muscle (abductor digiti minim or abductor pollicis brevis), a reference electrode over a tendon or other electrically inactive site, and stimulating the nerve (ulnar or median) at the wrist. These muscles are convenient to test, easy to activate maximally, and usually well tolerated.

For stimulation of the spinal accessory nerve, the active electrode is placed over the trapezius muscle at the angle between the neck and shoulder, with the reference electrode placed over the acromion. The spinal accessory nerve is stimulated in the neck at the posterior border of the sternocleido-mastoid muscle. Since the trapezius is a tonically active axial muscle, it is difficult to maximally exercise this muscle making determinations of PAF or PAE technically challenging.

Facial muscles are tested with the active electrode over either the nasalis or inferior orbicularis oculi muscles with the reference electrode either lateral to the eye or on the contraleteral orbicularis oculi muscle, respectively. The facial nerve is stimulated below the ear. Patients tend to find repetitive stimulation of the facial nerve uncomfortable and movement artifact typically obscures interpretation of the results.

The musculocutaneous nerve can be stimulated in the axilla while recording from the biceps muscle. A technique for repetitive stimulation of the phrenic nerve with recording of the responses over the diaphragmatic muscle has been described (23). This technique is often poorly tolerated, and recording of the normally low amplitude diaphragmatic compound muscle action potentials may not be possible in obese individuals.

The ulnar, median, and musculocutaneous nerves are useful if the patient's symptoms are most prominent in the extremities. The facial and spinal accessory nerves are probably of higher yield in patients with predominantly ocular or bulbar weakness. Most laboratories require testing of at least three muscles for an examination to be considered a complete evaluation for NMJ disease. However, once a proximal or facial muscle is tested and is negative in a patient with oculobulbar symptoms, one may elect to proceed directly to single-fiber electromyography (see below). A reproducible decrement of greater than 10% in two muscles constitutes a definite electrodiagnosis of a defect in neuromuscular transmission, as long as primary disorders of nerve and muscle are ruled out.

In order for RNS of a particular muscle to be abnormal, there must be *failure* of neuromuscular transmission at a sufficient number of endplates to cause a decrease in the size of the recorded CMAP (see Fig. 3.2). Neuromuscular transmission failure at a small number of endplates or instability of neuromuscular transmission *without failure* will not result in a decremental response during RNS. For this reason, RNS is unlikely to be abnormal in mild NMJ disease, particularly in the absence of clinical weakness or fatigability. Several methods of enhancing or provoking a decremental response in mild NMJ disease have been described.

The production of ischemia in tested muscles may enhance the sensitivity of RNS. Harvey and Masland (17) first described the effects of ischemia on neuromuscular transmission. A provocative technique called the "double-step" RNS test involves prolonged distal nerve stimulation before and after ischemia of the limb. This technique was found to be slightly more sensitive than RNS of the trapezius and only 60% as sensitive as single-fiber electromyography of a forearm muscle (24).

Mild abnormalities of neuromuscular transmission may also be revealed by regional infusions of small doses of curare given in association with performance of RNS studies (25,26). The use of a neuromuscular blocking agent like curare will increase the sensitivity of RNS studies, particularly in muscles that are only mildly affected. Abnormal curare sensitivity may also be seen in primary nerve disease, and this diagnostic possibility must be considered and excluded if a curare test is positive. Neither of these provocative techniques (ischemia, curare) are in common use today given the development of more sensitive diagnostic techniques, particularly single-fiber eletromyography.

Repetitive Nerve Stimulation in Specific Neuromuscular Junction Disorders

Myasthenia Gravis: In MG, the typical pattern seen with at 2–5 Hz is a progressive decrement of the second through the fourth or fifth response with some return toward the initial CMAP size during the subsequent responses to a train of stimuli, the so-called U-shaped pattern (Fig. 3.5). The baseline CMAP amplitude in affected muscles is typically normal. Most laboratories use stimulation trains of 9–10 for the measurement of the decremental response at rest. Subsequently, trains of 5–6 are sufficient for determination of PAF and PAE.

Voluntary activation of the tested muscle by sustained contraction for 30–60 s or longer will produce characteristic RNS findings in patients with postsynaptic disorders like MG. Immediately after activation of a muscle in a patient with MG, one may see a modest increase in the size of the baseline CMAP and a "repair of the decrement" (Fig. 3.6). After 2–5 min, a worsening of the decremental response compared to pre-exercise values or PAE is seen. In some muscles, particularly in patients with mild disease, an abnormal decrement may be seen only during the PAE stage (Fig. 3.7).

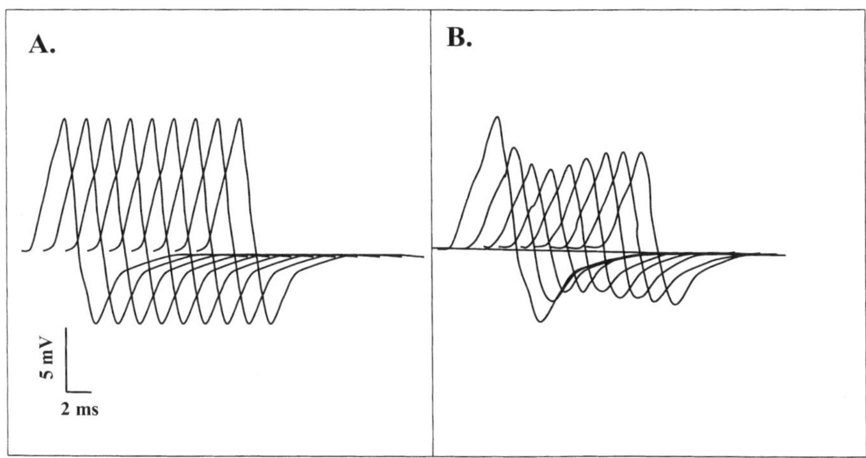

Figure 3.5 Tracings from a normal control subject (A) and a patient with myathenia gravis (B) illustrating a classic decremental response. Responses were obtained with repetitive stimulation of the ulnar nerve at 3 Hz, recording from the abductor digiti minimi muscle. The maximal decrement in CMAP amplitude occurs after the fourth stimulation (−39.7%), producing the classic U-shaped or saddle-shaped pattern.

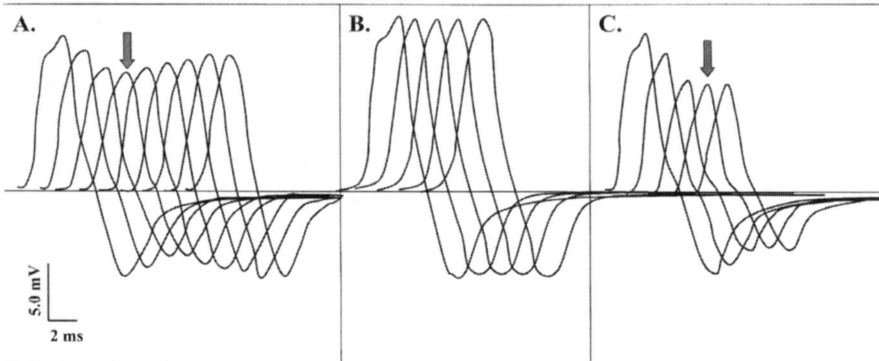

Figure 3.6 Tracings of the responses to repetitive stimulation in a patient with myasthenia gravis. (A) A prominent decrement is seen with 3 Hz stimulation of the ulnar nerve recording from the abductor digit minimi muscle at rest. Comparing the amplitude of the first potential with the fourth potential (arrow), there is a 23.6% decrement. (B) Immediately after 30 s of exercise, the decrement is now much less ("repair of the decrement") and there has been a slight increase in the baseline CMAP amplitude. (C) Four minutes after exercise the decrement is now worsened (32%) compared to the resting baseline (postactivation exhaustion).

RNS studies demonstrate an abnormal decrement in an extremity muscle (hand or shoulder) in approximately 60% of patients with MG, being more sensitive in generalized disease (27). When signs or symptoms are limited to ocular or bulbar muscles, it is not unusual for RNS studies to be completely normal if only extremity muscles are tested. The yield may be improved by testing facial or even diaphragmatic muscles. However, the technical difficulty and poor patient tolerance of these procedures often preclude their use. Thus, RNS is a very useful test in generalized MG and in muscles that are clinically weak and fatigable to demonstrate that the observed weakness is due to a defect in neuromuscular transmission. On the other hand, RNS is of limited diagnostic utility in patients with mild MG or in patients with predominantly oculobulbar symptoms. Normal RNS studies, even if performed in multiple muscles, do not rule out the diagnosis of MG in these patients.

Lambert-Eaton Syndrome: The pattern of abnormality on RNS in LES is characteristic and forms the basis for the clinical diagnosis. The typical findings are low-amplitude baseline CMAPs with an abnormal decrement at rest (28). Immediately after a brief period of exercise, there is a marked

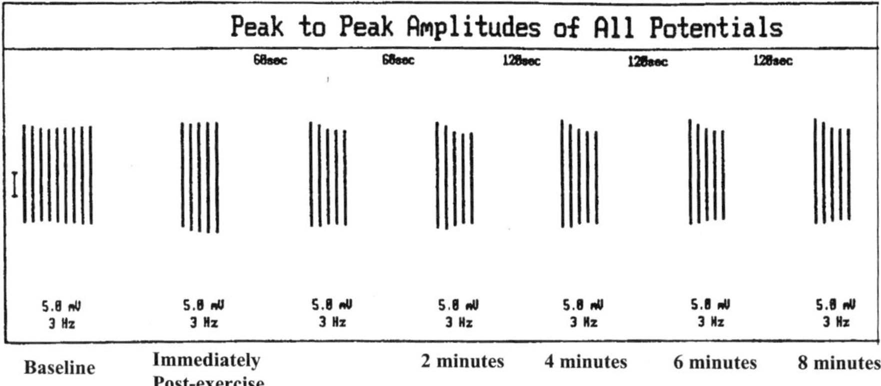

Figure 3.7 Stimulation paradigm in a patient with mild MG. The vertical lines represent CMAP amplitudes obtained with stimulation of the ulnar nerve at 3 Hz, recording from the abductor digiti minimi muscle; the results of eight trains of stimuli are shown. In the first train, nine stimuli were applied to the ulnar nerve and the responses were recorded from the abductor digiti minimi muscle. Subsequent trains consist of five stimuli. All stimuli were given at a rate of 3 Hz. The second train was obtained immediately after 30 s of maximal voluntary contraction. Subsequent trains were obtained with the timing shown in the figure. Note that the decremental response at rest was not abnormal (8%). Maximal postactivation exhaustion occurred with the fifth stimulation train (18.6%) obtained 4 min after the exercise period.

facilitation of CMAP amplitude (200–1000% or more) (Fig. 3.8). Practically speaking, it is preferable to assess for the presence of facilitation after sustained voluntary exercise of the muscle rather than after high-frequency RNS since it is less painful and just as effective for demonstrating PAF (29).

RNS is the most specific test to confirm the clinical diagnosis in patients with suspected LES. The most common finding is a decremental response at low rates of stimulation performed in a hand muscle (22,30). Care must be taken not to exercise the muscle for too long as this may deplete neurotransmitter release and blunt the facilitory response. It is also very important to make sure that the tested muscle is adequately stabilized to minimize movement artifact when determining baseline CMAP amplitudes and assessing for a decrement at rest. In contrast to postsynaptic disorders in which at least 1 min of exercise is best to demonstrate PAE, 10–15 s is all that is required to best elicit PAF in LES.

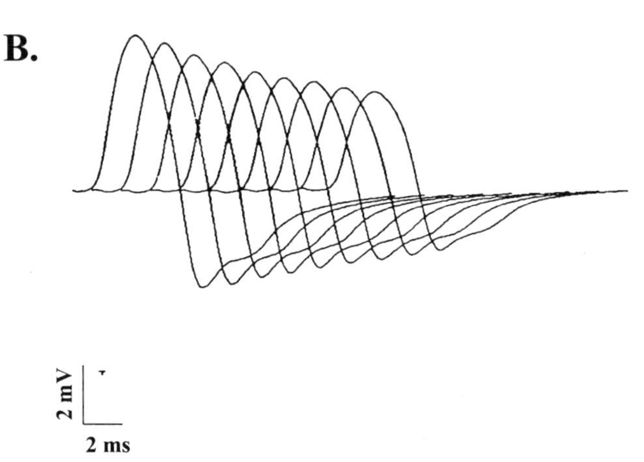

Figure 3.8 Classic RNS findings in LES. (A) CMAP responses obtained with repetitive stimulation of the median nerve recording from the abductor pollicis brevis muscle. Note the low resting CMAP amplitude. A decremental response is also present but is somewhat difficult to visualize due to the low baseline amplitudes. (B) Results of repetitive stimulation immediately after 10 s of maximal voluntary contraction. Marked postactivation facilitation of greater than 200% is demonstrated.

A few additional technical notes merit consideration when performing RNS in suspected LES. First, as with all NMJ disorders, it is important to ensure adequate warming of the tested muscle. The skin surface temperature should be maintained at a minimum of 36° Centigrade during testing. Second, complete muscle relaxation is crucial prior to stimulation for determination of baseline CMAP amplitudes and pre-exercise decremental responses. Any subliminal activation of the tested muscle may facilitate neuromuscular transmission at a number of endplates and affect the results. Selection of muscles is also important. Unlike MG, the intrinsic hand muscles are the most frequently involved electrophysiologically in LES and are also the easiest to exercise maximally. Finally, although pronounced PAF is the signature finding for LES, a decremental response to slow-rate RNS is the most sensitive finding (29,30) and may be the only abnormality in a patient with early or mild disease.

CASE 3.2 A 59-year-old man presents for electrodiagnostic testing. He has experienced progressive lower extremity weakness and fatigue with walking for the past 10 months. He has no ocular or bulbar complaints. As part of his diagnostic workup, he had an MRI of the lumbar spine, which showed degenerative changes and multilevel spinal stenosis. He is referred for evaluation of lumbar polyradiculopathy. The electrodiagnostic technician finds that performing nerve conduction studies on this patient is "technically difficult." He is unable to get "a stable, supramaximal CMAP." He thinks this is because the patient is "too tense."

The neurologist examines the patient and finds mild proximal lower extremity weakness and diffuse hyporeflexia. He performs a motor nerve conduction study stimulating the ulnar nerve and recording from the abductor digiti minimi muscle. He delivers a single stimulus after the patient has completely relaxed the muscle for 60 s. He then asks the patient to contract the muscle maximally for 10 s and delivers a single stimulus immediately after exercise. The results are shown in Fig. 3.9.

Discussion The PAF illustrated in the figure is consistent with a presynaptic NMJ disorder. The diagnosis of LES was confirmed in this patient by RNS studies and serologic testing. The technician's inability to obtain a consistent CMAP amplitude was due to the fact that the tested muscle was being activated to varying degrees during the course of the study. The patient was, in effect, autofacilitating by sustaining contraction (albeit mild) in the muscle and producing calcium accumulation in the nerve terminal facilitating the release of increased amounts of ACh. This illustrates the importance of ensuring complete relaxation of the muscle during RNS studies so that accurate baseline CMAP amplitudes and, subsequently, accurate PAF measurements may be obtained.

Botulism: Several patterns of RNS abnormalities may be observed in botulism depending on the severity of the disease and whether the patient is an adult or an infant. There are four characteristic RNS findings that may be encountered. These are (a) reduced resting CMAP amplitude, (b) at least

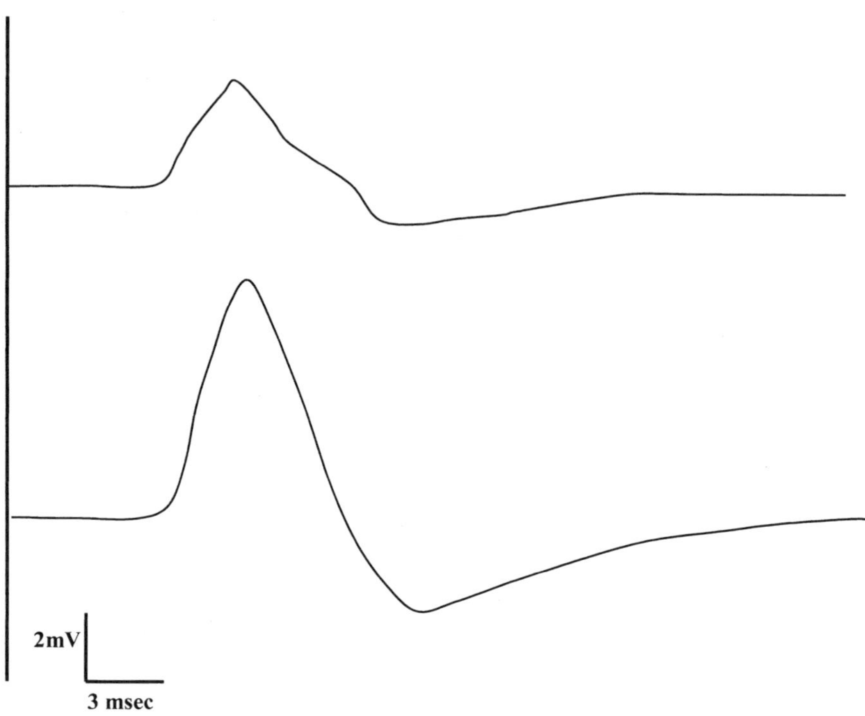

Figure 3.9 Single supramaximal stimulation of the median nerve recording from the abductor pollicis brevis muscle at rest (top) and immediately after 10 s of maximal voluntary contraction (bottom).

40% facilitation of CMAP amplitude after tetanic stimulation, (c) persistence of facilitation for at least 2 min after activation, and (d) the absence of PAE. The presence of all four of these electrophysiologic features is virtually diagnostic of botulism, although hypermagnesemia (31) must be considered and ruled out.

In infants, the baseline CMAP amplitude is reduced (less than 2 mV) in virtually all cases. A decrement at low rates of stimulation is seen in only about half, in contrast to the findings in LES. PAF in excess of 40% compared to baseline is present in the majority of cases. An important characteristics of this facilitation is that it persists for 4–20 min (32,33), a feature virtually unique to botulism compared to other endplate disorders.

In adults, the electrophysiologic findings depend very much on the severity of the disease (34). Patients with mild disease may have practically normal resting CMAP amplitudes, no decrement with low rate stimulation, and a modest degree of PAF. A decrement at low rates of stimulation is less common in adult botulism than in the infantile form. In more severe disease, the electrodiagnosis is usually more straightforward since most patients will have low-amplitude resting CMAPs and, consequently, more pronounced PAF. It is very important to examine clinically weak muscles in botulism, since the electrophysiologic abnormalities may be restricted to these muscles. PAF is observed in only approximately 60% of adult cases (33). As in the infantile form, this facilitation may be prolonged, lasting at least 2 min. Facilitation may require prolonged stimulation and may be absent in severe cases due to functional denervation. No PAE is seen. This is predictable based on the pathophysiology of botulism. The impaired release of synaptic vesicles prevents significant vesicle depletion with sustained stimulation.

Congenital Myasthenic Syndromes: The specific electrodiagnostic findings in the different congenital myasthenic syndromes will be detailed in Chapter 6. In most congenital myasthenic syndromes, the electrodiagnostic findings resemble those in autoimmune MG (35). However, in many of these disorders, a progressive CMAP decrement is noted that increases with stimulation rate, a finding that differs from the "repair of the decrement" seen in MG. In disorders that cause an increased duration of the endplate potential (congenital AChE deficiency and slow-channel syndrome) a repetitive CMAP (35) is observed (Fig. 3.10). This occurs when a single electrical stimulus elicits two or more consecutive CMAPs. This is due to the fact that the prolonged depolarization at the endplate remains above threshold for longer than the absolute refractory period of the muscle fiber action potential. The repetitive CMAPs are smaller in amplitude compared to the initial CMAP and they decrement faster. As in MG, the yield of RNS is improved by testing clinically affected, weak muscles. The decremental response in certain congenital myasthenic syndromes may be seen only with prolonged stimulation (or exercise) of the tested muscle (see Chapter 6).

2. Needle Electromyography

Needle electromyography (EMG) allows one to record the electrical activity generated by muscle fibers. During voluntary contraction of a muscle, the EMG needle records the summation of the electrical activity (within its recording territory) of the muscle fibers belonging to an active motor unit. This recorded electrical activity is termed a motor unit action potential (MUP). The amplitude, duration, morphology, stability of configuration, and recruitment characteristics of an MUP are affected by diseases of the motor unit. Specific alterations in these parameters may be indicative of primary nerve or muscle disease.

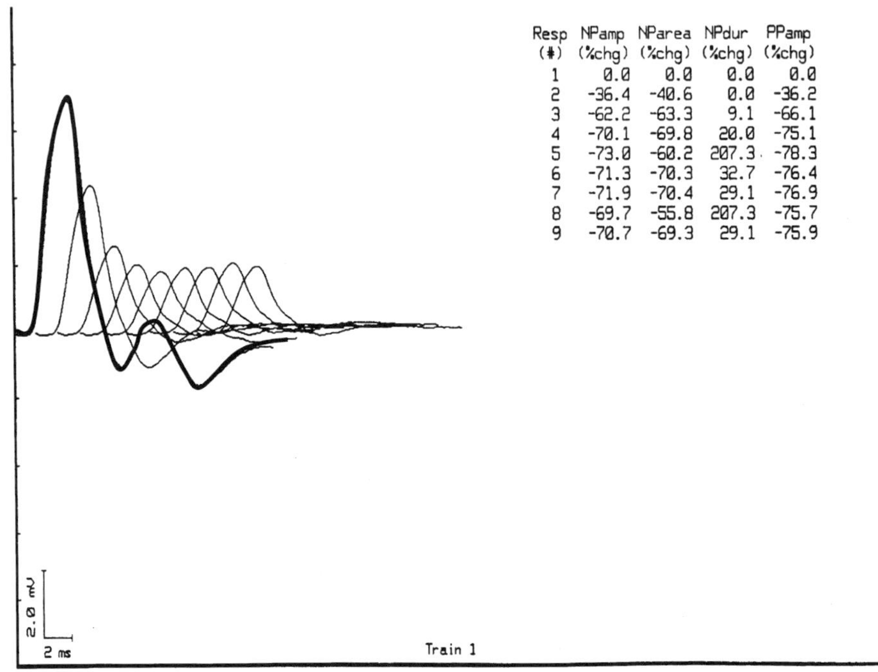

Figure 3.10 Repetitive CMAP. A repetitive CMAP in response to a single supramaximal stimulation may be observed in congenital maysthenic syndromes in which there is a prolongation of the duration of the endplate potential (i.e., endplate AChE deficiency and congenital slow-channel syndrome). The repetitive CMAP is smaller than the initial CMAP and decrements very quickly.

In disorders of the NMJ, the MUP amplitude, duration, recruitment, and morphology are usually within normal limits. During sustained contraction of a muscle in a patient with NMJ disease, failure of neuromuscular transmission may occur at a number of endplates. This may result in a change in the shape and size of the recorded MUP. Less severe disruptions in neuromuscular transmission will result in differences in the time that single muscle fibers reach threshold, also potentially changing the configuration of the MUP on consecutive firing. This phenomenon is called MUP instability or "jiggle" (36) and is illustrated in Fig. 3.11. Obviously, unstable MUPs may also be seen in primary nerve or muscle disease, but in these situations there are associated abnormalities in MUP duration, morphology, and recruitment that clarify the diagnosis.

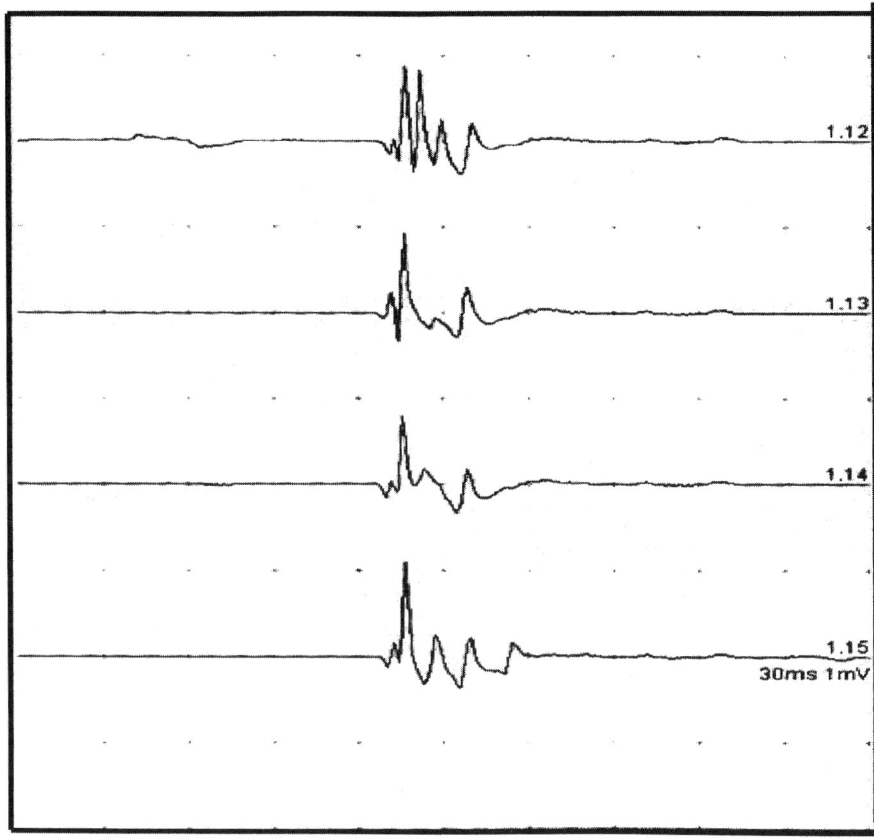

Figure 3.11 Unstable motor unit action potential (MUAP) recorded with a concentric electromyography needle in a patient with MG. Notice the changing morphology of the MUAP on consecutive firings.

3. Single-Fiber Electromyography

Single-fiber EMG (SFEMG) is a selective recording technique in which a specially constructed concentric needle is used to identify and record action potentials from individual muscle fibers. The technique was originally developed in 1964 by Erik Stalberg and Jan Ekstedt to investigate muscle fatigue (37). The monograph by Drs. Stalberg and Trontelj, *Single Fiber Electromyography*, is an essential reference for anyone interested in the technique (38).

The selectivity of the recording results from the small recording surface (25 μm in diameter compared to 120 mm for a standard concentric needle) of the recording needle electrode and the use of a high-pass filter of 500 Hz. The amplitude of an action potential (AP) recorded with an SFEMG electrode falls to approximately 10% of the maximal value when the electrode is 350 μm from the muscle fiber. The amplitude of the AP recorded with a SFMEG electrode from an average muscle fiber decreases to 200 μV when the electrode is approximately 300 μm from the muscle fiber (39). Thus, it follows that APs greater than 200 μV arise from muscle fibers within 300 μm of the recording surface.

By positioning an SFEMG electrode to record consecutive firings of two or more single muscle fiber APs belonging to the same motor unit, one can measure the variation in time interval between the firing of one potential in relation to the other (Fig. 3.12). This variation is the *neuromuscular jitter* and is produced by fluctuations in the time it takes for the EPP at the NMJ to reach the threshold for AP generation. These fluctuations are in turn due to the normally varying amount of ACh released from the nerve terminal after a nerve impulse. A small amount of jitter is seen in normal muscles due to this phenomenon. An increase in the magnitude if this jitter is the most sensitive electrophysiologic sign of a defect in neuromuscular transmission. Jitter is increased when the safety factor of neuromuscular transmission is reduced.

When the defect in neuromuscular transmission is more severe, some nerve impulses fail to elicit APs and SFEMG recordings demonstrate intermittent impulse blocking. SF EMG recordings demonstrate this as an intermittent absence of one or more single muscle fiber action potentials on consecutive firings (Fig. 3.13). When impulse blocking occurs at a sufficient number of endplates, clinical weakness is observed in the affected muscle. As we have seen, in order for a muscle to demonstrate an abnormal decrement on RNS, a critical number of NMJs must demonstrate impulse blocking. SFEMG allows one to detect milder defects in neuromuscular transmission (as increased jitter without blocking) in muscles that are clinically normal and have no decrement on RNS.

Activation and Recording Technique   SFEMG studies are performed either during mild voluntary activation of the muscle under study or with axonal microstimulation.

Voluntary Activation: Jitter measurements performed during voluntary activation of the muscle are less subject to technical problems but are more dependent on patient cooperation. As the patient minimally contracts the muscle under study, the examiner positions the recording electrode to record two or more time-locked APs. A constant recording

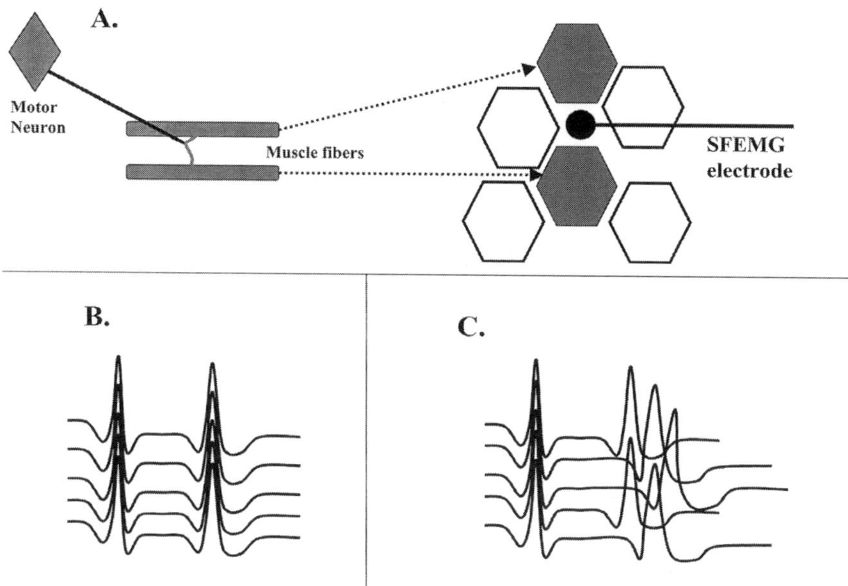

Figure 3.12 Method of single-fiber electromyography (SFEMG) obtained with voluntary activation. (A) The single-fiber needle is inserted into voluntarily activated muscle and is positioned so that recordings are obtained form two or more single muscle fibers belonging to the same motor unit. One of the single muscle fiber action potentials serves as a reference point and the interpotential interval is measured after consecutive discharges. (B) There is minimal variation of the IPI on consecutive firings in normal muscle (normal jitter). (C) In disorders of the NMJ, there may be marked variability of the IPI (abnormal jitter).

position is maintained until at least 50 discharges are recorded (Fig. 3.14). APs should have an amplitude of at least 200 μV with a steep rising phase. At least 20 potential pairs from different areas in the muscle should be sampled, taking care not to measure the same pair of potentials more than once. This usually requires three to four separate skin insertions.

Electrical Stimulation: Stimulation jitter studies are particularly useful in patients who have difficulty maintaining constant voluntary contraction of a muscle, in patients who are lethargic or comatose, and in young children. For limb muscles, intramuscular axonal stimulation is delivered using a monopolar needle inserted near the endplate region; another monopolar needle or a surface electrode serves as the anode (40). Stimulation is delivered at a rate of 2–10 Hz and the intensity is adjusted to

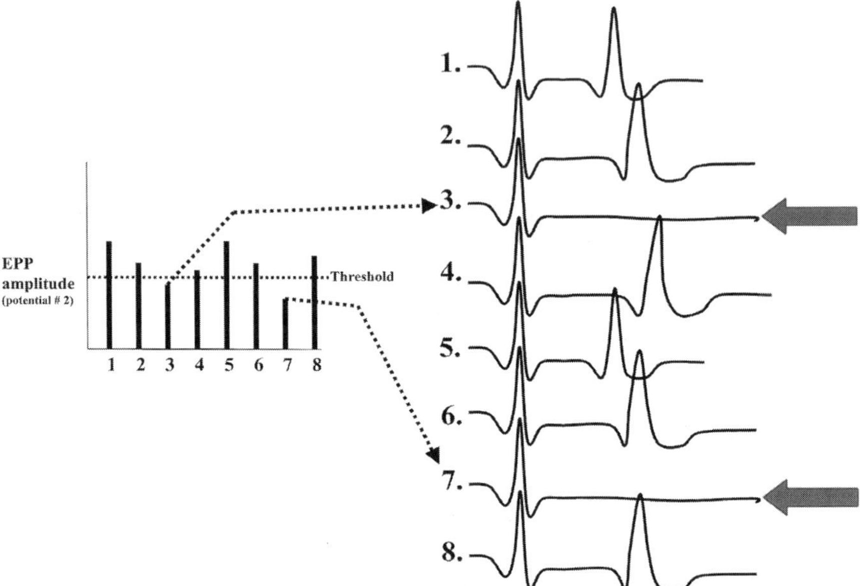

Figure 3.13 Neuromuscular transmission failure, impulse blocking. Diagrammatic representation of neuromuscular transmission failure causing impulse blocking during an SFEMG recording. When the endplate potential (EPP) fails to reach the threshold for action potential generation in the muscle fiber of the second recorded fiber pair, the initial fiber potential triggers the oscilloscope screen, but no potential is recorded from the second muscle fiber (arrows).

produce a slight twitch of the muscle. The SFEMG needle is inserted in the twitching portion of the muscle and positioned to record APs. With increasing stimulus intensity, increasing number of single muscle fiber APs appear, initially with high jitter and blocking. This is due to subliminal stimulation and should not be mistaken for true neuromuscular jitter. In addition, if the muscle fiber is stimulated directly, recordings with unusually low jitter (less than 5 µs) will result (40). Data from these responses should not be included. Failure to recognize these sources of technically produced

Figure 3.14 Voluntary jitter recordings obtained from the extensor digitorum communis muscle in (A) a normal control subject (100 consecutive discharges are superimposed), and (B) a patient with MG (52 consecutive discharges are superimposed).

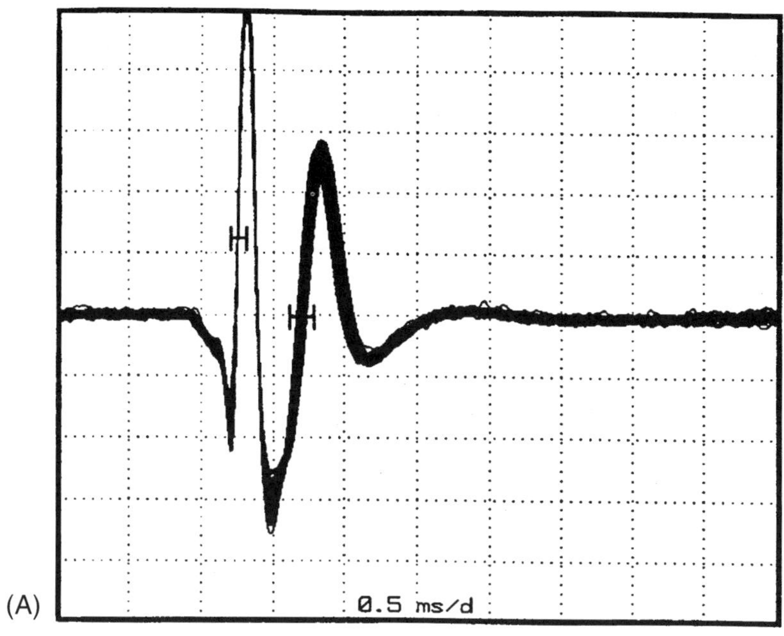
0.5 ms/d
(A)

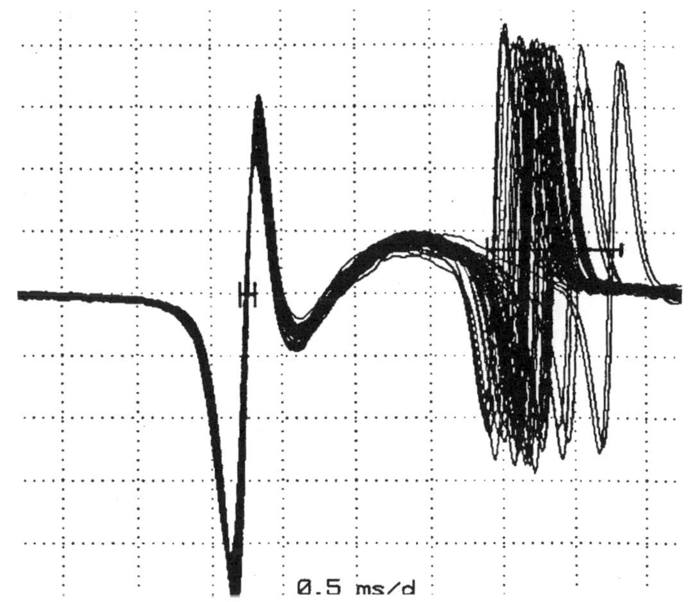
0.5 ms/d
(B)

jitter will obviously affect the final results. For this reason, stimulation jitter studies should be performed only by those experienced in the performance of this technique.

The motor nerve may be stimulated proximal to its entry into the muscle, or individual motor nerve branches may be stimulated as described above. Many motor units are activated when a surface electrode is used for stimulation, making it difficult to identify responses of single muscle fibers. In addition, artificial jitter may be introduced by variations in the intensity of the stimulus that reaches the individual axons particularly when surface stimulation is used.

Jitter Analysis   For recordings made during voluntary activation of the tested muscle, jitter is measured as the variation in the time interval between the two APs in the pair. This is called the interpotential interval (IPI) and represents the combined jitter in two endplates. The variation in IPIs can be expressed as the standard deviation of a series of intervals. However the intervals may slowly increase or decrease due to electrode movement or other factors. To minimize the effects of such slow trends, the mean consecutive differences (MCDs) of successive IPIs may be calculated from the following formula:

$$MCD = \frac{IPI_1 - IPI_2 + \ldots + IPI_{n-1} - IPI_n}{n - 1}$$

where IPI is the interpotential interval (or stimulus–response interval when nerve stimulation is used) and n is the number of discharges where IPIs were measured.

In voluntarily activated jitter studies, the IPI may be influenced by variations in firing rate that may introduce changes in the velocity of AP propagation in the muscle fibers (40). This is not a factor with stimulation jitter studies if the first 10 intervals of each train are excluded from the jitter calculation. This effect can be minimized in jitter studies obtained with voluntary activation by sorting the IPIs according to the length of the preceding interdischarge interval (IDI) and then calculating the mean of the consecutive IPI differences. This is called the mean sorted-data difference or MSD. If the ratio MCD/MSD is greater than 1.25, variations in firing rate have contributed to the measured jitter, and the MSD should be used in the final calculations.

The following parameters are calculated and reported for each muscle tested:

- The mean jitter (MCD) of all potential pairs tested
- The percentage of potential pairs in which jitter is normal

- The percentage of potential pairs in which jitter is abnormal
- The percentage of potential pairs in which impulse blocking is seen

A study is ***abnormal*** if one of the following criteria is met:

1. The mean jitter of all potential pairs exceeds the upper limit of normal for that muscle, or
2. More than 10% of pairs or endplates have jitter that exceeds the upper limit of normal for jitter in that muscle.

These criteria are valid for patients younger than 60 years. Above age 60, criterion 1 is not used and a study is defined as abnormal if more than 10% of fiber pairs have jitter greater than that defined by criterion 2.

Reference values for jitter during voluntary activation have been determined for a number of muscles in a multicenter collaborative study (Table 3.2) (41). Reference values for jitter during axonal stimulation have been determined for the extensor digitorum communis and orbicularis oculi muscles (42,43).

In Myasthenia Gravis Single-fiber electromyography demonstrates increased jitter in virtually all patients with MG. In patients with MG, jitter is greatest in weak muscles but is usually increased even in muscles with normal strength. There is no one muscle that will be most abnormal in every patient with MG although the extensor digitorum communis (EDC) is abnormal in most. The muscle or muscles to be tested should be selected based on the distribution of weakness in the individual patient. It is reasonable to test the EDC muscle first unless the signs and symptoms of weakness are limited to the ocular or facial muscles, in which case starting with the orbicularis oculi muscle may be of higher yield. If the EDC is normal, the orbicularis oculi or frontalis is tested. If the first of these facial muscles tested is normal, the other should be tested before one can conclude that the study is normal. If any limb muscle is weak, it should be tested. *The finding of normal jitter in a clinically weak muscle essentially rules out a primary defect in neuromuscular transmission as a cause for the weakness.*

It is important to understand that jitter is increased in primary disease of nerve and muscle. Thus, although SFEMG is a highly sensitive technique for demonstrating abnormalities in neuromuscular transmission, it is not specific for MG (or other *primary* NMJ diseases). Diseases of nerve and muscle must be excluded by the appropriate electrophysiologic and clinical examinations before one can conclude that the patient has MG. If primary nerve or muscle disease is present, increased jitter does not indicate that MG is also present.

Table 3.2 Reference Values for Jitter Measurements in Control Subjects During Voluntary Muscle Activation Given in Microseconds[a]

Muscle	10 years	20 years	30 years	40 years	50 years	60 years	70 years	80 years	90 years
Frontalis	33.6/49.7	33.9/50.1	34.4/51.3	35.5/53.5	37.3/57.5	40.0/63.9	43.8/74.1		
Orbicularis oculi	39.8/54.6	39.8/54.7	40.0/54.7	40.4/54.8	40.9/55.0	41.8/55.3	43.0/55.8		
Orbicularis oris	34.7/52.5	34.7/52.7	34.9/53.2	35.3/54.1	36.0/55.7	37.0/58.2	38.3/61.8	40.2/67.0	42.5/74.2
Tongue	32.8/48.6	33.0/49.0	33.6/50.2	34.8/52.5	36.8/56.3	39.8/62.0	44.0/70.0		
Sternocleido-mastoid	29.1/45.4	29.3/45.8	29.8/46.8	30.8/48.4	32.5/52.4	34.9/58.2	38.4/62.3		
Deltoid	32.9/44.4	32.9/44.5	32.9/44.5	32.9/44.6	33.0/44.8	33.0/45.1	33.1/45.6	33.2/46.1	33.3/46.9
Biceps	29.5/45.2	29.6/45.2	29.6/45.4	29.8/45.7	30.1/46.2	30.5/46.9	31.0/57.2		
EDC	34.9/50.0	34.9/50.1	35.1/50.5	35.4/51.3	35.9/52.5	36.3/54.4	37.7/57.2	39.1/61.1	40.9/66.5
ADM	44.4/63.5	44.7/64.0	45.2/65.5	46.4/68.6	48.2/73.9	51.0/82.7	54.8/96.6		
Tibialis Anterior	49.4/80.0	49.3/79.8	49.2/79.3	48.9/78.3	48.5/76.8	47.9/74.5	47.0/71.4	45.8/67.5	44.3/62.9

[a] 95% confidence limits for upper limit of mean MCD/95% confidence limit for MCD values of individual fiber pairs (41).

Single-Fiber Electromyography in Lambert-Eaton Syndrome, Botulism, and Congenital Myasthenic Syndromes SFEMG demonstrates abnormal jitter in virtually all patients with LES, usually with prominent impulse blocking. The magnitude of the increased jitter is often quite out of proportion to the relatively mild degree of clinical weakness. Jitter typically decreases with increasing firing rate in LES, although this effect is not seen in all patients (44). Neuromuscular jitter, as measured by SFEMG, in botulism and congenital myasthenic syndromes is usually increased, with impulse blocking occurring particularly in clinically weak muscles.

Quality Control A number of factors affect normal jitter and may lead to false-positive or false-negative studies. These factors include criteria for acceptance of a potential, failure to account for the effect of firing rate on jitter, distinguishing true impulse blocking from "pseudoblock" due to loss of the triggering potential, and failure to recognize potentials arising from a damaged muscle fiber. Further technical pitfalls are encountered when jitter is measured during intramuscular axonal stimulation. The examiner must have considerable experience with SFEMG to perform adequate studies on the majority of patients.

CASE 3.3 A 63-year-old man complains of progressive ptosis, blurred vision, and dysarthria for the past 12 years. His examination reveals bilateral, relatively symmetric ptosis and severe ophthalmoparesis. He has a flaccid dysarthria, mild tongue weakness, and moderate facial weakness. He has been diagnosed with "seronegative" myasthenia gravis and presents for a second opinion.

Repetitive stimulation studies are normal in the hypothenar and trapezius muscles. Single-fiber electromyography recorded during voluntary activation of the frontalis muscle reveals increased neuromuscular jitter (25% of fiber pairs have abnormal jitter). However, fiber density measurements are also abnormal with an average of 3.8 single muscle fiber potentials per recording site (normal < 1.76). Genetic testing confirms the diagnosis of oculopharyngeal muscular dystrophy.

Discussion This case illustrates a number of important points regarding the diagnosis of NMJ disorders. None of the diagnostic tests described thus far are specific for a diagnosis of a *primary* defect in neuromuscular transmission. The enhanced sensitivity of SFEMG comes at the price of diagnostic specificity. Because the technique is so sensitive, it is more likely to detect neuromuscular transmission problems caused by primary neurogenic or, as in this case, myopathic disorders. Fiber density measurements yield information analogous to fiber type grouping on muscle biopsy and should be normal in MG. They are quite useful in determining when increased jitter is due to primary disease of nerve or muscle. Finally, "seronegative" MG refers to autoimmune MG in which antibodies to AChE are not detected (see next chapter). Alternatively, "seronegativity" may be an indication of an erroneous diagnosis.

C. Serologic (Immunologic) Testing

The commercial availability of immunologic assays for the diagnosis of MG and LES has provided relatively sensitive and specific tests for the evaluation of these particular NMJ disorders. However, both false-positive and, more commonly, false-negative results may occur. Furthermore, these assays do not appear to correlate with the functional status of the NMJ as determined by the patient's disease severity. Recently, a number of antibodies to different skeletal muscle antigens have been reported to be detectable in certain subgroups of patients with acquired myasthenic syndromes. These new antibodies may not only facilitate the diagnosis in patients previously classified as "seronegative", but may also help to clinically define specific subtypes of myasthenia gravis.

1.   Anti-Acetylcholine Receptor Antibodies

Antibodies that react with AChR proteins are generally regarded as specific serologic markers for acquired MG. The AChR binding antibody (AChR-ab) assay has become a widely utilized diagnostic test for MG. The most commonly available AChR-ab assay is one using purified human AChRs. This test is positive in approximately 80% of patients with acquired generalized MG but in only approximately 55% of patients with purely ocular muscle weakness (45,47). Diagnostic sensitivity may be modestly increased by adding AChR blocking and modulating antibody assays, but this increase is minimal (4%) (48).

The serum concentration of AChR-ab varies widely among patients with similar degrees of weakness. AChR-abs cannot predict the severity of disease in individual patients. The concentration of AChR-abs may be low at symptom onset and become elevated later; thus, repeat testing may be appropriate when initial values are normal. In general, an elevated concentration of AChR-abs in a patient with compatible clinical features essentially confirms the diagnosis of MG. However, normal antibody concentrations do not exclude the diagnosis (see below). AChR binding antibodies may rarely be found in autoimmune liver disease, systemic lupus erythematosus, inflammatory neuropathies, amyotrophic lateral sclerosis, patients with rheumatoid arthritis receiving penicillamine, patients with thymoma without MG, and in first-degree relatives of patients with acquired autoimmune MG (49). Up to 13% of patients with LES may have anti-AChR or antistriational antibodies (Table 3.3).

2. Anti-Striated Muscle Antibodies or Striational Autoantibodies

Antibodies to striated muscle (StrAb) were the first autoantibodies discovered in patients with MG (50). They are reactive with contractile elements of skeletal muscle. They are positive in 30% of all cases of adult-onset MG. They are highly associated with thymoma, being positive in 80% of MG patients with thymoma and 24% of patients with thymoma without MG (51). Seronegativity does not exclude thymoma, and seropositivity is not absolutely indicative of thymoma particularly in elderly patients (52). StrAbs are most useful as a marker of thymoma in patients with MG onset before age 40. A progressive rise in StrAbs titer after resection of thymoma is a good indicator of tumor recurrence (51). StrAbs may be a valuable marker in middle-aged or elderly patients with mild MG, where they may be the only serologic abnormality. False positives are rare in patients without MG and/or thymoma. They sometimes occur in patients with rheumatoid arthritis who are treated with penicillamine, in 3–5% of patients with LES, and in recipients of bone marrow allografts with graft vs. host disease (51).

3. Acetylcholine Receptor–Modulating and Blocking Antibodies

AChR-modulating antibodies bind to exposed segments of the AChR on skeletal muscle membranes (53). Elevated levels of these antibodies are

Table 3.3 Serologic Diagnosis of Neuromuscular Junction Disorders (%)

Diagnosis	AChR binding	Anti-striational	AChR modulating	AChR blocking	Anti-VGCC
MG (all)	75–86	30	86	52	<5
MG (ocular)	70	—	72	30	—
MG (thymoma)	100	80	69*	54	—
LEMS	7–13	3–5	—	—	50–100

*80–100% loss.
Source: Data from Ref. 54.

typically found in generalized MG and MG associated with thymoma (48). A positive result is most useful when the AChR binding assay is negative, which occurs in about 3–4% of patients (48). Therefore, for general clinical purposes the AChR-modulating antibody test should be reserved for patients with undetectable AChR-binding antibodies. It is important to realize that false-positive results may arise due to hemolysis, bacterial contamination, and exposure of the serum to ambient heat (54). Thus, if it is the only serologic abnormality in a patient, the test should be repeated with a freshly drawn serum sample.

AChR-blocking antibodies bind at or near the neurotransmitter binding site on the skeletal muscle AChR and are detectable by a modified immunoprecipitation assay (54,55). They are found in approximately 52% of MG patients, but in only 1% of MG patients without AChR-binding antibodies (48). For this reason, the assay is not useful as an initial screening test for MG, but may have some utility in the serial monitoring of patients with positive AChR modulating antibodies, since the blocking antibodies provide a measure of the percentage of blocked receptor sites that may increase during disease exacerbation.

4. Antibodies to Other Skeletal Muscle Proteins

Antibodies directed against the intracellular striated muscle protein, titin, were originally believed to be a potentially sensitive marker for detecting the presence of thymoma in patients with MG (56). However, antititin antibodies were subsequently also detected in patients with late-onset MG without thymoma but appeared to be relatively uncommon in early-onset MG (57). Similarly, antibodies to the ryanodine receptor (RyR) are found primarily in late-onset MG with thymoma and are correlated with severe MG symptoms (58). AChR binding antibodies are typically detectable in patients with either or both of these non-AChR antibodies. The role of these antibodies in the clinical diagnosis and management of MG remains to be determined, although patients with antititin and/or anti-RyR antibodies may be less responsive to treatment (59).

As we have learned in Chapter 1, the development of the NMJ involves the interaction of a number of muscle membrane molecules. The muscles-pecific tyrosine kinase (MuSK) plays an important role in the clustering of AChRs and other important elements of the NMJ. Recently, antibodies to MuSK have been reported to be involved in the pathogenesis of AChR antibody–negative MG (60). In this study, 70% of AChR antibody–negative MG patients were found to have serum autoantibodies to MuSK. These autoantibodies were not found in seropositive patients. Thus, MuSK antibody–positive patients may represent a distinct subtype of autoimmune myasthenia both pathophysiologically and clinically, and the measurement of MuSK antibodies may aid in diagnosis and treatment of this subgroup of autoimmune MG patients (61).

5.   Seronegativity in Patients with Clinically Suspected Myasthenia Gravis

The diagnosis of MG ultimately depends on the clinical history and examination. Approximately 15–20% of patients with acquired autoimmune MG do not have detectable antibodies to AChR (62,63). Repeat testing in these patients is often useful since "seroconversion" is not uncommon, particularly within the first 6 months of disease onset (63). Diagnostic confirmation in patients who are consistently seronegative primarily depends on the results of electrophysiologic testing. In seronegative patients with childhood-onset MG, the diagnosis of a congenital myasthenic syndrome should be considered.

In patients with generalized MG who are AChR antibody negative, there is convincing evidence that their disease is autoimmune in nature (63,64). Patients with seronegative MG improve after immunotherapy. Serum from patients with seronegative MG causes abnormal neuromuscular transmission when injected into mice (65). Finally, babies born to mothers with seronegative MG may develop transient neonatal MG (see Chapter 4). Nevertheless, there are differences that may distinguish seropositive from seronegative patients. It is likely that for at least some of the seronegative patients, a distinct pathogenesis may be operative such that the immune response is directed against nonAChR determinants (i.e., MuSK) at the NMJ.

6.   Antibodies to the Voltage-Gated Calcium Channel

Fifty to one hundred percent of patients with LES have antibodies directed against the voltage-gated calcium channel on the presynaptic nerve terminal (66–68). The sensitivity and specificity of the test depends on the source of antigen and the specific laboratory measuring the antibody. Antibodies to the voltage-gated calcium channels are found more frequently in patients with LES who have an underlying small cell lung cancer. In fact, in one study, anti-P/Q type channel antibodies were found in all 32 tested cases of LES with a diagnosis of cancer, and in 91% of the 32 cases of LES without cancer (68). As is the case for MG, there is no correlation between the antibody titer and disease severity, and seronegativity does not exclude the diagnosis. Anti-voltage-gated calcium channel antibodies are rarely found in patients with MG (69) but may be found in up to 25% of patients with lung cancer without LES. Patients treated with immunosuppressive agents may become seronegative. Thus, it is important to obtain these serologic tests prior to instituting immunotherapy.

As will be discussed in Chapter 5, the diagnosis of LES requires a high index of suspicion. Patients who present with the complaints of proximal weakness, gait abnormalities, dry mouth, or impotence should be screened for LES using the appropriate electrodiagnostic procedures (see above), particularly if there is a history of tobacco abuse. While antibodies to the voltage-gated calcium channels are a useful diagnostic aid in LES, the principal diagnostic test remains RNS.

IV. COMPARISON OF DIAGNOSTIC TESTS IN MYASTHENIA GRAVIS

When assessing the sensitivity of the various diagnostic tests in the most common NMJ disorder, MG, one must be aware of how the patient population is defined and what is used as the "gold standard" for inclusion into the population. In many of the studies comparing the sensitivity of the different diagnostic techniques in MG, the diagnosis was based on one of the techniques being positive, which obviously affects the results of the comparison.

The edrophonium (tensilon) test is abnormal in most patients with ocular MG but is not entirely objective, and false-positive results do occur. Elevated serum levels of AChR-abs are the most specific test for MG, but levels are normal in 15–20% of patients with generalized MG and in up to 50% of patients with purely ocular weakness. RNS tests are the least sensitive of the diagnostic techniques, but have the advantage of being widely available and relatively simple to perform. Although SFEMG is clearly the most sensitive technique, it also demonstrates abnormalities in neuromuscular transmission in primary disorders of nerve and muscle, and these must be excluded before a diagnosis of MG is made. SFEMG is most valuable in patients with mild or purely ocular disease, particularly when AChR-abs are negative. It is also valuable in excluding a disorder of neuromuscular transmission, since the finding of normal jitter in a weak muscle indicates the weakness is *not* due to a defect in neuromuscular transmission. An algorithm for the diagnostic approach to a patient with suspected MG is given in the following chapter.

V. OVERVIEW

The various diagnostic procedures for confirming the clinical suspicion of an NMJ disorder were discussed in this chapter. Pharmacologic tests such as the edrophonium test are useful to make a quick diagnosis. Unfortunately, interpretation of these tests is subjective, and more objective tests are usually required to confirm the diagnosis in most cases. Electrophysiologic tests are designed to expose the reduced safety factor of neuromuscular transmission in disorders of the NMJ. The results of electrophysiologic tests often reveal characteristic patterns (particularly repetitive nerve stimulation studies) that facilitate the diagnosis of a particular NMJ disorder. Single-fiber electromyography is the most sensitive test to detect a disorder of neuromuscular transmission. However, its sensitivity comes at the cost of diagnostic specificity, as abnormalities may occur with primary nerve and muscle disease.

Serologic (immunologic) tests are used to confirm the diagnosis in NMJ disorders that are immune mediated, i.e., myasthenia gravis and LES. These tests are disease specific and essentially confirm the diagnosis in patients with a suggestive clinical presentation. Seronegativity in certain patients may be explained by immune targeting of different NMJ antigens. Further investigation of these seronegative patients may reveal a distinct immunopathogenesis perhaps leading to improved treatment strategies.

REFERENCES

1. Osserman KE, Kaplan LI. Rapid diagnostic test for myasthenia gravis. JAMA 1952; 150:265–268.
2. Katz B, Miledi R. The binding of acetylcholine to receptors and its removal from the synaptic cleft. J Physiol 1973; 231:549–574.
3. Daroff RB. The office tensilon test for ocular myasthenia gravis. Arch Neurol 1986; 43:843–844.
4. Scopetta C, Casali C, D'Agostini S, La Cesa I, Parisi L. Repetitive stimulation in myasthenia gravis: decrementing response revealed by anticholinesterase drugs. EEG Clin Neurophysiol 1990; 75:122–124.
5. Dirr LY, Donofrio PD, Patton JF, Troost BT. A false-positive edrophonium test in a patient with a brainstem glioma. Neurology 1989; 39:865–867.
6. Fierro B, Croce G, Filosto L, Carbone N, Lupo I. Ocular pseudomyasthenia: report of a case with a pineal region tumor. Ital J Neurol Sci 1991; 12:593–596.
7. Branley MG, Wright KW, Borchert MS. Third nerve palsy due to cerebral artery aneurysm in a child. Aust N Z J Ophthalmol 1992; 20:137–140.
8. Osserman KE, Genkins G. Studies in myasthenia gravis: review of a 20-year experience in over 1200 patients. Mt Sinai J Med 1971; 38:497–537.
9. Kelly JJ, Daube JR, Lennon VA, Howard FM, Younge BR. The laboratory diagnosis of mild myasthenia gravis. Ann Neurol 1982; 12:238–242.
10. Phillips LL, Melnick PA. Diagnosis of myasthenia gravis in the 1990s. Semin Neurol 1990; 10:62–69.
11. Rowland LP. Prostigmine-responsiveness and the diagnosis of myasthenia gravis. Neurology 1955; 5:612–624.
12. Viets HR, Schwab RS. Prostigmine in the diagnosis of myasthenia gravis. N Engl J Med 1935; 213:1280–1283.
13. Rowland LP, Aranow II, Hoefer PF. Observations on the curare test in the

differential diagnosis of myasthenia gravis. In: Viets HR, ed. Myasthenia Gravis. Springfield, IL: Charles C Thomas, 1961:411–434.

14. Kennedy F, Wolf A Experiments with quinine and prostigmine in treatment of of myotonia and myasthenia. Arch Neurol Psychiatry 1937; 37:68.

15. Harvey AM, Whitehill MR. Quinine as an adjuvant to prostigmine in the diagnosis of myasthenia gravis. Bull Johns Hopkins Hosp 1937; 61:216.

16. Jolly F. Ueber myasthenia gravis pseudoparalytica. Berl Klinische Wochenschrift 1895; 32:1–7.

17. Harvey AM, Masland RL. A method for the study of neuromuscular transmission in human subjects. Bull Johns Hopkins Hosp 1941; 68:81–93.

18. Kimura J. Principles of nerve conduction studies. In: Kimura J, ed. Electrodiagnosis in Diseases of Nerve and Muscle. Philadelphia: F.A. Davis, 1989:78–101.

19. Desmedt JE. The neuromuscular junction in myasthenia gravis, 1: Electrical and mechanical response to nerve stimulation in hand muscles. In: Desmedt JE ed. New Developments in Electromyography and Clinical Neurophysiology. Basel: Karger, 1973:241–304.

20. Howard JF, Sanders DB, Massey JM. The electrodiagnosis of myasthenia gravis and the Lambert-Eaton myasthenic syndrome. Neurol Clin 1994; 12:305–329.

21. Slomic A, Rosenfalck A, Buchthal F. Electrical and mechanical responses of normal and myasthenic muscle. Brain Res 1968; 10:1–78.

22. Borenstein S, Desmedt JE. Local cooling in myasthenia: improvement in neuromuscular failure. Arch Neurol 1975; 32:152–157.

23. Zifko UA, Nicolle MW, Griswold W, Bolton CF. Repetitive phrenic nerve stimulation in myasthenia gravis. Neurology 1999; 53:1083–1087.

24. Gilchrist JM, Sanders DB. Double-step repetitive stimulation in myasthenia gravis. Muscle Nerve 1987; 10:233–237.

25. Horowitz SH, Genkins G, Kornfield P, et al. Electrophysiologic diagnosis of myasthenia gravis and the regional curare test. Neurology 1976; 26:410–417.

26. Ricker KW, Hertel G, Reuther P. Repetitive proximal nerve stimulation and systemic curare test in myasthenia gravis. Ann NY Acad Sci 1981; 377:877–878.

27. Howard JF Jr, Sanders DB, Massey JM. The electrodiagnosis of myasthenia gravis and the Lambert-Eaton myasthenia syndrome. Neurol Clin 1994; 12:305–330.

28. Maselli RA. Electrodiagnosis of disorders of neuromuscular transmission. Ann NY Acad Sci 1998; 841:696–711.

29. Tim RW, Sanders DB. Repetitive nerve stimulation studies in the Lambert-Eaton myasthenic syndrome. Muscle Nerve 1994; 17:995–1001.

30. Tim RW, Massey JM, Sanders DB. Lambert-Eaton myasthenic syndrome: electrodiagnostic findings and response to treatment. Neurology 2000; 54:2176–2178.

31. Grand'Maison F. Methods of testing neuromuscular transmission in the intensive care unit. Can J Neurol Sci 1998; 25:S36–S39.

32. Fakadej A, Gutmann L. Prolongation of post-tetanic facilitation in infant botulism. Muscle Nerve 1982; 5:727–729.

33. Cornblath DR, Sladky JT, Sumner AJ. Clinical electrophysiology of infant botulism. Muscle Nerve 1983; 6:448–452.
34. Cherington M. Electrophysiologic methods as an aid in diagnosis of botulism: a review. Muscle Nerve 1982; 5:528–529.
35. Engel AG. The investigation of congenital myasthenic syndromes. Ann NY Acad Sci 1993; 681:425–434.
36. Stalberg EV, Sonoo M. Assessment of the variability in the shape of the motor unit action potential, the "jiggle" at consecutive discharges. Muscle Nerve 1994; 17:1135–1144.
37. Ekstedt J. Human single muscle fiber action potentials. Acta Neurol Scand 1964; 61:1–96.
38. Stalberg EV, Trontelj JV. Single Fiber Electromyography: studies in Healthy and Diseased Muscle, 2nd ed. New York: Raven Press, 1994.
39. Sanders DB, Stalberg E. AAEM Minimonograph No. 25: Single-Fiber Electromyography. Muscle Nerve 1996; 19:1069–1083.
40. Trontelj JV, Stalberg EV. Jitter measurement by axonal micro-stimulation: guidelines and technical notes. Electroencephalogr Clin Neurophys 1992; 85: 30–37.
41. Gilchrist JM. ad hoc Committee: Single fiber EMG reference values: a collaborative effort. Muscle Nerve 1992; 15:151–161.
42. Trontelj JV, Khuraibet A, Mihelin M. The jitter in stimulated orbicularis oculi muscle: technique and normal values. J Neurol Neurosurg Psychiatry 1988; 51:814–819.
43. Trontelj JV, Mihelin M, Fernandez JM, Stalberg E. Axonal stimulation for endplate jitter studies. J Neurol Neurosurg Psychiatry 1986; 49:67–685.
44. Sanders DB. The effect of firing rate on neuromuscular jitter in Lambert-Eaton myasthenic syndrome. Muscle Nerve 1992; 15:256–258.
45. Lindstrom J. An assay for antibodies to human acetylcholine receptor in serum from patients with myasthenia gravis. Clin Immunol Immunopathol 1977; 7:36–43.
46. Lindstrom JM, Seybold ME, Lennon VA, Whittingham S, Duane DD. Antibody to acetylcholine receptor in myasthenia gravis: prevalence clinical correlates, and diagnostic value. Neurology 1976; 26:1054–1059.
47. Vincent A, Newsom-Davis J. Acetylcholine receptor antibody as a diagnostic test for myasthenia gravis: results in 153 validated cases and 2967 diagnostic assays. J Neurol Neurosurg Psychiatry 1985; 48:1246–1252.
48. Howard FM, Lennon V, Finley J, Matsumoto J, Elveback LR. Clinical correlations of antibodies that bind, block or modulate human acetylcholine receptors in myasthenia gravis. Myasthenia gravis: biology and treatment. Ann NY Acad Sci 1987; 505:526–538.
49. Sanders DB, Howard JF. Disorders of neuromuscular transmission. In: Bradley WG Daroff RB, Fenichel GM, Marsden CD, eds. Neurology in Clinical Practice. Boston: Butterworth, 1991:1819–1842.
50. Strauss AJ, Seegal BC, Hsu KC, Burkholder RM, Nastuk WL, Osserman KE. Immunofluorescence demonstration of a muscle binding, complement fixing

serum globulin fraction in myasthenia gravis. Proc Soc Exp Biol Med 1960; 105:184–191.

51. Cikes N, Momoi MY, Williams CL, et al. Striational autoantibodies: quantitative detection by enzyme immunoassay in myasthenia gravis, thymoma, and recipients of D-penicillamine or allogeneic bone marrow. Mayo Clin Proc 1988; 63:474–481.

52. Lennon VA, Howard FM. Serological diagnosis of myasthenia gravis. In: Nakamura M O'Sullivan MB, eds. Clinical Laboratory Molecular Analysis: New Strategies in Autoimmunity, Cancer and Virology. New York: Grune & Stratton, 1985:29–44.

53. Lennon VA, Jones G, Howard FM, Elveback L. Autoantibodies to acetylcholine receptors in myasthenia gravis. N Engl J Med 1983; 308:402–403.

54. Lennon, VA. Serological Diagnosis of Myasthenia Gravis and Lambert-Eaton Myasthenic Syndrome. In: Lisak RP, ed. Handbook of Myasthenia Gravis and Myasthenic Syndromes. New York: Marcel Dekker, 1994:49–164.

55. Lennon VA, Griesmann GE. Evidence against acetylcholine receptor having a main immunogenic region as target for autoantibodies in myasthenia gravis. Neurology 1989; 39:1069–1076.

56. Gautel M, Lakey A, Barlow DP, Holmes Z, Scales S, Leonard K, Labeit S, Mygland A, Gilhus NE, Aarli JA. Titin antibodies in myasthenia gravis: identification of a major immunogenic region of titin. Neurology 1993; 43: 1581–1585.

57. Skeie GO, Mygland A, Aarli JA, Gilhus NE. Titin antibodies in patients with late onset myasthenia gravis: clinical correlations. Autoimmunity 1995; 20:99–104.

58. Skeie GO, Lunde PK, Sejersted OM, Mygland A, Aarli JA, Gilhus NE. Autoimmunity against the ryanodine receptor in myasthenia gravis. Acta physiol Scand 2001; 171:379–384.

59. Romi F, Gilhus NE, Varhang JE, Mygland A, Skeie GO, Aarli JA. Thymectomy and anti-muscle autoantibodies in late-onset myasthenia gravis. Eur J Neurol 2002; 9:55–61.

60. Hoch W, McConville J, Helms S, Newsom-Davis J, Melms A, Vincent A. Auto-antibodies to the receptor tyrosine kinase MuSK in patients with myasthenia gravis without acetylcholine receptor antibodies. Nature Medicine 2001; 7:365–368.

61. Liyanage Y, Hoch W, Beeson D, Vincent A. The agrin/muscle-specific kinase pathway: new targets for autoimmune and genetic disorders at the neuromuscular junction. Muscle Nerve 2002; 25:4–16.

62. Soliven BC, Lange DJ, Penn AS, Younger D, Jaretzki A, Lovelace RE, Rowland LP. Seronegative myasthenia gravis. Neurology 1988; 38:514–517.

63. Sanders DB, Andrews PI, Howard JF, Massey JM. Seronegative myasthenia gravis. Neurology 1997; 48(suppl 5):S40–S51.

64. Miller RG, Milner-Brown HS, Dau PC. Antibody-negative acquired myasthenia gravis: successful therapy with plasma exchange. Muscle Nerve 1981; 4:255.

65. Burges J, Vincent A, Molenaar PC, Newsom-Davis J, Peers C, Wray D. Passive

transfer of seronegative myasthenia gravis to mice. Muscle Nerve 1994; 17: 1393–1400.
66. McEvoy KM. Diagnosis and treatment of Lambert-Eaton myasthenic syndrome. Neurol Clin 1994; 12:387–399.
67. Sher E, Carbone E, Clementi F. Neuronal calcium channels as target for Lambert-Eaton myasthenic syndrome autoantibodies. Ann NY Acad Sci 1993; 681:373–381.
68. Lennon VA, Kryzer TJ, Griesmann GE, O'Suilleabhain PE, Windebank AJ, Woppman GP, Lambert EH. Calcium-channel antibodies in the Lambert-Eaton syndrome and other paraneoplastic syndromes. N Engl J Med 1995; 332:1467–1474.
69. Lennon VA. Serological profile of myasthenia gravis and distinction from Lambert-Eaton myasthenic syndrome. Neurology 1997; 48(suppl 5):S23–S27.

4

Myasthenia Gravis

I. INTRODUCTION

Although autoimmune myasthenia gravis (MG) is a relatively uncommon clinical disorder, it is one of the most extensively studied and best understood autoimmune diseases. Advances in our understanding of the pathophysiology and the immunopathogenesis of MG have allowed for the development of increasingly selective and targeted therapeutic interventions. The prognosis of the disease has been dramatically altered over the last 50 years, from a disorder that was marginally treatable and often fatal to one in which treatment is very successful in the majority of cases.

The symptoms of MG are known to be due to an antibody-mediated, T-cell-dependent, autoimmune attack directed against the acetylcholine receptors (AChRs) at the neuromuscular junction (NMJ). The clinical manifestations and options for treatment are well described. Despite this, there is still no consensus among experts on a number of therapeutic issues. This is largely due to the paucity of evidence-based data derived from well-designed clinical trials. In fact, at the time of the writing of this chapter, only two adequately controlled therapeutic trials had been performed (1,2). Table 4.1 lists a number of unanswered questions regarding the pathophysiology and management of MG. The information in this chapter will not answer these

Table 4.1 Unanswered Questions About Myasthenia Gravis

1. Where does the breakdown of immune tolerance to self acetylcholine receptor occur?
2. What is the cause of this breakdown of tolerance?
3. What is the precise role of the thymus gland in disease initiation and maintenance?
4. Does the role of the thymus gland in disease development differ in thymomatous and nonthymomatous MG?
5. Is thymectomy beneficial in autoimmune MG?
6. If the answer to no. 5 is "yes," which patients with nonthymomatous MG are likely to benefit from thymectomy?
7. Why are the extraocular muscles "selectively" involved in MG?
8. Which of the available immunosuppressive agents are most effective from a risk–benefit point of view for long-term management of MG?
9. Which group of patients are most likely to have a milder clinical course or have a spontaneous remission of symptoms without the use of immuno-suppressive drugs?
10. What is the optimal dose and method of administration (daily vs. alternate-day) of prednisone in the management of MG?
11. Is it possible to completely discontinue immunosuppressive treatment once remission of signs and symptoms has been achieved?
12. Is "seronegative" MG a distinct disease(s) in terms of clinical features and pathogenesis?

questions but will provide the reader with a summary of the current under-standing of the etiology, diagnosis, and management of autoimmune MG.

II. HISTORY

Sir Thomas Willis is credited by many with the first description of a patient with MG in 1672 (3). He reported a "woman who temporarily lost her power of speech and became 'mute as a fish'" (3). In 1892, Friedrich Jolly used the term "myasthenia gravis pseudoparalytica" to describe patients with fatiga-ble muscle weakness that often led to death (4). The term "myasthenia" is de-rived from the Greek term for muscle weakness; "gravis" is derived from the Latin meaning "grave." Early descriptions of symptom complexes consistent with MG emphasized the cardinal features of fatigable muscle weakness often affecting the bulbar and respiratory muscles leading to respiratory failure.

The first treatment for MG was described in 1934 when Mary Broadfoot Walker introduced the use of the acetylcholinesterase (AChE) inhibitor phy-sostigmine in a patient with MG (5). She correctly surmised that physostig-mine, a curare antidote, would be effective since MG was characterized by symptoms very similar to curare poisoning. She subsequently described the beneficial effect of neostigmine in MG in 1935 (6). In 1939, Alfred Blalock, a Baltimore surgeon, reported a patient with MG and a thymic tumor who improved after thymectomy (7). He subsequently reported similar results in other patients (8), and the procedure quickly gained acceptance as a therapy for MG. Thus, up to the 1950s, the options for management of MG were limited to AChE inhibitors and thymectomy, and MG remained a very "grave" disease. Many patients developed permanent, fixed weakness and eventually were bedridden. Infections led to severe exacerbations of the disease often resulting in death due to acute respiratory failure or as a consequence of aspiration.

The first discovery leading to the hypothesis of an autoimmune cause for MG came in 1944 when Wilson et al. (9) reported that a circulating factor was inhibiting neuromuscular transmission in patients with MG. Simpson and Nastuk independently hypothesized that this "circulating factor" may be composed of muscle-binding autoantibodies (10,11). Finally, in 1973, Patrick and Lindstrom immunized rabbits with AChRs purified from eel electric organs, and found that these rabbits developed symptoms of MG as well as circulating anti-AChR antibodies (12). With its establishment as an antibody-mediated autoimmune disease, further characterization of the immunopathogenesis of acquired MG (see below) has made it the best understood human autoimmune disease. This has led to the development of immune therapies which, in addition to technical improvements in the care of critically ill patients, has resulted in a drastic change in the prognosis of MG. Today, with the appropriate therapy, the vast majority of patients with the disease can expect to achieve complete control of symptoms with few or no functional limitations.

III. EPIDEMIOLOGY AND NATURAL HISTORY

A. Epidemiology

Myasthenia gravis is a rare disease. Based on published prevalence rates there are anywhere from 3.05 to 175 people with MG per million population, depending on the location of the epidemiologic study (13–20). The incidence of MG is thought to be in the range of 2.0–10.4 cases per million per year (17). Based on these numbers there are an estimated 20,000–70,000 patients with MG in the United States. Both the prevalence and incidence of MG appear to be steadily increasing worldwide (17). This increase is mostly attributable to improved diagnosis and prolonged survival with the disease.

MG may occur at any age. However, onset tends to be earlier in females than males. Patients with disease onset before the age of 40 are more likely to be female (70:30); both sexes are equally affected between the ages of 40 and 50; and males are more frequently affected (3:2) after age 50 (21,22).

B. Natural History

Grob and colleagues (21,22) studied more than 1400 patients with MG from 1940 to 1985. The patients reported in these studies were treated with AChE inhibitors alone. Thus, the results of these extensive reports are an important source of information regarding the natural history of MG. The course of the MG varies considerably, but in most patients the disease is usually characterized by gradual deterioration. Maximal severity occurs within the first year of onset in 65% and in the second or third year in 19% (21,22). Thus, the severity of the disease is largely determined during the first 3 years, and it would make sense that this is the crucial period for institution of definitive therapy. After this, the disease tends to become more stable with fewer severe exacerbations and a more constant or fixed level of weakness. About one third of patients with generalized symptoms develop severe weakness and bulbar manifestations such as a weak cough or dysphagia. The average time from onset of disease to the first severe episode is 8 months. Roughly 20% of patients treated with cholinesterase inhibitors alone have a complete or near-complete remission of symptoms lasting at least 6 months (21). The mean duration of remission is 5 years, but some patients have long-term remissions lasting for more than 20 years.

Mortality due to MG has fallen from 31% in the 1940s and 1950s (21,22) to below 5% currently. Death is usually due to weakness leading to failure of the bulbar and respiratory muscles. Improved care of critically ill patients has likely had the most significant effect on the improved mortality rate. Recognition of the autoimmune nature of MG, which led to the eventual use of corticosteroids and other immunosuppressant medications, has also contributed to the drop in mortality and the improved therapy and management of MG (23–25).

IV. ETIOLOGY AND IMMUNOPATHOGENESIS

Effective management of MG requires a knowledge of the immunopathogenesis of the disease (Chapter 2). It is widely accepted that MG is an antibody-mediated disease in which the target autoantigen is the nicotinic AChR of skeletal muscle (26). Although the production of antibodies is directly attributable to B lymphocytes, there is extensive evidence that T lymphocytes play a critical role in the autoimmune response in MG in both humans and animal models (27–29). T lymphocytes are directly involved and required for both the induction and development of autoimmune MG. A breakdown in tolerance toward the AChR is the critical event leading to T-cell-dependent autoantibody production. The cause or trigger for this breakdown in tolerance is not known.

As discussed in Chapter 1, the AChR is composed of two α, one β, one δ, and either a γ or an ε subunit. Numerous antigenic determinants are present in each subunit, but the majority of determinants recognized by B and T lymphocytes are located on the α subunit (30), and in particular on a specific region on the extracellular loop of the α subunit called the main immunogenic region. Different antigenic determinants are immunodominant in different patients, and subsequently the B- and T-cell responses are very heterogeneous among patients with MG.

The development of a T-cell-dependent autoimmune disease requires the loss of self-tolerance to a particular self antigen. The mechanism for the breakdown of tolerance to the AChR in MG is not understood. However, there are several lines of evidence that point to a prominent role for the thymus gland in at least a subgroup of patients with MG. The thymus is critically involved in the induction of T-cell tolerance to self antigens (31). Myoid cells that express muscle proteins (including AChR subunits) are present in normal and hyperplastic thymus glands of MG patients, but are not found in MG patients with thymoma (32,33). This could very well provide a source for sensitization of T cells to the skeletal muscle AChR in non-thymomatous MG patients. In MG patients with thymoma, epithelial cells composing the tumor bind AChR antibodies and express parts of the α subunit, although functional AChRs are not expressed. Clinical evidence in favor of a role for the thymus gland in the immunopathogensis of MG includes the apparent clinical benefit of thymectomy on the disease course and the finding of pathologic abnormalities (neoplasia or hyperplasia) of the thymus in the majority of patients with MG.

Once there is a break in tolerance to the AChR, the sensitized B lymphocytes (with help from T lymphocytes) produce autoantibodies that bind to the AChR of skeletal muscle. Although AChR antibodies are the immunologic hallmark of MG, there is little correlation between the concentration of serum antibodies and clinical disease severity. AChR antibodies induce a neuromuscular transmission defect by one of four main mechanisms (Table 4.2). The most significant mechanism is probably the initiation of a complement-mediated lysis of the postsynaptic muscle membrane (34). AChR antibodies may also directly block neuromuscular transmission by occupying the AChR binding site or they may cross-link AChRs. Mainly as a result of the complement-mediated autoimmune attack, the postsynaptic muscle membrane loses its normal morphology and becomes simplified (Fig. 4.1) with smaller junctional folds and fewer numbers of functioning AChRs. There is evidence to suggest that once there is damage of this type to

Table 4.2 Proposed Immunologic and Inflammatory Mechanisms of Endplate Injury and Dysfunction in Myasthenia Gravis

1. Direct block of neuromuscular transmission by binding of antibodies at or near the ACh binding site on the AChR.
2. Cross-linking of AChRs by AChR antibodies, accelerating their internalization and degradation.
3. Bound AChR antibodies activate complement and produce lysis of the AChR and subsequent degeneration and postsynaptic membrane injury.
4. Non-AChR antibodies binding to junctional components and causing either membrane injury or blockade of non-AChR ion (i.e., Na^+) channels.

the postsynaptic muscle membrane, other antigenic determinants become exposed initiating a distinct autoimmune response, a phenomenon called *epitope spreading* (35,36). This is an important concept because if *epitope spreading* is indeed an important occurrence, one may argue that MG patients should be treated aggressively and early with immunomodulating therapy to prevent "broadening" of the immune derangement. The functional conse-

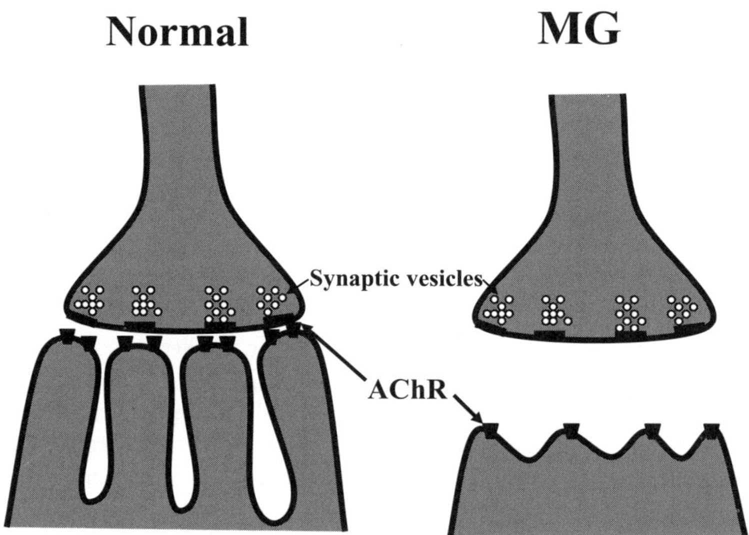

Figure 4.1 Schematic representation of ultrastructural abnormalities occurring at the postsynaptic membrane in MG. The extensively folded pattern seen in normal endplates is lost, and there is simplification of postsynaptic folds and widening of the synaptic cleft.

quences of the destruction and simplification of the postsynaptic membrane are obvious and were covered in detail in Chapter 2. The safety margin of neuromuscular transmission is reduced due to loss of functional AChRs as well as loss of voltage-gated sodium channels (37).

As discussed in Chapter 1, AChRs have a normal half-life of approximately 8 days. As AChRs degrade and are internalized, they are replaced by newly synthesized AChRs that are inserted into the postsynaptic junctional membrane. It is likely that the rate of synthesis increases in response to a more rapid loss of AChRs. When the synthesis of new AChRs cannot keep up with the rate of degradation and internalization, the safety margin of neuromuscular transmission is reduced. The destructive changes in the junctional postsynaptic membrane, largely induced by complement, restricts the membrane surface available for insertion of newly synthesized AChRs. When these destructive changes are severe, the clinical result may be "fixed" weakness in the affected muscles. This may be the explanation for the refractoriness to treatment observed in patients with long-standing, largely untreated MG and makes an argument in favor of early definitive immunotherapy.

V. CLINICAL PRESENTATION

The clinical hallmark of myasthenia gravis is the presence of fatigable muscle weakness. It is useful to distinguish fatigable muscle weakness from general fatigue or exhaustion. Patients with fluctuating, fatigable muscle weakness due to MG will specifically describe weakness in a specific group of muscles that is brought on by activity and improves with rest. In contrast, patients with general fatigue/exhaustion due to any number of causes will typically complain of "all-over-weakness," "tiredness," "lack of energy," and malaise. Patients with MG may have symptoms and signs only after exertion or at the end of the day. This may result in little detectable objective weakness at the time of examination, often delaying the diagnosis. Maneuvers that fatigue specific muscle groups can be very useful in eliciting signs of weakness in patients with MG, as will be discussed below.

A. Symptoms

Initial symptoms involve the ocular muscles in the majority of patients (21). Most patients complain of ptosis, intermittent diplopia, or both. Occasionally, patients complain of "blurred" vision rather than diplopia, prompting them to change their eyeglasses in an attempt to correct the problem. Ptosis may not be noticed until it obscures vision. Patients with ptosis will note that the severity of the eyelid droop varies during the course of the day, often worsening after exercise, reading, while driving, and with exposure to direct sunlight. Nearly all patients with MG develop ocular manifestations at some point during the course of their illness. Thus, the diagnosis of MG should be questioned if ocular symptoms do not develop within 1–2 years (38).

Approximately 20% of patients with MG present with prominent bulbar symptoms, including dysarthria, dysphagia, and difficulty chewing (21). Weakness of palatal muscles may result in a nasal quality to the voice. Speech may become slurred with prolonged talking, i.e., talking on the telephone or giving a speech or presentation. Swallowing complaints may be limited to mild difficulty with solid foods, i.e., "feels like the food gets stuck." More serious symptoms, such as nasal regurgitation of liquids and aspiration, are indicators of severe disease. Patients with MG who have difficulty chewing often describe progressively weaker chewing force with each successive bite. The difficulty is worse with solid foods, particularly steak. There is no associated pain, differentiating this complaint from jaw claudication due to temporal arteritis.

Rarely, patients with MG may present with respiratory muscle weakness without other prominent MG symptoms (39). However, the vast majority of patients with respiratory muscle weakness usually have ocular and bulbar symptoms. Patients with diaphragmatic weakness often have orthopnea as an early symptom. This may lead to respiratory failure when the patient is placed in the supine position. Patients with MG and respiratory muscle weakness may complain of the inability to draw a full breath. They often describe their breathing as rapid and shallow, which may be misinterpreted as hyperventilation due to anxiety.

Fatigable extremity weakness in MG may affect any muscle group and may be asymmetric. Rarely, weakness may be very focal affecting distal limb muscles or neck extensors selectively (40). As previously noted, muscles are noted to weaken with repeated use, and strength improves with rest. Patients have noted the development of a foot drop with prolonged walking, hip extension weakness with climbing several flights of stairs, shoulder muscle fatigue with activities that require holding the arms above the head, and weakness of finger flexors and extensors with prolonged typing. Symptoms may worsen with exposure to extreme heat or severe stress. Patients may report that they plan activities for early in the day when their strength is at its peak. On the other hand, severe disease may cause prominent muscle weakness in which fatigability is not necessarily apparent.

The initial symptoms may occur after a specific precipitating event. Most often, this event is a systemic illness or infection. Patients have also developed symptoms after insect bites or vaccinations. The disease may manifest itself after exposure to any one of a number of drugs that may exacerbate MG (see Chapter 7). Finally, initial presentation after pregnancy or other surgical procedures may occur.

B. Signs

The classical physical signs of MG include ptosis, ophthalmoparesis, bulbar weakness, and fatigable extremity weakness. Unfortunately, the clinical presentation in individual patients is often quite variable, and the diagnosis may be difficult. A history of fatigable weakness in specific muscle groups should prompt further investigation for a neuromuscular junction defect (Chapter 3) regardless of whether clinical signs of weakness are observed on examination. In a patient with suspected MG, the following muscle groups should be specifically tested: facial, ocular, oropharyngeal, respiratory, axial, and limb muscles.

1. Facial Muscles

Many patients with MG have a characteristic facial appearance. Facial weakness may produce a "sagging" appearance and loss of facial expression. Often patients will elevate their eyebrow by contracting the frontalis muscle in an attempt to compensate for ptosis. One may observe fatiguing of the frontalis muscle as the eyebrows come down after sustained elevation. With blinking or eyelid closure, the sclera may not be completely covered due to weakness of the orbicularis oculi muscle (Fig. 4.2). Weakness of eyelid closure is seen in the vast majority of patients with MG and should be specifically looked for by asking patients to forcefully close their eyes while the examiner attempts to manually open the eyelids. Weakness of the orbicularis oris muscle may produce a horizontal or "snarling" appearance with attempts to smile. Patients may also have difficulty puffing their cheeks or pursing their lips. With attempts to purse the lips, a "horizontal pucker" is frequently observed due to the inability to approximate the sides of the mouth because of orbicularis oris weakness.

2. Ocular Muscles

As noted, most patients with MG have ocular muscle weakness. The extra-ocular muscles and the eyelid elevators are involved to different degrees in individual patients. Pupillary responses are normal. Eyelid ptosis is usually asymmetric and may vary considerably during the course of the examination. Ptosis is worsened with sustained upgaze. Resting the lids by having the patient close the eyes for 30 s may reduce the ptosis for a time. Patients with little or no ptosis at rest may develop ptosis after sustained upgaze for 60–180 s. There may be a brief correction of ptosis when gaze is directed from low to high; one may also observe an excessive elevation of the eyelid with this maneuver (Cogan's eye twitch). Manual elevation of the more ptotic lid may worsen ptosis on the contralateral side, a phenomenon known as "enhanced

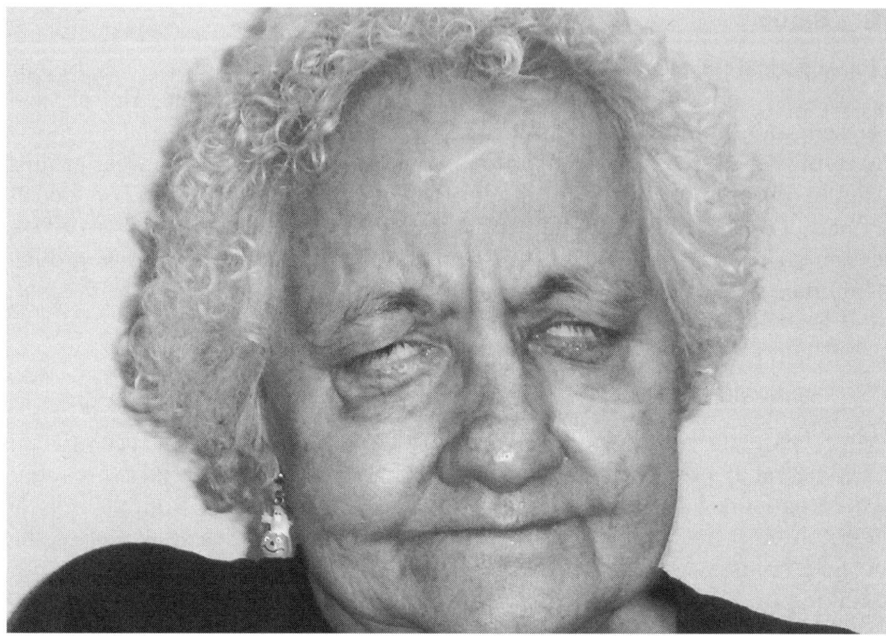

Figure 4.2 Severe facial weakness in a woman with long-standing MG. Note incomplete eyelid closure and prominent Bell's phenomenon.

ptosis" (41) or the "see-saw effect." Finally, ptosis may improve in response to local cooling of the lid (42).

The pattern of extraocular muscle weakness in MG is typically asymmetric and not isolated to the distribution of a single cranial (III, IV, VI) nerve. The pattern of weakness may fluctuate and change even during the course of a single examination. The medial rectus muscle is most frequently affected, followed by the superior and lateral rectus muscles. Rarely, weakness may be isolated to the lateral recti. Examination of extraocular movements should include a minimum of 15–30 s of lateral and superior gaze holding. The cover/uncover test may elicit mild weakness of a specific extraocular muscle by causing shifting fixation in the direction of action of the weak muscle. Red glass testing is useful if diplopia is present without observable dysconjugate gaze. Sustained lateral gaze produces fatigable weakness of the medial or lateral rectus muscles. With attempted lateral gaze, the adducting eye may not move, and the abducting eye may demonstrate nystagmus, which becomes coarser as the lateral rectus muscle fatigues—a phenomenon called *pseudointernuclear ophthalmoplegia*.

Sustained upgaze for 30 s is usually sufficient to produce weakness of the medial rectus muscles and the eyelid elevator muscles in MG. It is important to be aware that holding the stimulus for upgaze too close elicits a failure of convergence alone that is not necessarily an abnormal finding. If diplopia or dysconjugate gaze is due to a failure of convergence alone, moving the target farther from the patient will improve the abnormality. Conversely, moving the target farther away will exacerbate the problem in MG and increase the apparent separation of the images.

3. Oropharyngeal Muscles

Weakness of the pharyngeal, laryngeal, lingual, tongue, or masticatory muscles is a serious sign in MG. The immediate concern is to ensure adequate protection of the airway as palatal weakness may place the patient at risk for aspiration. Nasal speech is an early sign of pharyngopalatal weakness. This may become apparent only after prolonged talking causes increasing palatal weakness and air escapes through the nose. More severe weakness may cause nasal regurgitation of liquids. The dysarthria in MG is also characterized by articulation abnormalities with labial and lingual consonant and vowel distortion due to facial and tongue weakness. Laryngeal weakness may cause speech output to be hypophonic (breathy, whispered). Again, these abnormalities are brought on (or worsened) by sustained talking. It is sometimes useful to ask MG patients with bulbar symptoms to count up to 50, and listen for the development of nasal speech and labial and lingual dysarthria.

Patients with dysphagia should be carefully examined for palatal weakness. As noted, an early sign of palatal weakness is nasal speech. The soft palate should be observed as the patient says "Ah" to make sure that it rises normally in the midline. Weakness of the tongue muscles may also cause dysphagia due to abnormal movement of the bolus of food in the oral cavity. Tongue protrusion should be checked by having the patient protrude the tongue into the cheek while the examiner applies resistance on the outside surface of the cheek. Some experience is required to determine the amount of resistance to apply and the force of protrusion that is normal.

Patients with MG who have difficulty chewing usually give a revealing history as described above. When these patients are examined, weakness of jaw closure due to masseter and temporalis muscle weakness may be present. Weakness of jaw opening due to pterygoid muscle weakness, on the other hand, is rarely seen in MG even with relatively severe weakness of the masseter muscles. This pattern of weak jaw closure and strong jaw opening is typical for MG. The masseter and temporalis muscles are checked by having the patient clamp the jaws together while the examiner attempts to separate them by applying downward pressure on the chin. It is best to sustain a moderate level of downward pressure for 30 s rather than applying momentary pressure forcefully. The pterygoid muscles are evaluated by having the patient open the jaw while the examiner applies upward pressure below the chin.

4. Respiratory Muscles

It is frequently difficult to distinguish the status of the respiratory muscles from the functional status of the lungs themselves. However, simple observation is often revealing. Patients with respiratory muscle weakness due to MG often present with tachypnea and shallow breathing. They may be anxious due to an inability to draw a full breath. Asking the patient to inspire quickly and loudly (inspiratory sniff) can give one a good indication of inspiratory muscle strength. To assess expiratory muscle function, the patient should be asked to cough or clear his or her throat. Outward protrusion of the abdomen against the examiner's hand is an indirect measure of diaphragmatic strength because the abdominal contents will be pushed upward instead of outward if the diaphragm is weak. A weak sniff and cough along with significant tachypnea are signs of severe respiratory muscle weakness.

Formal measurements of pulmonary function, such as forced vital capacity, may be useful but are also dependent on pulmonary factors. Arterial blood gas measurements are a relatively insensitive measure of impending respiratory decompensation in MG since the initial changes are consistent with hyperventilation and are usually attributed to anxiety. By the time CO_2 retention occurs, the respiratory muscles have already begun to decompensate. Very often MG patients with respiratory muscle weakness also have weakness of neck flexion, which may be a useful association if there is doubt that the respiratory decompensation is due to myasthenic weakness.

5. Axial/Limb Muscles

Myasthenia gravis patients may have weakness in many different patterns affecting the limb and truncal muscles. Patients with mild disease may have weakness limited to the neck flexor muscles. Typically, neck flexion is weaker than neck extension in patients with MG. In general, upper extremity muscles are more severely involved than lower extremity muscles. Finger and wrist extensors and shoulder abductor muscles are most likely to be affected in the upper limb. In the lower extremity, the foot dorsiflexors and hip flexors are most frequently involved. Weakness may be asymmetric, and is rarely focal. Fatigable muscle weakness may be demonstrated by having the patient sustain arm abduction for a period of time or by having him or her raise one leg at an angle of 30–40 degrees while lying supine and maintain this position against gravity. Patients may be tested in this way until they fatigue, or the muscles may be manually tested after 1–2 min of fatiguing exercise.

Arising from a low chair without using the arms 10 times repeatedly is a good test for hip extensor muscle fatigue.

CASE 4.1   A 32-year-old man presents with the complaint of fatigable lower extremity weakness for the past 4 months. He is a recreational distance runner and has noted a progressive worsening of his ability to complete his "usual workouts." He states that his legs tire and feel "like they weigh a ton." He is able to perform better if he stops and rests "for a while." He reports a single episode of "slurred speech" after a particularly long run on a hot day. He has had no other bulbar or ocular symptoms. He has been seen by two neurologists who told him he may have "chronic fatigue syndrome" and referred him to a rheumatologist.

On examination, aside from mild weakness of eyelid closure, he has no other facial or oropharyngeal weakness. With sustained upgaze, mild bilateral medial rectus weakness is detected. There is no objective weakness in the extremities. He is able to perform 25 deep knee bends without difficulty. Arm abduction is manually overcome only after 2 min of holding the arms outstretched. The diagnosis of myasthenia gravis is confirmed on the basis of abnormal single-fiber electromyography and elevated AChR-binding antibodies.

Discussion   This case illustrates the fact that a "normal" neurologic examination does not necessarily rule out the diagnosis of MG. Objective signs in MG may not be apparent unless maneuvers designed to elicit fatigable weakness are used. This patient's complaints were very suggestive of the diagnosis given the clearly fatigable muscle weakness, which worsened with activity and improved with rest. Testing designed to elicit muscle fatigability resulted in the demonstration of objective signs and led to the appropriate diagnosis.

As previously stated, weakness in MG becomes worse with repeated effort and improves with rest. Thus, patients are at their best early in the morning and weakest in the evening. This should be taken into account when examining patients. In a few patients, weakness does not vary to any considerable degree. Muscle atrophy may occur in muscles that have been severely affected for a long period of time. Muscle pain and soreness are occasionally noted perhaps due to the increased stress of stronger muscles compensating for weak muscles. It is important to remember that in individual patients different muscles will be affected to varying degrees and some muscles may not be affected at all.

VI. DIAGNOSIS

As with all neurologic illnesses, the diagnosis of MG depends on the recognition of a suggestive clinical history followed by a complete but focused neurologic examination. Once the clinical diagnosis is made, there are a number of tests that are available for diagnostic confirmation (Chapter 3). The sensitivity of the various diagnostic tests in MG is given in Table 4.3. In general, increased AChR-binding antibody titers in a patient with a history consistent with MG essentially confirms the diagnosis. However, up to 20% of patients will not have these antibodies (43–45). In a few of these patients, titers are increased on repeat testing performed 6–8 months later. As discussed in the previous chapter, there are three AChR autoantibody tests. For general clinical purposes, these tests should be obtained in a selective manner. In a patient with suspected MG, the AChR-binding antibody should be obtained first because it is the most sensitive test. If this is negative, the AChR-modulating antibody test may increase the yield slightly. Striational antibodies may also aid in making the diagnosis if the AChR-binding antibodies are negative, particularly in later onset (>50 years) disease where they may be the only serologic abnormality. In early-onset disease, the presence of antistriational muscle antibodies increases the likelihood of an underlying thymoma. AChR-blocking antibodies are not helpful in making the diagnosis and should not be ordered routinely.

Although the AChR antibodies are the most specific diagnostic test, in most cases it is desirable to confirm the diagnosis as soon as possible, and antibody testing may take several days to weeks before results are available. The edrophonium test may be helpful in confirming the diagnosis of MG (particularly MG with prominent ocular signs) quickly, but, as discussed in

Table 4.3 Sensitivity of Various Diagnostic Tests in Myasthenia Gravis

Test	Generalized MG (% abnormal)	Ocular MG (% abnormal)
AChR antibodies	80	60
RNS	75	48
SFEMG	99	97

RNS, repetitive nerve stimulation; SFEMG, single-fiber electromyography.

Chapter 3, the results are entirely subjective. Thus, most patients will have electrodiagnostic studies performed. Single-fiber electromyography is the most sensitive diagnostic test for MG, but abnormalities are not specific for a primary defect in neuromuscular transmission. However, in a patient with a clinical presentation consistent with MG, single-fiber electromyography showing abnormal jitter in the setting of normal nerve conduction studies and conventional needle electromyography is confirmatory. An algorithm for the electrodiagnostic approach to MG is shown in Fig. 4.3.

All patients with a new diagnosis of MG should have serologic testing of thyroid function and computed tomography of the chest to determine if there is a thymoma. With regard to the mediastinal imaging, contrast is not needed and may exacerbate weakness in MG. There is no evidence that magnetic resonance imaging is superior for evaluation of thymoma. Furthermore, thymoma cannot be distinguished from thymic hyperplasia on the basis of imaging studies alone. As noted above, the presence of elevated striational antibodies is suggestive, although not diagnostic, of an underlying thymoma,

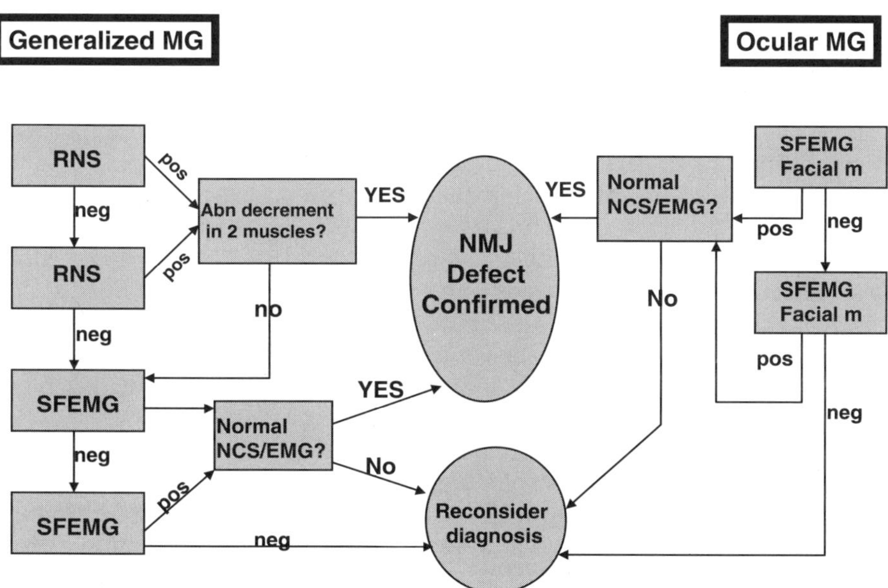

Figure 4.3 Algorithm for the electrodiagnostic approach to a patient with suspected MG. In general, the diagnostic yield is increased if clinically weak muscles are tested. pos, positive; neg, negative; SFEMG, single-fiber electromyography; EDC, extensor digitorum communis muscle; NCS/EMG, nerve conduction studies/ conventional electromyography.

particularly in younger patients. Sudden and severe onset of MG in patients older than 50 is particularly suggestive of an underlying thymoma, but histopathologic examination is required for definitive evaluation of an enlarged gland.

VII. TREATMENT AND MANAGEMENT

The outlook for patients with MG has improved considerably in recent years largely due to the use of immunosuppressive agents. Despite this success, considerable differences of opinion remain regarding the optimal use of these agents. This is complicated by the fact that few therapies have been tested by rigorous, prospective, placebo-controlled studies. The goal of therapy is to return the patient to normal function as rapidly as possible while minimizing the side effects of treatment. The art of providing optimal medical care for patients with MG often lies in deciding when it is appropriate to treat aggressively and when it is not. The discussion below provides guidelines for the practical management of patients with MG, emphasizing the pharmacology and judicious use of immunosuppressants.

A number of clinical factors need to be taken into account when considering the optimal choice of treatment in individual patients. The severity and distribution of weakness, the rate of progression and the impact of the disease on the functional capabilities of the patient are important factors for immediate therapeutic decisions. In addition, the age, sex, and general health of the patient and the presence of coexisting medical conditions, such as diabetes mellitus, thyroid disease, and the potential presence of thymoma or history of other malignancy, are important variables that may affect the long-term therapeutic plan. Finally, an assessment needs to be made regarding each patient's ability to comply with a given therapy and the surveillance required to monitor for the adverse effects of immunosuppression. Management of MG is a long-term commitment requiring ongoing communication between patient and physician.

The current therapeutic options for MG may be divided into (a) symptomatic therapy with acetylcholinesterase inhibitors, and (b) immunotherapy consisting of thymectomy and the use of immunosuppressive agents. These options are discussed below and a review of therapeutic strategies is presented.

A. Acetylcholinesterase Inhibitors

Traditionally, AChE inhibitors have been used as the first line of treatment in patients with MG. These agents prolong the action of ACh at the NMJ resulting in improved neuromuscular transmission. Although these drugs relieve symptoms in most patients with MG, it is important to remember that this beneficial effect is temporary, often incomplete, and has no effect on the course of the illness because it does not affect the underlying dysimmune process.

Pyridostigmine bromide (Mestinon) and neostigmine bromide (Prostigmine) are the most commonly used cholinesterase inhibitors in MG. Pyridostigmine bromide has become the preferred agent because of its longer duration of action (3–6 h) and higher tolerability. The initial oral dose in adults is 30 mg every 4–6 h. This initial dose may be adjusted as needed to maximize benefit and minimize side effects. Doses exceeding 120 mg every 4 h are rarely effective and potentially dangerous since higher doses may overexpose remaining functional AChRs to ACh, thereby desensitizing them and causing increased weakness. Patients usually report the onset of a beneficial response 30–40 min after administration of pyridostigmine and a wearing off of benefit approximately 3–6 h later. Patients can often be instructed to adjust the dosage schedule themselves to determine the optimal regimen, keeping in mind that excessively high doses may exacerbate weakness. Patients with oropharyngeal weakness should be instructed to take pyridostigmine 30 min before meals. A timed-release preparation of pyridostigmine (Mestinon Timespan) may be used at bedtime for patients who have prominent symptoms upon awakening. Unfortunately, its absorption is variable and unreliable, frequently leading to either an insufficient response or overdosage. It is preferable to have patients awaken at the appropriate times and take the standard preparation if nighttime or early morning weakness is a problem.

It is important to stress that treatment with cholinesterase inhibitors will not prevent a patient with severe bulbar and respiratory muscle weakness from experiencing a worsening of symptoms and requiring intubation (myasthenic crisis). In fact, the increased bronchial and oral secretions frequently associated with cholinesterase inhibitors may cause a serious problem in patients with bulbar and respiratory muscle weakness.

CASE 4.2 A 59-year-old man was diagnosed with MG at age 28 when he developed ptosis, diplopia, and mild generalized weakness. The diagnosis was based on a positive edrophonium test. He was treated with cholinesterase inhibitors alone and noted mild symptomatic improvement. Although he continued to have symptoms, he "learned to deal with (my) limitations." He had general anesthesia for a cholecystectomy and developed prolonged paralysis requiring ventilatory support. He was eventually weaned off the ventilator but complained of persistent symptoms of generalized weakness, fatigability, and swallowing difficulties. He was on pyridostigmine at a dose of 120

mg every 4 h, which caused frequent diarrhea. His examination revealed bilateral fatigable ptosis, bilateral medial rectus weakness, moderate facial weakness, poor tongue protrusion into the cheek, and mild
neck flexion and proximal extremity weakness. He also had mild weakness of finger extension and foot dorsiflexion. He had a reduced inspiratory sniff and cough.

The patient responded to a course of plasmapheresis and was
started on high-dose daily (60 mg) prednisone. Six months later, he had
few or no myasthenic symptoms on 30 mg of prednisone every other
day. He no longer required pyridostigmine. More importantly, he underwent a prostatectomy under general anesthesia and was extubated
without difficulty. He had no further exacerbations and was eventually
weaned to a stable prednisone dose of 15 mg every other day.

Discussion   This case illustrates an important point regarding symptomatic management of MG with cholinesterase inhibitors. While
symptoms may be controlled and patients may adapt to their reduced
level of function, patients treated with cholinesterase inhibitors alone
are at risk for severe MG exacerbations during times of stress, i.e.,
systemic infections, surgical procedures, etc. This may occur even after
prolonged periods of apparent disease stability as exemplified by this
patient. Definitive immunotherapy of MG not only improves baseline
function but also decreases the risk of significant disease exacerbation
during periods of stress. Once patients have achieved an optimal response to definitive immunotherapy, there is often no further need for
treatment with cholinesterase inhibitors.

Equivalent doses of the available cholinesterase inhibitors are given in
Table 4.4. The indications for use cholinesterase inhibitors other than
pyridostigmine are rare. Occasionally, cholinesterase inhibitors may be given
parenterally (intramuscularly and intravenously) when patients have severe
dysphagia preventing oral intake. Muscarinic side effects are the most
common adverse reactions of cholinesterase inhibitors and include stomach
cramps, diarrhea, sweating, nasal and bronchial secretions, bradycardia,
nausea, and vomiting (46). When these side effects occur, it is an indication
that the dose is too high. Suppressing gastrointestinal side effects with agents
such as loperamide is rarely necessary. It is preferable to identify the maximal
cholinesterase dose tolerated and initiate definitive immunotherapy if this
dose does not control myasthenic symptoms. Patients taking large amounts of
pyridostigmine bromide rarely develop bromism, which may present with
acute psychosis (47). Some patients are allergic to bromide and develop a skin
rash. These patients may be treated with ambenonium chloride (Mytelase).

Table 4.4 Equivalent Doses of Anticholinesterase Drugs

Drug	Oral	Intramuscular	Intravenous
Neostigmine bromide (*Prostigmine bromide*)	15 mg		
Neostigmine methyl sulfate (*Prostigmine methylsulfate*)	—	1.5 mg	0.5 mg
Pyridostigmine bromide (*Mestinon*)	60 mg	2.0 mg	0.7 mg
Mestinon Timespan	90–180 mg	—	—
Ambenonium chloride (*Mytelase*)	7.5 mg	—	—

B. Immunotherapy of MG

Immunosuppressive treatment of MG can be divided into long- and short-term strategies (Table 4.5). Thymectomy, corticosteroids, azathioprine, cyclosporine, and other immunosuppressive agents are used in an effort to induce long-term improvement. Plasmapheresis and intravenous immunoglobulin induce short-term improvement with rapid onset in most patients with MG.

1. Long-Term Immunotherapy

Thymectomy Thymectomy has been a well-accepted treatment for generalized myasthenia gravis with age of onset between 18 and 60 years despite the absence of controlled studies demonstrating long-term benefit. Clearly, all patients with thymoma should undergo surgical removal since

Table 4.5 Immunotherapy of Myasthenia Gravis

Long-term immunotherapies
Thymectomy
Corticosteroids (prednisone)
Azathioprine
Cyclosporine
Cyclophosphamide
Mycophenolate mofetil
Short-term immunotherapies
Plasmapheresis (plasma exchange)
Intravenous immune globulin

these tumors may spread locally and become invasive. The therapeutic use of thymectomy in nonthymomatous MG is based primarily on the presumed role of the thymus gland in initiation and/or maintenance of the autoimmune process. At least 80% of MG patients have pathologic thymic abnormalities, either hyperplasia or thymoma (48). Thymic hyperplasia is often found in early-onset (<40 years) MG, and cultured thymic cells from such patients can produce anti-acetylcholine receptor antibody (49). However, in late-onset patients as well as in other (i.e., seronegative) patients, thymic pathology is normal for age (50) and antibody production usually cannot be detected (51). Nevertheless, these patients may have an observed beneficial response to thymectomy.

Clinical support for the beneficial effect of thymectomy is found in published controlled but nonrandomized studies in which the incidence of clinical remission and improvement are increased in patients undergoing thymectomy. An evidence-based review of thymectomy in nonthymomatous MG analyzed 21 controlled but nonrandomized studies conducted between 1953 and 1998 (52). The authors found a positive association between thymectomy and MG remission or improvement. Patients undergoing thymectomy were twice as likely to attain a medication-free clinical remission than patients who did not have thymectomy. However, the authors also concluded that the efficacy of thymectomy could not be conclusively established on the basis of these data. mainly because of confounding factors including differences in baseline characteristics between the thymectomy and nonthymectomy patient groups in the studies analyzed.

Despite the lack of controlled data, a number of observations can be made based on the therapeutic use of thymectomy in MG over the past 50 years or so. First, the apparent beneficial effect of thymectomy may be enhanced when the procedure is performed early in relation to onset of symptoms (53,54). The potential benefit of thymectomy decreases and the risk of surgery increases as the adult patient gets older. Second, the onset of beneficial effect is delayed, occurring 6–12 months post procedure but potentially requiring as long as 2–5 years for maximal benefit (55). Finally, disease severity, AChR-Ab levels, and thymic pathology have no clear relationship to outcome (52,56). Significant controversy exists regarding the role of thymectomy in late-onset (older than 60 years) disease, ocular or mild generalized MG, and childhood MG. Consideration of thymectomy in these patients needs to be individualized, with the risks of surgery weighed against the potential benefit. Since the benefit of thymectomy has not been established conclusively by controlled randomized studies, this determination may be difficult and thymectomy should be viewed as an option to increase the probability of drug-free remission, induce clinical improvement, or potentially reduce the cumulative exposure to immunosuppressive agents.

Multiple techniques have been employed for removal of the thymus gland in MG (57,58) (Table 4.6). Although "total thymectomy" (i.e., removal of all tissue in the anterior mediastinum and neck that may contain thymic tissue) is generally accepted to be the goal of the procedure, it has not been conclusively demonstrated to be necessary. This has led some to pursue a less aggressive approach (i.e., transcervical thymectomy) in the hope of reducing risk and morbidity. Two basic types of transcervical thymectomy have been performed. The "basic" resection involves using a central cervical incision to remove the central mediastinal thymic tissue (59). The second or "extended" transcervical technique employs a manubrial retractor for improved exposure and allows for removal of more laterally located thymic tissue and fat (60). The video-assisted techniques employ a cervical incision with either unilateral or bilateral thorascopic exposure of the mediastinum allowing for the removal of mediastinal thymus and perithymic fat (61).

The transsternal approaches remove the central cervical and all visible mediastinal thymic tissue with the different variations distinguished by the extent of mediastinal and cervical fat removal (58). Whether there is a relationship between the specific resectional technique used and the rate of remission or improvement is not clearly established. However, a number of retrospective studies report lower remission rates with the transcervical technique or partial sternotomy compared to extended transsternal thymectomy (62–64). Furthermore, transsternal reexploration of patients who did not improve after transcervical thymectomy has yielded substantial amounts of residual thymic tissue and in several cases has resulted in clinical improvement (65,66). Thymomas have been found upon reexploration in patients previously undergoing the transcervical resection (67). For these reasons and to maximize the likelihood of remission, most centers employ the transsternal technique.

Perioperative mortality rates of thymectomy performed in MG patients after 1970 are consistently less than 3% (68–70), but the procedure is not

Table 4.6 Thymectomy Techniques

Transcervical thymectomy
Basic
Extended
Videoscopic
Transsternal thymectomy
Standard
Extended ("transsternal radical thymectomy")
Transsternal and transcervical thymectomy

without risk. Potential complications include acute respiratory failure from crisis, infection, and recurrent laryngeal or phrenic nerve injury. The main determinant of the immediate postoperative course of MG patients undergoing thymectomy is their preoperative clinical status. It is important to recognize that thymectomy is an elective procedure, and patients must have management of their MG optimized prior to the procedure. A preoperative pulmonary function test is useful to help identify patients with borderline respiratory muscle function. If significant bulbar or respiratory muscle weakness is present (i.e., forced vital capacity <2 L), a course of plasmapheresis is recommended prior to the surgery. There is no question that patients with moderately severe to severe bulbar or respiratory muscle weakness should be pretreated with plasmapheresis and/or corticosteroids prior to thymectomy. The question is whether all patients with any active myasthenic signs or symptoms should be pretreated. In the absence of controlled data, we elect to treat all patients with significant bulbar or respiratory signs as we would any MG patient *not* undergoing thymectomy. We then schedule the procedure after these signs have responded to therapy.

After thymectomy, the patient should be closely monitored for myasthenic signs and symptoms by a neurologist. Most patients tolerate the procedure quite well if symptoms are well controlled going into the procedure. The most common complaint following surgery is pain. The use of thoracic epidural analgesia maximizes postoperative pain control. Pyridostigmine may be given intramuscularly if the patient is unable to swallow immediately after thymectomy. Myasthenic weakness not controlled by cholinesterase inhibitors alone should be treated optimally with the use of immunosuppressive agents (corticosteroids, plasmapheresis, intravenous immune globulin), as will be discussed below.

Thymectomy for Thymoma: Virtually all patients with a known or suspected thymoma should undergo thymectomy. Patients must be stabilized prior to surgery in the manner described for nonthymomatous MG. A transsternal approach with exploration for mediastinal spread of tumor is required. Because malignant tumors may not be resected totally, postoperative radiation therapy is employed to suppress tumor spread or recurrence in cases in which there is spread of tumor beyond the thymic capsule. Postoperatively, the treatment of signs and symptoms of MG is no different than that for MG without thymoma.

Corticosteroids   Corticosteroid drugs (i.e., prednisone) are the most widely used form of immunotherapy in patients with MG. Their effects on the immune system are numerous, complex, and incompletely understood. The most important effect with regard to autoimmune disease is likely the interference with the production or function of numerous lymphokines, including interleukin-1, interleukin-2, and tumor necrosis factor (71). These actions potently inhibit the accumulation of leukocytes and macrophages in an immune response. Antibody production may be reduced by large doses of prednisone but is generally unchanged by moderate (20 mg/day) doses (72).

Corticosteroids have generally been used as the first choice for immunosuppressive therapy in MG. They are indicated when generalized or ocular MG symptoms are not adequately controlled by cholinesterase inhibitors alone. It is important to inform patients of the long list of steroid-related side effects prior to initiation of treatment (Table 4.7). Relative contraindications include severe obesity, poorly controlled diabetes mellitus, ulcer disease, uncontrolled hypertension, osteoporosis, and active systemic infections.

Considerable disagreement exists regarding the optimal dosing regimen for initiation of steroid therapy. There have been no controlled studies comparing the efficacy and safety of the different steroid induction regimens

Table 4.7 Side Effects of Corticosteroids

Side effect	Prevention
Sodium retention	Sodium-restricted diet
Fluid retention	Sodium-restricted diet
Potassium loss	Supplement as needed
Hypertension	Monthly checks, treat
Obesity	Low-calorie, low-fat diet; exercise
Impaired glucose tolerance	Monitor fasting blood sugar, treat
Peptic ulcer	Antacids, H_2 blockers
Osteoporosis	Calcium supplementation, vit D, alendronate, female hormone replacement
Steroid myopathy	Exercise
Impaired wound healing	Use minimal dose that controls disease
Skin friability/easy bruising	Use minimal dose that controls disease
Cushingoid appearance	Use minimal dose that controls disease
Acne	
Personality change	
Mood swings	
Menstrual irregularities	
Suppression of growth in children	
Reduced resistance to infection	Prompt recognition and management of systemic infections
Cataracts	Regular ophthalmologic evaluation
Glaucoma	Regular ophthalmologic evaluation

in MG. One method is to begin treatment with high-dose daily prednisone (60–100 mg/day). This dose produces a prompt, predictable response with sustained improvement usually occurring within 2–3 weeks. Roughly one-third of patients have an exacerbation of weakness after starting high-dose daily prednisone. This usually occurs within the first 7–10 days and may last for as long as 6 days (73). This worsening is usually mild but may cause symptomatic bulbar or respiratory muscle weakness. Thus, patients with moderate or severe weakness, particularly involving bulbar or respiratory muscles, should be hospitalized for initiation of steroid treatment. Often, patients receive a course of plasmapheresis prior to initiation of steroids. This may be done on an outpatient basis with steroid treatment being initiated once there is a clear objective response to plasmapheresis. This approach may also produce a more rapid response.

Daily steroid treatment may also be started at a low dose (10 mg/day) to minimize the risk of exacerbation. The dose is then increased by 5–10 mg/day on a weekly basis until improvement occurs. This is a regimen favored by many clinicians for steroid initiation in MG with purely ocular symptoms. A disadvantage of this approach is that the anticipated onset of clinical benefit as well as the timing of the possible transient worsening is less predictable.

Prednisone may also be started with high-, moderate-, or low-dose alternate-day therapy. The main reasons for opting for the initiation of prednisone therapy with the alternate-day regimen are to avoid steroid-induced worsening and to lessen side effects. No data are available for the incidence of steroid-induced worsening when treatment is started with a low-dose alternate-day regimen, but it is believed to be a rare occurrence. Furthermore, there are no data directly comparing the incidence of side effects during the first year of treatment in patients started on a low-dose alternate-day regimen vs. a high-dose daily regimen. With the low-dose alternate-day regimen, a dose of 20 mg every other day is started, with gradual increments (5–10 mg qod) every 2–5 days until there is improvement or a dose of 100–120 mg qod is reached. Advantages and disadvantages of the high-dose daily and low-dose alternate-day incrementing induction schemes are listed in Table 4.8.

High-dose daily or alternate-day prednisone is given until there is a sustained (1–3 days) improvement. The dose is then decreased gradually (and converted to an alternate-day regimen for patients started on daily prednisone) to the lowest dose needed to maintain disease control. Frequent clinical observations are necessary as the prednisone dose is decreased to monitor for return of weakness. Should weakness return, the dose must be increased to a level that maintains an optimal clinical response. Many patients require long-term maintenance therapy (20–25 mg qod or less) to prevent return of myasthenic weakness. Patients requiring more than 25 mg qod to maintain

Table 4.8 High-Dose Daily vs. Low-Dose Alternate-Day Corticosteroid Initiation in Myasthenia Gravis

Induction regimen	Advantages	Disadvantages
High-dose daily	Prompt, predictable response Reduces time to maximal benefit Timing of SI exacerbation more predictable Lessens long-term exposure?	Increased number of SI exacerbations Hospitalization or pretreatment w/short-term therapy required
Low-dose alternate-day, incrementing	Decreased risk of SI exacerbation Hospitalization or pretreatment not required Reduces side effects?	Beneficial response and SI exacerbation less predictable

SI, Steroid induced.

improvement, patients who fail to respond, and patients in whom toxicity exceeds benefit are candidates for other forms of immunotherapy.

Potential side effects of chronic corticosteroid administration are significant and numerous (Table 4.7). As many as 66% of patients experience one or more side effects of steroid administration (74,75). Preventive treatment (summarized in Table 4.9) includes exercise, calcium supplementation (1500 mg/day), vitamin D (50,000 units once or twice weekly), and replacement of gonadal hormones in postmenopausal women. The use of calcitonin

Table 4.9 Corticosteroid Collateral Program

- Diet: A strict low-carbohydrate, low-salt, high-protein diet is recommended.
- Antacids: To counter possible gastrointestinal discomfort, a calcium-containing antacid (Tums) should be taken between meals.
- Calcium and vitamin D: Postmenopausal patients are candidates for a calcium supplement (1 gr/day) and vitamin D (500 U/week) when long-term corticosteroid treatment is required.
- Reassurance: Patients need reassurance that common symptoms, including "flushing" or redness of the face, insomnia, and tremor, are transient and resolve when the steroid dose is lowered.
- TB prophylaxis: Patients at high risk of tuberculosis exposure or those with a recently documented "positive" PPD skin test should be given prophylaxis with isoniazid.

or alendronate should be considered in treated patients who develop osteopenia and in all postmenopausal women (76). There may be an increased incidence of premature ovarian failure in young female MG patients (personal observations) which may be autoimmune in etiology. Thus, female patients of childbearing age should be questioned regarding possible abnormalities in their menstrual cycles prior to initiation of steroid treatment. These women may need hormonal replacement and/or alendronate. Antacids and/or H_2 receptor antagonists should be given to susceptible individuals but probably need not be administered as routine prophylaxis.

Azathioprine   Azathioprine (AZA), a purine analogue that inhibits DNA synthesis, has been used as an immunosuppressive agent since the 1960s (77). The use of AZA in MG was pioneered in Europe (78) in the late 1960s. Uncontrolled retrospective studies have demonstrated its apparent efficacy and safety in MG (79,80). A recent randomized double-blind trial of prednisolone alone vs. prednisolone plus AZA revealed fewer treatment failures, longer remissions, and fewer side effects in patients who received AZA as an adjunct to prednisolone (81).

AZA has had three main indications in MG: (a) as a steroid-sparing agent, (b) as combination therapy in patients with an insufficient response to corticosteroids, and (c) as an initial immunosuppressive agent in patients for whom corticosteroids are contraindicated or poorly tolerated. Its therapeutic action in MG is quite delayed, with clinical benefit expected within 4–6 months, but maximal improvement often requires up to a year. This must be accounted for when initiating therapy with AZA, and another mode of treatment (i.e, corticosteroids) must maintain disease stability until AZA takes effect.

Treatment is typically initiated with a dose of 50 mg/day for a week. If this is tolerated, it is increased by 50 mg/week to a target dose of 2–3 mg/kg/day. Azathioprine may be taken as a single daily dose or given two or three times a day if the full dose causes gastrointestinal upset. Complete blood counts and liver enzymes should be monitored closely (every other week for the first 2–3 months of therapy and monthly thereafter).

Although long-term treatment with AZA is usually well tolerated, some adverse effects limit its use. Approximately 15–20% of patients develop an idiosyncratic reaction consisting of fever, malaise, and myalgias that precludes the use of AZA. Other common side effects are hematologic (consisting of leukopenia, anemia, and thrombocytopenia) and gastrointestinal (including nausea, anorexia, abdominal discomfort, and diarrhea) (82,83). AZA should be discontinued if the absolute neutrophil count falls below 1000 per mm^3 and the dose reduced if the white blood cell count (WBC) falls below 3000 per mm^3. An increase of the mean corpuscular volume (MCV), often to greater than 10 units above baseline, does not require discontinuation of therapy and may parallel the therapeutic response (84). Hepatic toxicity usually takes the form of elevation of liver enzymes, but cholestatic jaundice (85) and acute liver failure (86) rarely occur. In 104 patients treated with AZA for a median period of 29 months, 35% had adverse reactions necessitating discontinuance of therapy in 11% (83).

The risk of neoplasia is often a major concern for patients on AZA. The specific risk of treatment in MG patients is not clearly known. An increased risk for lymphoma has been reported for AZA treatment in rheumatoid arthritis (87,88). A possible increased risk was also identified in multiple sclerosis after 10 years or more of continuous AZA therapy (89), but no clear enhanced risk was found for inflammatory bowel disease managed with AZA (90). In a series of 159 MG patients treated with AZA for a median of 3.4 years, two patients developed primary central nervous system lymphoma after 6 and 12 years of AZA treatment (91). This occurrence was significantly increased compared with the general population. Thus, there may be an increased risk of lymphoma in MG patients treated with AZA, and this risk may be dose and duration related. Is it therefore appropriate to discontinue AZA therapy after a stable period of remission? The answer to this question requires consideration of another question.

Do most patients require life-long AZA therapy? If treatment is stopped abruptly, MG exacerbations are likely to occur, based on the current limited literature. Eight of 15 patients experienced relapse after discontinuation of AZA in the only study looking at the incidence of disease exacerbation after stopping AZA (92). In the absence of substantial data regarding AZA tapering, it is advisable to reduce AZA doses gradually after a long symptom-free period (>1 year) in an effort to identify a minimal effective maintenance dose. Complete discontinuation of therapy should probably be limited to patients with hematologic or hepatic side effects or to very young patients in whom life-long treatment may increase the risk of malignancy.

Cyclosporine Cyclosporine is a potent immunomodulating agent that has been shown to be effective in the management of MG in a controlled, double-blind clinical trial (93). Cyclosporine binds cyclophylin and inhibits calcineurin, which leads to inhibition of interleukin-2 production and, subsequently, T-lymphocyte proliferation and amplification (94). It has been used effectively in MG mainly in patients whose conditions are refractory to other forms of therapy. It may be used as a steroid-sparing agent in combination with prednisone. The recommended dose is 5 mg/kg/day in divided doses given 12 h apart. At this dose, trough levels of 90–150 µg/L are attained, usually corresponding to clinical improvement. Onset of clinical improvement is 4–8 weeks after initiating therapy. Regular monitoring (at least monthly) of blood pressure, serum creatinine, and plasma trough cyclosporine levels is advisable. If the baseline serum creatinine increases over 30% of baseline, treatment should be stopped. Because of numerous potential drug interactions, printed materials listing medications that may affect serum cyclosporine levels should be provided to patients (Table 4.10).

Common side effects associated with cyclosporine treatment include nephrotoxicity, hypertension, headaches, hirsutism, and tremors (94,95). The nephrotoxicity of cyclosporine appears to be dose and duration related. In a retrospective analysis of the use of cyclosporine in MG, the authors found that 95% of 57 patients had clinical improvement with a median time to best clinical response of 7 months (96). However, major side effects included ele-

Table 4.10 Cyclosporine Drug Interactions

Drugs that may cause kidney damage when combined with cyclosporine:
    Antibiotics: aminoglycosides, vancomycin, trimethoprim, and fluoroquinolones
    Antifungals: amphotericin B (Fungizone), ketoconazole
    Antivirals: acyclovir (Zovirax)
    Antiulcer: cimetidine (Tagamet), ranitidine (Zantac)
    Nonsteroidal anti-inflammatory drugs
    Chemotherapy: melphalan (Alkeran), etopside (VePesid)
    Cardiac/blood pressure: Captopril (Capoten), acetazolamide (Diamox), furosemide (Lasix), disopyramide (Norpace)
Drugs that may raise cyclosporine levels:
    Antibiotics: erythromycin
    Antifungals: ketoconazole, difluconazole, iatroconazole
    Stomach/ulcer: metoclopramide (Reglan), cimetidine (Tagamet)
    Cardiac/blood pressure: diltiazem (Cardizem), nicardipine (Cardene), verapamil
    Hormones: danazol (Danocrine), oral contraceptives, methylprednisolone
    Misc.: bromocriptine (Parlodel)
Drugs that may reduce cyclosporine levels:
    Antibiotics: rifampin, imipenem (Primaxin), nafcillin, trimethoprim
    Epilepsy: phenytoin, phenobarbital, carbamazepine
Drugs that may accumulate in the blood when taken with cyclosporine:
- Steroids: prednisone
- Cardiac: digoxin
- Cholesterol: HMG-CoA reductase inhibitors may cause myopathy when combined with cyclosporine
- Sildenafil (Viagra)

There are many conflicting reports about potential interactions when these and other drugs are used with cyclosporine. It is probably wise to monitor kidney function and cyclosporine levels frequently whenever a new medication is started.

vation of serum creatinine (28%) and malignancy (11%). This highlights the need for regular monitoring of renal function, and also argues that the use of cyclosporine should be reserved for patients with MG in whom cortico-steroids and azathioprine are ineffective, poorly tolerated, or contraindicated.

Mycophenolate Mofetil   Mycophenolate mofetil (MM) is a novel and potent immunosuppressive agent. It blocks purine synthesis in activated T and B lymphocytes and selectively inhibits their proliferation (97). An open-label pilot study to assess the efficacy and safety of MM in patients with refractory or steroid-dependent MG (98) showed that 8 of 12 patients improved within 2 months of treatment initiation. No significant side effects were observed. In addition, a retrospective case series of MM treatment in MG (among other autoimmune neuromuscular diseases) supported these findings (99). A double-blind, placebo-controlled pilot trial of MM in suboptimally treated MG demonstrated greater improvement in MM-treated patients on all four efficacy criteria compared to those treated with placebo (100). No severe adverse effects were observed. Taken together, these studies indicate that MM may be an important advance in the management of MG, but larger controlled studies are needed to confirm these preliminary findings. Despite this, MM is being used more and more by clinicians to manage MG.

The usual starting dose of MM is 1 g twice a day, but doses as high as 3 g/day have been used. There are no data regarding the use of mycophenolic acid serum levels to help to determine the most effective dose in an individual patient. There are no safety data regarding the concomitant use of AZA and MM, suggesting that these two agents should not be used in combination. Cyclosporine has been used extensively in combination with MM in organ transplantation and the combination has a favorable safety profile. The common side effects of MM include diarrhea, nausea, vomiting, and abdominal cramping. Recurrent upper respiratory or urinary tract infections may occur. Leukopenia, anemia, and thrombocytopenia, and sepsis are potential serious side effects. The risks associated with long-term use (i.e., malignancy) are not known.

Based on the studies performed to date, the beneficial response to MM has its onset as early as 6 weeks after initiation of treatment but may be delayed for as long as 6 months. The specific role of MM in the management of MG remains to be determined. There is little experience with its use as the initial form of immunotherapy in MG. Pending further clinical trials, the use of MM should probably be reserved for patients who are either intolerant or unresponsive to AZA, since it may be a less toxic alternative to cyclosporine.

Cyclophosphamide   Because of its significant toxicity, cyclophospha-mide's use in MG is limited to the most seriously ill patients whose disease is refractory to azathioprine, corticosteroids, and cyclosporine. An oral dose of 3–5 mg/kg is used, often preceded by an initial intravenous dose of 200 mg daily for 5 days (101). Serious adverse effects include leukopenia, hemorrhagic cystitis, anorexia, and infections (97). Alopecia is a common (75%) but less serious complication. Intravenous pulsed cyclophosphamide may be considered in severe, refractory, generalized MG, based on the results of a recently published study (102).

2. Short-Term Immunotherapy

Plasmapheresis (Plasma Exchange) Plasmapheresis or plasma exchange (PE) is an effective short-term therapy for MG (103–105) that is primarily used in three clinical situations: (a) in myasthenic crisis, (b) in severe exacerbations of myasthenic weakness, and (c) prior to surgery in patients undergoing thymectomy. It may also be used when initiating treatment with high-dose corticosteroids to reduce the risk of transient worsening, as discussed above. The mechanism of action is believed to be removal of circulating AChR antibodies and immune complexes. PE is given three times per week (removing 2–3 L of plasma per treatment) for a total of five or six treatments over a 2-week period. The onset of improvement is rapid, frequently beginning after the third treatment, and often correlating in individual patients with a reduction in AChR antibodies. Despite this, patients with seronegative MG also appear to derive benefit from the procedure (106).

In centers with sufficient experience, PE is usually very well tolerated. Complications include hypotension, altering of clotting mechanisms, hypoalbuminemia, hypocalcemia, and difficulty with vascular access (107). Careful clinical monitoring during the procedure is essential to avoid unexpected volume shifts into and out of the intravascular space. Transient worsening of symptoms of MG after the first one or two exchanges has been observed perhaps due to the removal of anticholinesterase drugs and corticosteroids. The benefit of PE must be weighed against the problems of vascular access, as well as the risks and high cost of the procedure.

Intravenous Immune Globulin (IVIg) The indications for use of intravenous immune globulin (IVIg) are essentially the same as for PE. Most patients with MG improve following administration of high doses of IVIg (108–110). In a randomized study, Gajdos et al. (111) treated 87 MG patients experiencing acute exacerbations with one of three treatments: (a) three courses of plasmapheresis; (b) IVIg, 0.4 g/kg/day (1.2 g/kg total dose) for 3 days; and (c) IVIg, 0.4 g/kg/day (2.0 g/kg total dose) for 5 days. The authors found no statistical difference among the three groups and concluded that IVIg was as effective as PE.

IVIg is usually administered at a dose of 2 g/kg over 2–5 days. Onset of improvement with this dose usually occurs within the first week and lasts for a mean period of 45 days (108–112). The mechanism of action is not known, although several possibilities have been advanced (113). Adverse reactions are usually mild, including headaches, chills, myalgias, nausea, and other gastrointestinal symptoms (114,115). Rare adverse effects include an acute anaphylactic reaction (116), aseptic meningitis (117), renal tubular toxicity (118), and stroke (119).

The precise role of IVIg in the treatment of MG has not been determined. Whether it is as effective (safer?) as PE in myasthenic crisis has not been conclusively determined. While offering the advantage of rapid onset of benefit with few side effects, it has the disadvantages of its high cost and the necessity of serial treatments. Further issues that have not been clarified include whether IVIg may have a role in the long-term immunosuppressive regimen in selected patients and, if so, when it should be used in relation to the other drugs. As is the case for many of the therapeutic agents in MG, the paucity of controlled clinical trials makes the effective and prudent use of these agents quite challenging.

3. Therapeutic Approach

When a clear diagnosis of MG is established, treatment must be tailored to the individual patient. Disease severity determines how aggressive the treatment plan should be. Often the first decision is whether or not to proceed with thymectomy. This decision requires consideration of a number of factors, including the patient's age, severity and distribution of disease, as well as the patient's overall medical health. In choosing a specific treatment plan, the physician must take into consideration the advantages and disadvantages of each treatment modality in the individual patient and carefully weigh the potential risks against the projected benefits (Table 4.11). The tolerated risk may vary considerably from one patient to another. For example, mild intermittent ptosis and diplopia may be tolerable in an 83-year-old retired steel worker but completely unacceptable in a 38-year-old pilot. In the latter case, the increased risk incurred by aggressively treating these recalcitrant symptoms is justifiable. An algorithm for the general approach to the treatment of a patient with generalized MG is given in Fig. 4.4.

The severity and stage of disease as well as the patient's age and general health are important variables needed to decide on an appropriate treatment plan. Close monitoring of the clinical course may call for changes in the initial treatment plan based on responses to therapeutic interventions as well as patient tolerance. Although there are a number of effective therapeutic options, the art of managing MG lies in identifying the treatment plan that

Table 4.11 Therapeutic Agents in Myasthenia Gravis

Treatment	Role/indications	Onset of benefit	Dose	Main advantages	Main disadvantages
Long-term immunotherapy					
Prednisone	1. Generalized MG—initial immunotherapy 2. Ocular MG—not controlled by cholinesterase inhibitors	2–3 weeks	60–80 mg/day	Rapid onset of action	Side effects—see Table 4.7
Azathioprine	1. Combination therapy—generalized MG not adequately controlled by thymectomy or corticosteroids 2. Steroid sparing 3. Initial immunotherapy in selected patients	4–6 months	2–3 mg/kg/day	Relative safety	1. Need for frequent blood monitoring 2. Delayed onset of benefit
Cyclosporine	1. Combination therapy—generalized MG not adequately controlled by thymectomy or corticosteroids 2. Steroid sparing 3. In patients with azathioprine toxicity, lack of efficacy	3–6 weeks	5 mg/kg/day	Prompt beneficial effect. Targeted immunomodulatory effects	1. Need for frequent blood monitoring 2. Renal toxicity with chronic use

Mycophenolate mofetil	1. Combination therapy (with cyclosporine)? 2. Steroid sparing? 3. Initial immunotherapy?	2–8 weeks	1 g BID	Rapid onset of benefit. Favorable side effect profile	More controlled trials in MG needed? Long-term risk of infection, malignancy
Cyclophosphamide	Severe MG unresponsive to all other therapies	??Rapid	2.5–3.0 mg/kg/day	Response rates up to 90%, but few studies and uncontrolled	Substantial toxicity— 1. myelosuppression 2. hemorrhagic cystitis 3. malignancy
Short-term immunotherapy					
Plasmapheresis	1. Myasthenic crisis 2. Short-term management of severe myasthenic weakness (preparation for thymectomy, surgery)	After 3rd–6th treatment	3–4 L exhanged qod × 6 treatments	Rapid onset of benefit within days of treatment initiation	1. Problems of vascular access 2. High cost
Intravenous Immunoglobulin	1. As for plasmapheresis 2. ?Maintenance therapy	Within 4–5 days	2 g/kg/day divided over 2–5 days	Rapid onset of benefit	1. Rare severe adverse reactions—ATN, stroke, aseptic meningitis, etc. 2. High cost

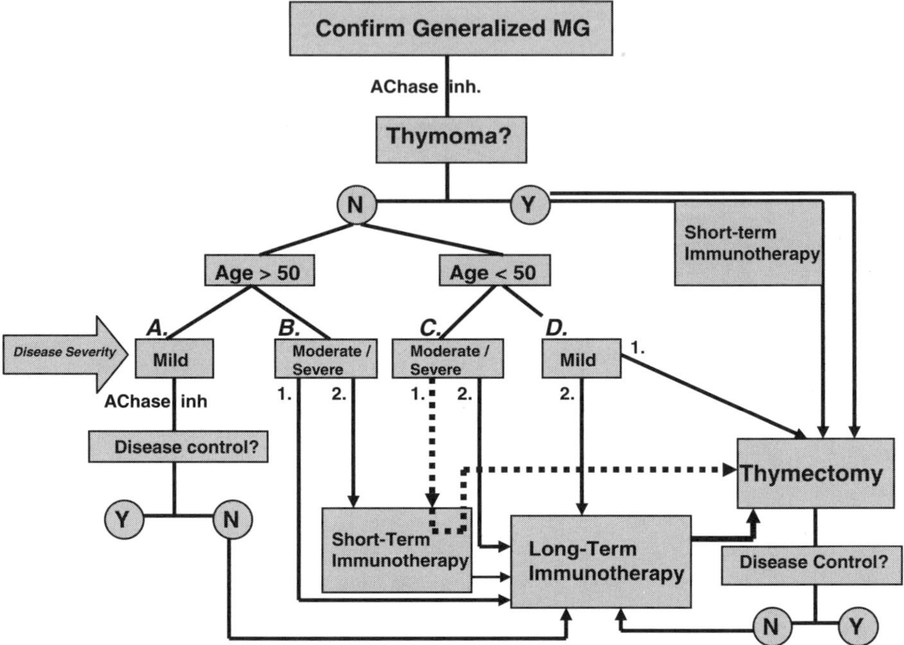

Figure 4.4 Algorithm for the therapy of generalized MG. The therapeutic approach must be individualized based on disease severity (as shown in the figure) and other factors described in the text. Consideration should be given to thymectomy in nonthymomatous, generalized MG primarily in patients with disease onset before the age of 50 (C and D). The therapeutic approach is similar in late-onset nonthymomatous MG (A and B) with the exception of thymectomy, which is not a first-line therapeutic intervention in these patients. Dotted line indicates short-term immunotherapy as preparation for thymectomy.

maximizes the likelihood of attaining remission of symptoms at the lowest possible risk.

VIII.   CLINICAL MANAGEMENT IN SPECIFIC SITUATIONS

A.   Exacerbations

Exacerbation of MG may occur under a variety of circumstances including systemic infection, surgery, thyroid hormone imbalance, pregnancy, exposure to drugs that affect neuromuscular transmission, and too rapid tapering of immunosuppressant medications. Thus, in managing an exacerbation, it is important to identify the trigger for the worsening of symptoms. If the trigger is modifiable (i.e., antibiotic treatment for a systemic infection) the appropriate action/treatment should be initiated. Drugs that adversely affect neuromuscular transmission should be discontinued. If the exacerbation is severe and produces bulbar or respiratory muscle impairment, hospitalization for a course of plasmapheresis will produce rapid improvement while the chronic immunosuppressive regimen is modified. In general, if a worsening is due to a decrease in an immunosuppressive medication, the dose prior to the worsening (at a minimum) should be reinstituted. It may be necessary to use a higher dose to ensure complete control of symptoms in patients with a moderate to severe exacerbation.

B. Myasthenic Crisis and Intensive Care of the MG Patient

Myasthenic crisis is defined as a severe worsening of symptoms involving bulbar and/or respiratory muscles, and requiring intubation for either respiratory failure or airway protection. There is an extreme variability in the reported incidence of myasthenic crisis ranging from 8% to 63% of patients with MG (120–126). Crisis is usually triggered by a specific antecedent event, although crises may occur without a clear precipitating cause, particularly early in the course of MG. Crisis occurs during the first 2 years of disease onset in the majority of patients (18). Rarely, a crisis occurs in a patient receiving high-dose cholinesterase inhibitors in which case the exacerbation of symptoms may represent a cholinergic crisis. This situation is rare, and it may be more likely that these patients have experienced a severe MG exacerbation that was made worse by the increased bronchial and oral secretions induced by cholinesterase inhibitors. Whatever the case, once a patient is intubated for MG crisis, cholinesterase inhibitors should be stopped as will be discussed below.

In general, respiratory assistance is required in an MG patient when the forced vital capacity is less than 15 mL/kg body weight. However, forced vital capacity measurements may be technically challenging since most of these patients have significant facial weakness preventing them from being able to maintain an adequate seal on the spirometer mouthpiece. Thus, bedside assessments, including the strength of cough and inspiratory sniff, are valuable aids in determining the need for intubation. As previously discussed, arterial blood gas measurements are a relatively insensitive measure of impending respiratory failure in MG.

Once it has been determined that a patient is in crisis, intubation and institution of mechanical ventilation should not be delayed. Cholinesterase inhibitors should be discontinued to prevent accumulation of excessive secretions. A search for a precipitating cause for the myasthenic crisis should be made. Any systemic infection that is identified should be treated aggressively with antibiotics, with care taken not to use agents known to worsen neuromuscular transmission (see Chapter 8).

Patients who are intubated due to severe exacerbations of MG are usually treated with a course of plasmapheresis or IVIg in an effort to improve respiratory and bulbar strength as rapidly as possible. High-dose corticosteroids are also given to maintain improvement on a long-term basis. Since the patient is intubated, there is no concern regarding corticosteroid-induced worsening of symptoms. If a patient experiences crisis while on corticosteroids, the dose should be increased and consideration should be given to starting other immunosuppressive treatments such as azathioprine, cyclosporine, or mycophenolate mofetil. It is important to realize that these agents have a delayed onset of beneficial effect, and another form of therapy (high-dose corticosteroids) must be instituted to maintain disease stability until the effects of these agents become manifest.

Patients should be examined daily to assess for improvement of muscle strength. Frequently, improvement in other muscle groups coincides with respiratory muscle improvement. Although examination of intubated patients in the intensive care unit is frequently limited, selection of specific sentinel muscles may be useful to follow the progress of an MG patient in crisis. For example, the ability to raise the head off the pillow may be assessed serially. With severe respiratory and bulbar weakness, the neck flexors are often quite weak and patients will be unable to lift their heads against gravity. The return of the ability to lift the head signifies a significant improvement in these patients. Respiratory mechanics may also be used to determine if extubation should be considered. An inspiratory pressure greater than -20 cm H_2O and an expiratory pressure greater than 35–40 cm H_2O are indicators that extubation should be attempted. Patients may be weaned from the ventilator for short periods of time increasing as tolerated. If patients complain of shortness of breath or fatigue during weaning, extubation should be delayed regardless of the inspiratory or expiratory pressures.

Prior to 1955, myasthenic crisis was fatal in up to 80% of cases. This situation has improved substantially as demonstrated by a more recent study (127) in which 3 of 73 patients (4%) died during crisis and four others died after extubation. All deaths in this series were due to serious medical comorbidities. Surprisingly, the authors reported that the median duration of intubation had changed remarkably little since the 1960s and suggested that prevention of complications may be the best strategy to improve outcome in the future. However, medical complications are closely associated with prolonged mechanical ventilation, and minimizing the duration of intubation is certainly a crucial factor in determining outcome. Until randomized, controlled clinical trials are performed to determine if plasmapheresis, intravenous immune globulin, or other forms of immunotherapy truly shorten the duration of crisis, clinicians must rely on judgment and anecdotal data to guide treatment decisions.

Another controversial issue is the preventability of myasthenic crisis. Does the incidence of crisis correlate with the aggressiveness of early immunotherapy, or will patients who are destined to have a crisis have one regardless of therapy? If the former is true, this may explain the wide range of crisis incidences among different reports and institutions. The majority of myasthenic crises occur after clinical worsening of MG symptoms. The interval between the onset of these symptoms and the onset of crisis ranges from 1 to 21 days, and most frequently occurs between 1 and 3 days (120). Thus, if these symptoms are recognized and managed in a timely manner, it is conceivable that crisis may be averted in these patients. Clearly, certain patients experience severe and acute exacerbations that will lead to crisis no matter what course of treatment is instituted. However, the incidence of crisis may be a measure of the effectiveness of therapy, and it is probably prudent to consider crisis as a preventable event requiring clinical vigilance leading to the prompt institution of therapy and/or the removal of triggering factors.

C. MG and Thymoma

Roughly 15% of patients with autoimmune MG have an underlying thymoma. It is well accepted that thymectomy should be performed in virtually all patients with thymoma. The only exceptions are patients with widespread locally invasive disease, patients who are very poor surgical risks, and elderly patients with small tumors who may be treated medically while the tumor size is monitored by serial chest computed tomography. Patients with significant bulbar or respiratory muscle weakness should be pretreated with a course of plasmapheresis until maximum improvement is attained. Thymectomy should follow within a week of the final exchange. Postoperative irradiation is performed on patients who have tumor spread beyond the thymic capsule. Subsequent (postsurgical) treatment of patients with thymoma is the same as for nonthymomatous MG.

CASE 4.3 A 58-year-old man presented to the emergency room with a 1-week history of progressive limb weakness, dysphagia, dyspnea, and ptosis. He had a transsternal thymectomy for resection of a "malignant thymoma" 5 weeks previously. He had no symptoms of weakness prior to the thymectomy. The thymoma was discovered by chest X-ray obtained as part of the workup for an upper respiratory infection. He received no postoperative radiotherapy and was on no medications other than analgesics at the time of discharge. He recently saw a neurologist who "did some blood tests" and placed him on pyridostigmine at a dosage of 60 mg every 3 h.

On examination, he was in obvious respiratory distress with a respiratory rate of 28. He had bilateral, asymmetric, fatigable ptosis and ophthalmoparesis most prominently affecting the medial and superior rectus muscles. Eyelid closure and cheek puff were very weak, as was neck flexion which could be overcome using two fingers. He had an inaudible inspiratory sniff and a poor cough. There was diffuse weakness in the extremities graded at 4/5, more prominent in proximal muscle groups.

A diagnosis of myasthenic crisis was made and the patient was immediately intubated. His pyridostigmine was stopped, plasmapheresis was initiated, and he was started on high-dose daily corticosteroids. Within 10 days, his strength improved and he was able to be extubated. The histopathologic slides from his thymectomy were obtained and reviewed. He indeed had a malignant thymoma with extension beyond the thymic capsule, and he received a course of radiation therapy. He continued to improve and by 5 months from the date of his presentation, was essentially in pharmacologic remission on an alternate-day prednisone regimen (50 mg every other day). Computed tomography (CT) of the chest was obtained and there was no evidence for thymoma recurrence.

A steroid-sparing agent (azathioprine) was added and his prednisone dose was slowly decreased without return of myasthenic symptoms. Two years from the date of his original presentation, he presented to the emergency room with severe chest wall pain. Chest imaging revealed recurrence of thymoma with metastases to the pleura and pericardium which was judged to be "inoperable." He received chemotherapy and radiation, but expired 3 months later.

Discussion   This case illustrates a number of important points. First, it is important to realize that patients with thymoma who do not have obvious signs of MG may have asymptomatic, subclinical disease that is prone to exacerbations particularly after significant stressors such as surgery. This is almost certainly what happened with this patient. The most common precipitant for MG exacerbation is surgery, particularly thymectomy, and it is not unusual for these exacerbations to be severe (often culminating in myasthenic crisis) and to occur several weeks after the surgical procedure.

Second, this patient had a malignant thymoma with disease beyond the thymic capsule, so plans for postoperative radiotherapy should have been arranged after his thymectomy. Once his condition was stabilized, he underwent a course of radiation and a follow-up chest CT was obtained 6 months later to determine if there was residual or recurrent thymoma. He subsequently (18 months later) developed recurrent malignant disease during a time when his myasthenia was under good control, emphasizing the importance of regular monitoring by chest CT even if there is clinical remission of MG symptoms. Tumor progression was not associated with disease deterioration in this case, as is usually expected.

It is reasonable to perform chest CT at least yearly in MG patients after invasive thymoma resection. An exacerbation of MG that does not respond adequately to immunosuppressive therapy may be evidence for thymoma recurrence. On the other hand, malignant thymomas may recur without significant exacerbation of MG (128). Thymoma recurrences may occur many years after thymectomy suggesting that surveillance should be prolonged. Furthermore, recurrences of encapsulated tumors have been rarely reported suggesting that postoperative surveillance should include patients with tumors limited to the thymic capsule (129).

Antibodies to muscle antigens (i.e., striational, titin, ryanodine) have been used to predict the presence of a thymoma but are of limited utility, as discussed in Chapter 3. When combined, the presence of ryanodine and titin antibodies is 70% sensitive and 70% specific for the presence of thymoma (130), with sensitivity and specificity improving in younger onset disease. Thus, in patients with early-onset MG, the presence of antimuscle antibodies is reasonably predictive of thymoma. However, in the majority of these cases, thymectomy is likely to be performed regardless. In late onset patients, the presence or absence of antimuscle antibodies is not useful in determining the presence of thymoma.

D. "Seronegative" MG

Approximately 15–20% of MG patients do not have detectable antibodies to AChR. Patients without AChR antibodies are more likely to have mild disease, "ocular MG" (see below), less likely to have thymoma, and more frequently have a normal thymus or thymic atrophy (131). Seronegative patients are otherwise clinically very similar to AChR-positive patients, and their treatment is no different. The diagnosis of autoimmune MG in these patients is usually based on single-fiber electromyography demonstrating a primary defect in neuromuscular transmission.

There is strong evidence that seronegative MG is caused by autoantibodies. Treatment of these patients with immunosuppressive medications results in clinical improvement. Immunoglobulin from affected patients causes a defect in neuromuscular transmission when transferred to mice (132), and sera from patients with seronegative MG inhibits the function of AChRs (133). There are three possible explanations for seronegative MG cases: (a) antibodies could be bound to the endplates without detectable circulating antibodies; (b) variation in antigenic determinants might result in antibodies that do not react with the assay antigen but still cause symptoms; or (c) the available assays are not sensitive enough to detect low levels of circulating antibody. More than one of these possibilities may be applicable depending on the individual case. Seronegative MG patients are clinically heterogeneous and may include patients with purely ocular symptoms, patients with mild generalized disease, or patients with severe generalized MG. It is likely that the reason for seronegativity differs among these individuals.

As noted in Chapter 3, antibodies to the muscle-specific receptor tyrosine kinase (MuSK) have been demonstrated in approximately 70% of seronegative MG patients with generalized symptoms, but *not* in patients with AChR-positive disease (134). MuSK is required for the normal formation and development of the neuromuscular junction, but its role in mature muscle is not clear. Thus, it is not known how the antibodies to MuSK affect neuromuscular transmission and lead to myasthenic weakness in these patients. Nevertheless, patients with MuSK antibodies appear to account for a significant number of seronegative patients with generalized MG, and disease pathogenesis in these patients differs from that of seropositive MG, suggesting a distinct disease entity. On the other hand, seronegativity in mild or purely ocular disease may more likely be explained by low-level disease activity, combined with the enhanced physiologic susceptibility of the extraocular muscles to mild disturbances in neuromuscular function.

E. "Ocular MG"

Ptosis and diplopia are among the most common symptoms in MG. In approximately 10–15% of patients, symptoms remain confined to the ocular muscles for an extended period. Roughly 50% of MG patients will have solely ocular symptoms at the time of presentation (135), and approximately 49–70% of these patients will develop generalized symptoms (18,135). The risk of generalization decreases with increasing duration of purely ocular symptomatology and is highest during the first 2 years from onset of symptoms. However, there are no clear clinical or electrophysiologic features that accurately predict generalization, including seropositivity. In other words, seropositive patients with purely ocular weakness are no more likely to go on to develop generalized disease than seronegative patients.

There are a number of factors that may explain the "selective" involvement of ocular muscles in MG, including the hypothesis that the autoimmune attack may be focused on distinct antigenic determinants unique to these muscles. Extraocular muscles have significant physiologic as well as immunologic differences compared to skeletal muscle (136). It may be likely that "ocular MG" represents a very mild form of autoimmune MG and that the ocular muscles are physiologically more sensitive to the effects of mildly impaired neuromuscular transmission.

Treatment of the MG patient with purely ocular symptoms requires an accurate assessment of the functional impairment and its effect on the patient's life. The physician needs to educate the patient regarding the possible complications of immunosuppressive treatment, particularly corticosteroids. These risks likely outweigh the benefits if treatment is being considered for purely cosmetic reasons. However, in other patients with diplopia having a profound bearing on their livelihood (i.e., pilots, surgeons), the risk–benefit ratio becomes more balanced. Patients should be started on cholinesterase inhibitors and the dose should be titrated for optimal control of symptoms. Cholinesterase inhibitors may control symptoms adequately in some patients. In others, corticosteroids are required, and should be started at a dose of 20 mg/day with gradual increases every 2–3 days until symptoms are controlled. Many patients experience a recurrence of symptoms with tapering of corticosteroids. If this occurs at a moderately high dose (i.e., greater than 25 mg every other day), a steroid-sparing agent should be added. Corticosteroid treatment may reduce the risk of generalization (137), but this observation needs to be confirmed.

F. MG and Pregnancy (Transitory Neonatal MG)

Pregnancy is not contraindicated in MG. However, the outcome may be affected by the course of the disease and its management. The course of MG is variable during pregnancy, but approximately 47% of women experience onset of disease or worsening during the first trimester or in the immediate postpartum period (138). Cholinesterase inhibitors and prednisone are safe to use in pregnancy. However, azathioprine and cyclosporine are potentially teratogenic and the effects of plasmapheresis and intravenous immune globulin are largely unknown, although there are case reports of plasmapheresis being used successfully during pregnancy (139). This makes for a number of challenging therapeutic decisions that are unique to this group of patients.

Immunosuppressive agents such as azathioprine and cyclosporine should be avoided when possible. When contemplating becoming pregnant, a woman with MG should have a discussion with her neurologist regarding the risk to herself and the fetus of various changes in her treatment regimen. Patients on azathioprine or cyclosporine may be taken off these medications prior to conception. In the case of azathioprine, it may be necessary to be completely off treatment for 6 months to effectively minimize risk. Patients in remission or with minimal clinical manifestations may be observed for worsening of symptoms. If worsening occurs, weakness can be controlled using cholinesterase inhibitors, corticosteroids, and/or plasmapheresis. The concerns regarding plasmapheresis involve the risk of removing the circulating factors important for the maintenance of a normal pregnancy, and the risk of the transient anticoagulated state predisposing to spontaneous abortions.

Although most MG experts advise discontinuance of azathioprine if a woman with MG becomes pregnant, there are reports of its use without significant fetal risk in transplantation patients (140). Discontinuing azathioprine may pose a greater risk to the mother and fetus than the potential teratogenicity due to disease exacerbation and respiratory compromise. A thorough discussion of the options for management of the potential risks of both continuing and stopping azathioprine should be initiated with the patient. It is also very important to communicate the agreed upon plan to the patient's obstetrician.

Since the uterus is composed of smooth muscle, it is not weakened by MG, and most women with MG have a normal vaginal delivery. Intravenous cholinesterase inhibitors may precipitate uterine contractions and should not be used. Magnesium sulfate is contraindicated due to its adverse effect on neuromuscular transmission. Postpartum exacerbation of MG symptoms should be anticipated, and patients should be monitored carefully because weakness can advance quite rapidly. In severe cases, postpartum exacerbation may lead to myasthenic crisis. The treatment of exacerbation or crisis in the postpartum period is the same as for exacerbation or crisis due to any other precipitating event.

Transient neonatal MG develops in approximately 20% of children born to myasthenic mothers (141). Antibodies to the AChR are transferred from mother to infant in all pregnancies of mothers with seropositive MG, but neonatal MG does not occur in the majority of cases. The pathogenic role of these antibodies is therefore questionable. In addition, transient neonatal MG also occurs in children of mothers with seronegative MG. There are no clinical or serologic features that are predictive of the development of transient neonatal MG. Affected infants will present with a weak cry, hypotonia, or respiratory failure. Symptoms usually begin within a few hours after birth, but may be delayed for up to 3 days. Accordingly, all infants born to myasthenic mothers should be carefully monitored for signs of myasthenic weakness for the first 3–4 days of life. The diagnosis is straightforward when the mother is known to have MG but may be difficult in asymptomatic mothers not carrying the diagnosis. There is evidence to suggest that antibodies to fetal AChR may be important in the development of transient neonatal MG (142). Once the diagnosis is made, supportive treatment is indicated since symptoms typically last for about 3 weeks, although recovery may not be complete for up to 2 months (141). Ventilatory support and nasogastric feeding may be necessary in severe cases. Anticholinesterase agents given prior to feedings may facilitate oral intake. Plasma exchange treatments have rarely been used and may accelerate clinical improvement (143).

G. Juvenile/Childhood MG

The occurrence of autoimmune MG prior to age 18 is well established (144,145). Childhood or juvenile MG patients account for approximately 10–15% of all patients with autoimmune MG (146). Fluctuating, fatigable weakness affecting the ocular, bulbar, respiratory, and extremity muscles is the hallmark of the disease, as is the case for adult-onset MG. AChR binding antibody levels are usually elevated in generalized disease. However, the highest proportion of "seronegativity" (36–50%) occurs among the youngest (prepubertal) patients (147). This makes diagnosis difficult because it is precisely these patients in whom the distinction between autoimmune MG and a congenital myasthenic syndrome is most difficult. Electrodiagnostic studies can help to identify a defect in neuromuscular transmission but cannot always distinguish between an autoimmune and congenital cause (see Chapter 6). A beneficial response to plasmapheresis or intravenous immune globulin may help to establish a diagnosis of autoimmune MG in some children where the diagnosis is not clear.

The options for management of childhood MG are not significantly different than those available for management of the adult disease. Treatment is initiated with pyridostigmine at an initial dose of 1 mg/kg every 4–6 h, which is then titrated to the optimally effective and tolerated dose. If symptoms are controlled, it is reasonable to continue to treat symptomatically and observe. Spontaneous remissions are relatively common particularly in prepubertal patients (144), so that subsequent treatment decisions require careful consideration of the risks and benefits. Several studies have indicated that thymectomy is generally effective in childhood MG, with remission rates ranging from 11% to 75% (144,145,148–151). However, given the rate of spontaneous remission in prepubertal disease, thymectomy likely produces little added benefit in this group of patients. In peripubertal or pubertal patients, it is reasonable to offer thymectomy within the first year of disease onset as a treatment option. Concern regarding enhancement of autoimmunity and the development of immune incompetence in neonatal mice undergoing thymectomy does not appear to be applicable to humans (152). Plasmapheresis is an effective short-term immunotherapy that can be used to prepare moderate to severely affected patients for thymectomy. The decision to initiate steroid treatment either prior to or after thymectomy needs to be made on an individual basis. Steroid-induced growth retardation is correlated with cumulative exposure and is maximal in peripubertal boys (153). Other forms of immunosuppression are used in more severe and refractory cases in a manner similar to that described in adult MG.

H. Late-Onset MG

Onset of autoimmune MG after the age of 50 has become more prevalent and is more common in males. The presenting features are no different than young-onset disease. The main immunologic difference is the increased finding of antibodies to non-AChR muscle proteins (titin and ryanodine) which can be detected in approximately 50% of patients with late-onset MG (154). Obviously, life expectancy and concurrent illnesses are important considerations in deciding on a treatment plan. If symptoms are not controlled with cholinesterase inhibitors, one may add azathioprine in patients who are relatively stable and do not require a more rapid onset of benefit. Mycophenolate mofetil monotherapy may turn out to be a very useful treatment strategy in elderly patients. The onset of benefit of mycophenolate mofetil appears to be shorter than that of azathioprine, and the side effect profile is attractive particularly in elderly patients. Alternatively, high-dose daily prednisone may be used as the initial immunosuppressive agent as has been described, followed by steroid-sparing agents (i.e., azathioprine, mycophenolate) if needed.

I. Medications/Situations to Avoid

A number of prescription and nonprescription drugs may potentially worsen symptoms of MG. A list of the implicated drugs may be found in Chapter 8. It is good practice to advise patients to be alert for any change in their MG symptoms following institution of a new medication regardless of whether that medication is on the list. The stress of surgery and some of the drugs used in the operating room may exacerbate myasthenic weakness. First of all, neuromuscular blocking agents should be used sparingly if at all because of the risk of prolonged paralysis in MG patients exposed to these agents. In general, it is preferable for a procedure to be performed under local anesthesia if possible. If general anesthesia is required, inhalation anesthetic agents without neuromuscular blocking drugs should be used. Patients with well-controlled MG usually tolerate most surgical procedures without difficulty and without the need for specific changes in their MG medication. Patients on prednisone should receive a "stress" dose of corticosteroids equivalent to twice their daily dose prior to surgery.

J. Familial Autoimmune Myasthenia Gravis and Other Genetic Factors

A minority of patients (3%) have family members with a history of auto-immune MG (155). Familial autoimmune MG is otherwise no different from the nonfamilial forms in terms of clinical manifestations and response to treatment. An association with autoimmune thyroid disease or other auto-immune illnesses is occasionally present (see below). All clinical manifestations of MG may occur, and different disease types and severities may be seen within families (156).

It is likely that several genetic and environmental factors are important in conferring a susceptibility to MG. Along these lines, associations between certain human leukocyte antigen (HLA) class II alleles and MG have been observed. In particular, HLA-A1, B8, and DRw3 alleles have been found in Caucasian MG patients with early-onset disease and no thymoma (157,158). Conversely, increased frequencies of HLA-A3, B7, and DRw2 have been demonstrated in older myasthenic with low AChR antibody levels (157,158). It is clear that the immunogenetics of MG is not linked to a single allele, and this genetic heterogeneity is likely responsible for the clinical and immuno-pathologic heterogeneity observed in MG patients.

K. Other Autoimmune Illnesses

Autoimmune thyroid disease is the most common associated autoimmune disease in MG patients. Onset or exacerbation of thyroid disease usually results in clinical worsening of MG. This is important since treatment of the thyroid derangement usually results in improvement of MG. Approximately 9–14% of MG patients develop other autoimmune diseases (159), including systemic lupus erythematosus, rheumatoid arthritis, Sjögren's syndrome, pernicious anemia, and polymyositis. MG patients with thymoma may have myositis, neuromyotonia, and myocarditis (160). MG patients may also have elevated serum levels of organ-specific autoantibodies in the absence of clinical manifestations of other autoimmune illnesses (161). These cases may best be explained by a basic, genetically determined predisposition to the development of immune dysregulation.

IX. OVERVIEW

Myasthenia gravis is one of the best understood human autoimmune diseases. Its signs and symptoms are caused by an autoimmune attack directed toward the AChRs of skeletal muscle, resulting in impaired function of these receptors and clinical muscle weakness. The recognition of the characteristic signs and symptoms of fatigable muscle weakness affecting the ocular, bulbar, respiratory, and limb muscles forms the basis for the diagnosis of MG. Treatment of patients with MG may be divided into symptomatic treatment and immunosuppressive treatment, which in turn may be divided into short- and long-term approaches. The selection of therapeutic agents in MG requires a careful consideration of the expected benefits of therapy vs. the potential adverse effects, and should be individualized based on disease course, severity, age of onset, and medical comorbidities. The prognosis of MG is very good, and with the appropriate treatment most patients achieve and maintain nearly complete control of myasthenic symptoms.

REFERENCES

1. Palace J, Newsom-Davis J, Lecky B, and the Myasthenia Study Group. A randomized, double-blind trial of prednisolone alone or with azathioprine in myasthenia gravis. Neurology 1998; 50:1778–1783.
2. Tindall RSA, Rollins JA, Phillips TJ, Greenles RG, Wells L, Belendiuk G. Preliminary results of a double-blind, randomized, placebo-controlled trial of cyclosporine in myasthenia gravis. N Engl J Med 1987; 316:719–724.
3. Viets HR. A historical review of myasthenia gravis from 1672 to 1900. JAMA 1953; 153:1273–1280.
4. Keynes G. The history of myasthenia gravis. Med Hist 1961; 5:313–326.
5. Walker MB. Treatment of myasthenia gravis with physostigmine. Lancet 1934; 1:1200–1201.
6. Walker MB. Case showing the effect of prostigmine on myasthenia gravis. Proc R Soc Med 1935; 28:759.
7. Blalock A, Mason MF, Morgan HJ, Riven SS. Myasthenia gravis and tumors of the thymic region: report of a case in which the tumor was removed. Ann Surg 1939; 110:544–561.
8. Blalock A. Thymectomy in the treatment of myasthenia gravis. J Thorac Surg 1944; 13:316.
9. Wilson A, Stoner HB. Myasthenia gravis: a consideration of its causation in a study of fourteen cases. Q J Med 1944; 13:1–18.
10. Simpson JA. Myasthenia gravis: a new hypothesis. Scot Med J 1960; 5:419–436.
11. Strauss AJL, Seegal BC, Hsu KC, Burkholder PH, Nastuk WL, Osserman KE. Immunofluorescence demonstration of a muscle-binding complement-fixing serum globulin fraction in myasthenia gravis. Proc Soc Exp Biol Med 1960; 105:184.
12. Patrick J, Lindstrom J. Autoimmune response to acetylcholine receptors. Science 1973; 180:871–872.
13. Giagheddu M, Puggioni G, Sanna G, et al. Epidemiologic study of myasthenia gravis in Sardinia Italy, (1958–1986). Acta Neurol Scand 1989; 79:326–333.

14. Hokkanen E. Epidemiology of myasthenia gravis in Finland. J Neurol Sci 1969; 9:463–478.

15. Kuroiwa Y. Epidemiologic aspects of myasthenia gravis in Japan. In: Satoyshi E, ed. Myasthenia Gravis: Pathogenesis and Treatment. Tokyo: University of Tokyo Press, 1981:9–17.

16. Kyriallis K, Hristova AH, Middleton LT. What is the real epidemiology of myasthenia gravis? Neurology 1995; 45(suppl 4):A351–A352.

17. Phillips LH, Torner JC. Epidemiologic evidence for a changing natural history of myasthenia gravis. Neurology 1996; 47:1233–1238.

18. Oosterhuis HJGH. The natural course of myasthenia gravis: a long term follow up study. J Neurol Neurosurg Psychiatry 1989; 52:1121–1127.

19. Sorenson TT, Holm E-B. Myasthenia gravis in the county of Viborg, Denmark. Eur Neurol 1989; 29:177–179.

20. Storm-Mathisen A. Epidemiological and prognostical aspects of myasthenia gravis in Norway. Ann NY Acad Sci 1966; 135:431–435.

21. Grob D. Course and management of myasthenia gravis. JAMA 1953; 153: 529–532.

22. Grob D, Brunner NG, Namba T. The natural course of myasthenia gravis and effects of therapeutic measures. Ann NY Acad Sci 1981; 377:652–669.

23. Grob D, Arsura EL, Brunner NG, Namba T. The course of myasthenia gravis and therapies affecting outcome. Ann NY Acad Sci 1987; 505:472–499.

24. Grob D, Namba T. Corticotropin in generalized myasthenia gravis. Effect of short intensive courses. JAMA 1966; 198:703–707.

25. Mertens HG, Balzereit F, Leipert M. The treatment of severe myasthenia gravis with immunosuppressive agents. Eur Neurol 1969; 2:321–339.

26. Drachman DB, De Silva S, Ramsey D, Pestronk A. Humoral pathogenesis of myasthenia gravis. Ann NY Acad Sci 1987; 505:90–105.

27. Hohlfeld R, Toyka KV, Michels M, Heininger K, Conti-Tronconi B, Tzartos SJ. Acetylcholine receptor-specific human T-lymphocyte lines. Ann NY Acad Sci 1987; 505:27–38.

28. Yi Q, Pirskanen R, Lefvert AK. Human muscle acetylcholine receptor reactive T and B lymphocytes in the peripheral blood of patients with myasthenia gravis. J Neuroimmunol 1993; 42:215–222.

29. Lennon VA, Lindstrom JM, Seybold ME. Experimental autoimmune myasthenia gravis: cellular and humoral immune responses. Ann NY Acad Sci 1976; 275:283–299.

30. Tzartos SJ, Lindstrom JM. Monoclonal antibodies used to probe acetylcholine receptor structure: localization of the main immunogenic region and detection of similarities between subunits. Proc Natl Acad Sci USA 1980; 77:755–759.

31. Goodnow CC. Cellular mechanisms of self-tolerance. Curr Opin Immunol 1989; 2:226–236.

32. Muller-Hermelink HK, Marx A, Geuder K, Kirchner T. The pathological basis of thymoma-associated myasthenia gravis. Ann NY Acad Sci 1993; 681: 56–65.

33. Kaminski HJ, Fenstermaker RA, Abdul-Karim FW, et al. Acetylcholine receptor subunit gene expression in thymic tissue. Muscle Nerve 1993; 16:1332–1337.

34. Engel AG, Fumagalli G. Mechanisms of acetylcholine receptor loss from the neuromuscular junction. Ciba Found Symp 1982; 90:197–224.

35. Curnow J, Corbett L, Willcox N, Vincent A. Presentation by myoblasts of an epitope from endogenous acetylcholine receptor indicates a potential role in the spreading of the immune response. J Neuroimmunol 2001; 115:127–134.

36. Vanderlugt CL, Miller SD. Epitope spreading in immune-mediated diseases: implications for immunotherapy. Nat Rev Immunol 2002; 2:85–95.

37. Ruff RL, Lennon VA. End-plate voltage-gated sodium channels are lost in clinical and experimental myasthenia gravis. Ann Neurol 1998; 43:370–379.

38. Daroff RB. Ocular myasthenia: diagnosis and therapy. In: Glaser J, ed. Neuro-Ophthalmology. St. Louis: Mosby, 1980:62–71.

39. Nagappan R, Kletchko S. Myasthenia gravis presenting as respiratory failure. N Z Med J 1992; 105:152.

40. Nations SP, Wolfe GI, Amato AA, Jackson CE, Bryan WW, Barohn RJ. Distal myasthenia gravis. Neurology 1999; 52:632–634.

41. Gorelick PB, Rosenberg M, Pagano RJ. Enhanced ptosis in myasthenia gravis. Arch Neurol 1981; 38:531.

42. Sethi KD, Rivner MH, Swift TR. Ice pack test for myasthenia gravis. Neurology 1987; 37:1383–1385.

43. Howard FM Jr, Lennon VA, Finley J, Matsumoto J, Elveback LR. Clinical correlations of antibodies that bind, block, or modulate human acetylcholine receptors in myasthenia gravis. Ann NY Acad Sci 1987; 505:526–538.

44. Lennon VA. Serological diagnosis of myasthenia gravis and the Lambert-Eaton myasthenia syndrome. In: Lisak RA, ed. Handbook of Myasthenia Gravis and Myasthenic Syndromes. New York: Marcel Dekker, 1994:149–164.

45. Vincent A, Newsom-Davis J. Anti-acetylcholine receptor antibodies. J Neurol Neurosurg Psychiatry 1980; 43:590–600.

46. Lisak RP, Barchi RL. Treatment and management. In: Lisak RP, ed. Myasthenia Gravis. Philadelphia: WB Saunders, 1982:184–190.

47. Rothenberg DM, Berns AS, Barkin R, Glantz RH. Bromide intoxication secondary to pyridostigmine bromide therapy. JAMA 1990; 263:1121–1122.

48. Hohlfeld R, Wekerle H. The thymus in myasthenia gravis. Neurol Clin 1994; 331–341.

49. Scadding GK, Vincent A, Newso-Davis J, Henry K. Acetylcholine receptor antibody synthesis by thymic lymphocytes: correlation with thymic histology. Neurology 1981; 31:935–943.

50. Myking AO, Skeie GO, Varhaug JE, Andersen KS, Gilhus NE, Aarli JA. The histomorphology of the thymus in late onset, non-thymoma myasthenia gravis. Eur J Neurol 1997; 5:401–405.

51. Newsom-Davis J, Wilcox N, Scadding G, Calder L, Vincent A. Anti-acetylcholine receptor antibody synthesis by cultured lymphocytes in myasthenia

gravis: thymic and peripheral blood cell interactions. Ann NY Acad Sci 1981; 377:393–402.

52. Gronseth GS, Barohn RJ. Thymectomy for non-thymomatous myasthenia gravis (an evidence-based review). Neurology 2000; 55:7–15.
53. Maggi G, Casadio C, Cavallo A, Cicanci R, Molinatti M, Ruffini E. Thymectomy in myasthenia gravis: results of 662 cases operated upon in 15 years. Eur J Cardiothorac Surg 1989; 3:453–458.
54. Durelli L, Maggi G, Casadio C, Ferri R, Rendine S, Bergamini L. Actuarial analysis of the occurrence of remissions following thymectomy for myasthenia gravis in 400 patients. J Neurol Neurosurg Psychiatry 1991; 54:406–411.
55. Masaoka A, Yamakawa Y, Niwa H, Fukai I, Kondo S, Kobayashi M, Fujii Y, Monden Y. Extended thymectomy for myasthenia gravis patients: a 20-year review. Ann Thorac Surg 1996; 62:853–859.
56. Olanow CW, Wechsler AS, Roses AD. A prospective study of thymectomy and serum acetylcholine receptor antibodies in myasthenia gravis. Ann Surg 1982; 196:113–121.
57. Jaretzki A, Wolff M. "Maximal" thymectomy for myasthenia gravis. Surgical anatomy and operative technique. J Thorac Cardiovasc Surg 1988; 96:711–716.
58. Jaretzki A. Thymectomy for myasthenia gravis: Analysis of the controversies regarding technique and results. Neurology 1997; 48(suppl 5):S52–S63.
59. Papatestas AE, Genkins G, Kornfeld P. Comparison of the results of transcervical and transsternal thymectomy in myasthenia gravis. Ann NY Acad Sci 1981; 377:766–778.
60. Cooper JD, Al-Jilaihawa AN, Pearson FG, Humphrey JG, Humphrey HE. An improved technique to facilitate transcervical thymectomy for myasthenia gravis. Ann Thorac Surg 1988; 45:242–247.
61. Klingen G, Johansson L, Westerholm CJ, Sundstrom C. Transcervical thymectomy with the aid of mediastinoscopy for myasthenia gravis: eight years' experience. ANN Thorac Surg 1977; 23:342–347.
62. Masaoka A, Monden Y. Comparison of the results of the transsternal simple, transcervical simple, and extended thymectomy. Ann NY Acad Sci 1981; 377:755–765.
63. Matell G, Lebram G, Osterman PO, Pirskanen R. Follow up comparison of suprasternal vs. transsternal method for thymectomy in myasthenia gravis. Ann NY Acad Sci 1981; 377:844–845.
64. Durelli L, Maggi G, Casadio C, Ferri R, Rendine S, Bergamini L. Actuarial analysis of the occurrence of remissions following thymectomy for myasthenia gravis in 400 patients. J Neurol Neurosurg Psychiatry 1991; 54:406–411.
65. Henze A, Biberfeld P, Christensson B, Matell G, Pirskanen R. Failing transcervical thymectomy in myasthenia gravis and evaluation of transsternal re-exploration. Scand J Thorac Cardiovasc Surg 1984; 18:235–238.
66. Masaoka A, Monden Y, Seike Y, Tanioka T, Kagotani K. Reoperation after transcervical thymectomy for myasthenia gravis. Neurology 1982; 32:83–85.
67. Austin EH, Olanow CW, Wechsler AS. Thymoma following transcervical thymectomy for myasthenia gravis. Ann Thorac Surg 1983; 35:548–550.

68. Blossum GB, Ernstoff RM, Howells GA, Bendick PJ, Glover JL. Thymectomy for myasthenia gravis. Arch Surg 1993; 128:855–862.

69. Jaretzki A III, Penn AS, Younger DS, Wolff M, Olarte MR, Lovelace RE, Rowland LP. "Maximal" thymectomy for myasthenia gravis: results. J Thorac Cardivasc Surg 1988; 95:747–757.

70. Mulder DG, Graves M, Hermann C. Thymectomy for myasthenia gravis: recent observations and comparisons with past experience. Ann Thorac Surg 1989; 48:551–555.

71. Haynes RC Jr. Adrenocorticotropic hormone: adrenocortical steroids and their synthetic analogues; inhibitors of the synthesis and actions of adrenocortical hormones. In: Gilaman AG, Rall TW, Nies AS, Taylor P, eds. The Pharmacological Basis of Therapeutics. New York: Pergamon Press, 1990: 1431–1462.

72. Goldfien A. Adrenocorticosteroids and adrenocortical antagonists. In: Katzung BG, ed. Basic and Clinical Pharmacology. Norwalk, CT: Appleton & Lange, 1992:543–558.

73. Miller RG, Milner-Brown HS, Mirka A. Prednisone-induced worsening of neuromuscular function in myasthenia gravis. Neurology 1986; 36:729–732.

74. Mann JD, John TR, Campa JF. Long-term administration of corticosteroids in myasthenia gravis. Neurology 1976; 26:729–740.

75. Pascuzzi RM, Coslett HB, Johns TR. Long-term corticosteroid treatment of myasthenia gravis: report of 116 patients. Ann Neurol 1984; 15:291–298.

76. Lane NE, Lukert B. The science and therapy of glucocorticoid induced bone loss. Endocrinol Metab Clin N Am 1998; 27:465–483.

77. Denton MD, Magee CC, Sayegh MH. Immunosuppressive strategies in transplantation. Lancet 1999; 353:1083–1091.

78. Mertens HG, Balzereit F, Leipert M. The treatment of severe myasthenia gravis with immunosuppressive agents. Eur Neurol 1969; 2:323–339.

79. Witte AS, Cornblath DR, Parry GJ, Lisak RP, Schatz NJ. Azathioprine in the treatment of myasthenia gravis. Ann Neurol 1984; 15:602–605.

80. Cornelio F, Peluchetti D, Mantegazza R, Sghirlanzoni A, Collarile C. The course of myasthenia gravis in patients treated with corticosteroids, azathioprine and plasmapheresis. Ann NY Acad Sci 1987; 505:517–525.

81. Palace J, Newsom-Davis J, Lecky B, and the Myasthenia Gravis Study Group. A randomized double-blind trial of prednisolone alone or with azathioprine in myasthenia gravis. Neurology 1998; 50:1778–1783.

82. Kissel JT, Levy RJ, Mendell JR, Griggs RC. Azathioprine toxicity in neuromuscular disease. Neurology 1986; 36:35–39.

83. Hohlfeld R, Michels M, Heininger K, Besinger U, Toyka KV. Azathioprine toxicity during long-term immunosuppression of generalized myasthenia gravis. Neurology 1988; 38:258–261.

84. Witte AS, Cornblath DR, Schatz NJ, Lisak RP. Monitoring azathioprine therapy in myasthenia gravis. Neurology 1986; 36:1533–1534.

85. Sparberg M, Simon N, DelGreco F. Intrahepatic cholestasis due to azathioprine. Gastroenterology 1969; 57:439–441.

86. Zarday Z, Verth FJ, Gliedman ML, Soberman R. Irreversible liver damage after azathioprine. JAMA 1972; 222:690–691.

87. Jones M, Symmons D, Finn J, Wolfe F. Does exposure to immunosuppressive therapy increase the 10 year malignancy and mortality risks in rheumatoid arthritis? A matched cohort study. Br J Rheumatol 1996; 35:738–745.

88. Asten P, Barret J, Symmons D. Risk of developing certain malignancies is related to duration of immunosuppressive drug exposure in patients with rheumatic diseases. J Rheumatol 1999; 26:1705–1714.

89. Confavreux C, Saddier P, Grimaud J, Moreau T, Adeleine P, Aimard G. Risk of cancer from azathioprine therapy in multiple sclerosis: a case-control study. Neurology 1996; 46:1607–1612.

90. Fraser AG, Orchard TR, Robinson EM, Jewell DP. Long-term risk of malignancy after treatment of inflammatory bowel disease with azathioprine. Aliment Pharmacol Ther 2002; 16:1225–1232.

91. Herrlinger U, Weller M, Dichgans J, Melms A. Association of primary central nervous system lymphoma with long-term azathioprine therapy for myasthenia gravis? Ann Neurol 2000; 47:682–683.

92. Hohlfeld R, Toyka KV, Besinger UA, Gerhold B, Heininger K. Myasthenia gravis: reactivation of clinical disease and of autoimmune factors after discontinuation of long-term azathioprine. Ann Neurol 1985; 17:238–242.

93. Tindall RS, Phillips JT, Rollins JA, Wells L, Hall K. A clinical therapeutic trial of cyclosporine in myasthenia gravis. Ann NY Acad Sci 1993; 681:539–551.

94. Kahan BD. Cyclosporine: the agent and its actions. Transplant Proc XVII,, (suppl 1):5–18.

95. Salmon SE. Immunopharmacology. In: Katzung BG, ed. Basic and Clinical Pharmacology. Norwalk, CT: Appleton & Lange, 1992:801–819.

96. Ciafaloni E, Nikhar NK, Massey JM, Sanders DB. Retrospective analysis of the use of cyclosporine in myasthenia gravis. Neurology 2000; 8:448–450.

97. Wierda D, Reasor MJ. Immunomodulating drugs. In: Raig CR, Stitzel RE, eds. Modern Pharmacology. Brown, Boston: Little, 1990:821–836.

98. Ciafaloni E, Massey JM, Tucker-Lipscomb B, Sanders DB. Mycophenolate mofetil for myasthenia gravis: an open-label pilot study. Neurology 2001; 56:97–99.

99. Chaudhry V, Cornblath DR, Griffin JW, O'Brien R, Drachman DB. Mycophenolate mofetil: a safe and promising immunosuppressant in neuromuscular diseases. Neurology 2001; 56:94–96.

100. Meriggioli MN, Rowin J, Richman JG, Leurgans S, Mycophenolate mofetil for myasthenia gravis: a double-blind, placebo-controlled, pilot study. Ann NY Acad Sci. In press.

101. Niakan E, Harati Y, Rolak LA. Immunosuppressive drug therapy in myasthenia gravis. Arch Neurol 1986; 43:155–156.

102. Gustavo De Feo L, Schottlander J, Martelli NA, Molfino NA. Use of intravenous pulsed cyclophosphamide in severe, generalized myasthenia gravis. Muscle Nerve 2002; 26:31–36.

103. Dau PC. Plasmapheresis therapy in myasthenia gravis. Muscle Nerve 1980; 3:468–482.

104. Dau PC, Lindstrom JM, Cassel CK, Denys EH, Shev E, Spitler LE. Plasmapheresis and immunosuppressive drug therapy in myasthenia gravis. N Engl J Med 1977; 297:1134–1140.

105. Howard JF. Treatment of myasthenia gravis with plasma exchange. Semin Neurol 1982; 2:273–279.

106. Miller RG, Milner-Brown HS, Dau PC. Antibody-negative acquired myasthenia gravis. Successful therapy with plasma exchange. Muscle Nerve 1981; 4:255.

107. Massey JM. Treatment of acquired myasthenia gravis. Neurology 1997; 48(suppl 5):S46–S51.

108. Arsura EL, Bick A, Brunner NG, Namba T, Grob D. High-dose intravenous immunoglobulin in the management of myasthenia gravis. Arch Intern Med 1986; 146:1365–1368.

109. Cosi V, Lombardi M, Piccolo G, Erbetta A. Treatment of myasthenia gravis with high-dose intravenous immunoglobulin. Acta Neurol Scand 1991; 84:81–84.

110. Gajdos P, Outin HD, Morel E, Raphael JC, Goulon M. High dose intravenous gamma globulin for myasthenia gravis: an alternative to plasma exchange? Ann NY Acad Sci 1987; 505:843–844.

111. Gajdos P, Chevret S, Clair B, Tranchant C, Chastang C. Clinical trial of plasma exchange and high-dose intravenous immunoglobulin in myasthenia gravis. Myasthenia Gravis Clinical Study Group. Ann Neurol 1997; 41:789–796.

112. Arsura E. Experience with intravenous immunoglobulin in myasthenia gravis. Clin Immunol Immunopathol 1989; 53:S170–S179.

113. Dwyer JM. Manipulating the immune system with immune globulin. N Engl J Med 1992; 326:107–116.

114. Brannagan TH III, Nagle KJ, Lange DJ, Rowland LP. Complications of intravenous immune globulin treatment in neurologic disease. Neurology 1996; 47:674–677.

115. Bertorini TE, Nance AM, Horner LH, Greene W, Gelfand MS, Jaster JH. Complications of intravenous gammaglobulin in neuromuscular and other diseases. Muscle Nerve 1996; 19:388–391.

116. Burks AW, Sampson HA, Buckley RH. Anaphylactic reactions after gamma globulin administration in patients with hypogammaglobulinemia. N Engl J Med 1986; 314:560–564.

117. Vera-Ramirez M, Charlet M, Parry GA. Recurrent aseptic meningitis complicating intravenous immunoglobulin therapy for chronic inflammatory demyelinating polyradiculoneuropathy. Neurology 1992; 42:1636–1637.

118. Tan E, Hajinazarian M, Bay W, Neff J, Mendell JR. Acute renal failure resulting from intravenous immunoglobulin therapy. Arch Neurol 1993; 50: 137–139.

119. Steg RE, Lefkowitz DM. Cerebral infarction following intravenous immunoglobulin therapy for myasthenia gravis. Neurology 1994; 44:1180–1181.

120. Berrouschot J, Baumann I, Kalischewski P, Sterker M, Schneider D. Therapy of myasthenic crisis. Crit Care Med 1997; 25:1228–1235.
121. Cohen MS, Younger D. Aspects of the natural history of myasthenia gravis: crisis and death. Ann NY Acad Sci 1981; 377:670–677.
122. Glaser GH. Crisis, precrisis and drug resistance in myasthenia gravis. Ann NY Acad Sci 1996; 135:335–345.
123. Gracey DR, Divertie MB, Howard FM. Mechanical ventilation for respiratory failure in myasthenia gravis. Mayo Clin Proc 1983; 58:597–602.
124. Osserman KE, Genkins G. Studies in myasthenia gravis: reduction in mortality after crisis. JAMA 1963; 183:99–101.
125. Osserman KE, Genkins G. Studies in myasthenia gravis: review of a twenty year experience in over 1200 patients. Mt Sinai J Med 1971; 38:497–537.
126. Tether JE. Management of myasthenic and cholinergic crisis. Am J Med 1955; 19:740–742.
127. Thomas CE, Mayer SA, Gungor Y, Swarup R, Webster EA, Chang I, Brannagan TH, Fink ME, Rowland LP. Myasthenic crisis: clinical features, complications and risk factors for prolonged intubation. Neurology 1997; 48: 1253–1260.
128. Evoli A, Batocchi AP, Lino MM, Tonali P, Lauriola L, Doglietto GB. Thymoma recurrences in myasthenia gravis patients. Ann NY Acad Sci 1998; 841:781–784.
129. Masunaga A, Sugawara I, Yoshitake T, Nakamura H, Itoyama S, Shimoyama N, Ishidate T. A case of encapsulated noninvasive thymoma (stage I) with myasthenia gravis showing metastasis after a 2-year dormancy. Surg Today 1995; 25:369–372.
130. Romi F, Skeie GO, Aarli JA, Gilhus NE. Muscle autoantibodies in subgroups of myasthenia gravis patients. J Neurol 2000; 247:369–375.
131. Sanders DB, Andrews PI, Howard JF Jr, Massey JM. Seronegative myasthenia gravis. Neurology 1997; 48(suppl 5):S40–S51.
132. Mossman S, Vincent A, Newsom-Davis J. Myasthenia gravis without acetylcholine receptor antibody: a distinct disease entity. Lancet 1986; 1:116–119.
133. Vincent A, Li Z, Hart A, Barret-Jolley R, Yamamoto T, Burges J, Wray D, Byrne N, Molenaar P, Newsom-Davis J. Seronegative myasthenia gravis: evidence for plasma factor(s) interfering with acetylcholine receptor function. Ann NY Acad Sci 1993; 681:529–538.
134. Hoch W, McConville J, Helsm S, Newsom-Davis J, Melms A, Vincent A. Autoantibodies to the receptor tyrosine kinase MuSK in patients with myasthenia gravis without acetylcholine receptor antibodies. Nature Med 2001; 7:365–368.
135. Bever CT, Aquino AV, Penn AS, Lovelace RE, Rowland LP. Prognosis of ocular myasthenia. Ann Neurol 1983; 14:516–519.
136. Ruff RL. More than meets the eye: extraocular muscle is very distinct from extremity skeletal muscle. Muscle Nerve 2002; 25:311–313.
137. Kupersmith MJ, Moster M, Bhuiyan S, Warren F, Weinberg H. Beneficial

effects of corticosteroids on ocular myasthenia gravis. Arch Neurol 1996; 53:802–804.

138. Eymard B, Morel E, Dulac O, Moutard-Codou ML, Jeannot E, Harpey JP, Rondot P, Bach JF. Myasthenia and pregnancy: a clinical and immunologic study of 42 cases (21 neonatal myasthenia cases). Revue Neurologique 1989; 145:696–701.

139. Levine SE, Keesey JC. Successful plasmapheresis for fulminant myasthenia gravis during pregnancy. Arch Neurol 1986; 43:197–198.

140. Haagsma EB, Visser GH, Klompmaker IJ, Verwer W, Sloof MJ. Successful pregnancy after orthotopic liver transplantation. Obstet Gynecol 1989; 74: 442–443.

141. Papazian O. Transient neonatal myasthenia gravis. J Child Neurol 1992; 7: 135–141.

142. Gardnerova M, Eymard B, Morel E, Faltin M, Zajac J, Sadovsky O, Tripon P, Dornergue G, Vernet-der Garabedian B. The fetal/adult acetylcholine receptor antibody ratio in mothers with myasthenia gravis as a marker of transfer of the disease to the newborn. Neurology 1997; 48:50–54.

143. Donat JF, Donat JR, Lennon VA. Exchange transfusion in neonatal myasthenia gravis. Neurology 1981; 31:911–912.

144. Andrews PI, Massey JM, Howard JF Jr, Sanders DB. Race, sex, and puberty influence onset, severity, and outcome in juvenile myasthenia gravis. Neurology 1994; 44:1208–1214.

145. Rodriguez M, Gomez MR, Howard FM Jr, Taylor WF. Myasthenia gravis in children: long-term follow-up. Ann Neurol 1983; 13:504–510.

146. Phillips LH, Torner JC, Anderson MS, Cox GM. The epidemiology of myasthenia gravis in central and western Virginia. Neurology 1992; 42:1888–1893.

147. Andrews PI, Massey JM, Sanders DB. Acetylcholine receptor antibodies in juvenile myasthenia gravis. Neurology 1993; 43:977–982.

148. Ryniewicz B, Badurska B. Follow-up study of myasthenic children after thymectomy. J Neurol 1977; 217:133–138.

149. Sarnat HB, et al. Effective treatment of infantile myasthenia gravis by combined prednisone and thymectomy. Neurology 1977; 27:550–553.

150. Seybold ME, Howard FM Jr, Duane DD, Payne WS, Harrison EG Jr. Thymectomy in juvenile myasthenia gravis. Arch Neurol 1971; 25:385–392.

151. Youssef S. Thymectomy for myasthenia gravis in children. J Pediatr Surg 1983; 18:537–541.

152. Sprent J, T lymphocytes and the thymus. Fundamental Immunology. 3rd ed. New York: Raven Press, 1993:75–109.

153. Rees L, et al. Growth and endocrine function in steroid sensitive nephrotic syndrome. Arch Dis Child 1988; 63:484–490.

154. Aarli JA. Late-onset myasthenia gravis: a changing scene. Arch Neurol 1999; 56:25–27.

155. Namba T, Brunner NG, Brown SB, Mugurama M, Grob D. Familial myasthenia gravis: report of 27 patients in 12 families and review 164 patients in 73 families. Arch Neurol 1971; 25:49–60.

156. Evoli A, Batocchi AP, Zelano G, Uncini A, Palmisani MT, Tonali P. Familial autoimmune myasthenia gravis: report of four families. J Neurol Neurosurg Psychiatry 1995; 58:729–731.
157. Compston DA, Vincent A, Newsom-Davis J, Batchelor JR. Clinical, pathological, HLA antigen, and immunological evidence for disease heterogeneity in myasthenia gravis. Brain 1980; 103:579–601.
158. Tournier-Lasserve E, Bach JF. The immunogenetics of myasthenia gravis, multiple sclerosis, and their animal models. J Neuroimmunol 1993; 47:103–114.
159. Christensen PB, Jensen TS, Tsiropoulos I, Sorensen T, Kjaer M, Hojer-Pedersen E, Rasmussen MJK, Lehfeldt E. Associated autoimmune diseases in myasthenia gravis. A population based study. Arch Neurol Scand 1995; 91:192–195.
160. Mygland A, Vincent A, Newsom-Davis J, Kaminski H, Zorzato F, Agius M, Gilhus NE, Aarli JA. Autoantibodies in thymoma-associated myasthenia gravis with myositis or neuromyotonia. Arch Neurol 2000; 57:527–531.
161. Lennon VA, Lambert EH, Whittingham S, Fairbanks V. Autoimmunity in the Lambert-Eaton myasthenic syndrome. Muscle Nerve, 1982, (suppl 9):S21–S25.

5

Lambert-Eaton Syndrome

I. INTRODUCTION

Lambert-Eaton syndrome (LES) is a rare acquired autoimmune disease in which pathogenic autoantibodies are directed against the voltage-gated calcium channels (VGCCs) on the presynaptic nerve terminal. As discussed in Chapter 1, the opening of these calcium channels is required for the influx of calcium into the presynaptic terminal, which leads to the exocytosis of synaptic vesicles and the release of acetylcholine. The pathogenic VGCC antibodies compromise presynaptic function by impairing the quantal release of acetylcholine.

LES is characterized clinically by the triad of muscle weakness, depressed muscle stretch reflexes, and autonomic dysfunction. There are two main groups of LES patients: (a) those with underlying neoplasms (small cell lung cancer in most) in which the autoimmune dysregulation is part of a paraneoplastic syndrome, paraneoplastic LES (P-LES); and (b) those without an underlying neoplasm in which the trigger for the autoimmune dysregulation is not known, nonparaneoplastic LES (NP-LES).

II. HISTORY

The first report of the occurrence of a myasthenic syndrome in a patient with a pulmonary neoplasm was published in 1953 (1). A 47-year-old man with fatigable proximal extremity weakness and absent tendon reflexes who experienced prolonged apnea after administration of succinylcholine was the subject of this report. The authors concluded that "such neoplasms might give rise to an unusual form of peripheral neoropathy, possibly similar to myasthenia gravis" (1). The first case series followed in 1956 with a report by Lambert, Eaton, and Rooke (2) and in 1957 with an article by Eaton and Lambert (3). The patients in these initial reports had fatigable muscle weakness that differed from the weakness of myasthenia gravis in its distribution and the associated clinical features of areflexia and autonomic dysfunction. By 1961, Lambert and colleagues had collected 17 cases (4), of which 7 involved small cell lung cancer (SCLC) and 3 involved other intrathoracic malignancies. Included in this case series were 7 patients who had no signs of cancer despite extended follow-up.

The pathophysiology of LES was first described by Elmqvist and Lambert (5,6) who demonstrated the presynaptic localization of dysfunction associated with reduced quantal release of acetylcholine. Doctor Lambert and colleagues also defined the clinical features and electrodiagnostic findings in a series of patients. The hypothesis that LES was an autoimmune disease was initially proposed by Gutmann et al. (7), who noted the occurrence of other autoimmue diseases in NP-LES. Other pertinent reports regarding the pathophysiology of LES will be discussed in the section "Etiology and Immunopathogenesis."

Vroom and Engel first reported a beneficial effect of corticosteroids in LES (8). In 1979, Lundh and colleagues reported clinical improvement in the symptoms of muscle weakness using 4-aminopyridine in six patients with MG (9). An analogue of 4-aminopyridine, 3,4-diaminopyridine (3,4-DAP), was reported to induce improvement in LES with fewer side effects due to its limited penetration into the central nervous system (10). Further experience with the use of 3,4-DAP in the management of LES was subsequently reported by McEvoy et al. in 1989 (11) and Sanders et al. in 1993 (12) Immunomodulating therapy in the form of plasmapheresis (13), intravenous immune globulin (IVIS) (14), and chronic immunosuppressive agents (13) were also reported to be effective in some LES patients.

III. EPIDEMIOLOGY AND NATURAL HISTORY

LES is a rare disease, and its true prevalence can only be estimated. It has been estimated that LES occurs in approximately 6% of all patients with small cell lung cancer (SCLC) (15–17), which would result in an annual incidence of LES associated with SCLC of roughly 8 per 1 million (18). Since roughly half of all LES patients have an underlying SCLC, the incidence of

LES should be twice this number, but in fact LES is diagnosed much less frequently. This is likely due to the fact that the disease probably goes undiagnosed in a significant number of patients. Particularly in P-LES (but also in NP-LES) the presenting symptoms may be dismissed and attributed to depression, deconditioning, or cachexia. This error is often encouraged by the finding of minimal weakness on physical examination (see below).

The natural history of LES obviously depends on whether or not there is an associated malignancy. The outcome for SCLC is poor with median survival of 10–16 months for patients with limited disease and 7–11 months for patients with extensive disease (19,20). Although SCLC is responsive to chemotherapy, most patients relapse and die from their disease, with a 5-year survival rate of 15% (2). In most patients, weakness does not affect muscles severely, and the main determinant of prognosis is the clinical response to management of the underlying tumor.

In LES patients without cancer, the long-term outlook is variable. Roughly half of these patients achieve sustained remission of symptoms, although most require substantial, long-term treatment with immunosuppressive medications (21). The remainder of patients have varying degrees of long-term disability. The only predictor of long-term outcome (clinical remission and/or independent ambulation) is the severity of weakness in proximal limb muscles. Prognosis is also determined by the side effects of immunosuppressive agents and the presence and severity of other auto-immune conditions.

IV. ETIOLOGY AND IMMUNOPATHOGENESIS

A. Immunopathogenesis and Pathophysiology of LES

Lambert-Eaton syndrome is an antibody-mediated neurologic disease in which the presumed autoantigen is the VGCC on the presynaptic nerve terminal VGCCs are found associated with all excitable tissues. A diagram of the structure of VGCCs is shown in Fig. 5.1. There are different types of VGCCs based on their pharmacology and biophysical properties (L type, N type, P/Q type, etc.), which are in a large part determined by the pore-forming α_1 subunit (22,23). The release of acetylcholine at the mammalian neuromuscular junction appears to be mediated by calcium influx through P/Q-type VGCCs (24), which are also present at preganglionic autonomic synapses.

The initial studies of Elmqvist and Lambert (3), in which detailed electrophysiologic studies were performed on a single patients, characterized the pathophysiology of LES. These findings were subsequently confirmed in a larger group of patients (4). Detailed microelectrode recordings revealed the nature of the neuromuscular transmission defect. Miniature endplate

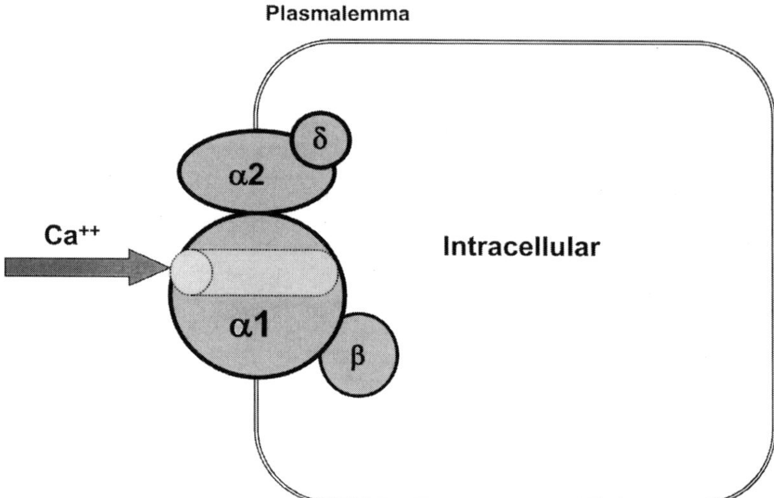

Figure 5.1 Schematic representation of the voltage-gated calcium channel (VGCC). VGCCs form pores across the cell membrane and consist of α1, α2-δ complex, and β subunits. VGCCs in skeletal muscle also have a membrane-spanning γ subunit. The subunits have different functions, but it is the α1 subunit that forms the transmembrane pore.

potential (MEPP) frequency and amplitude were normal, but the quantal content and subsequently the endplate potential (EPP) amplitude were reduced, causing a decrease in the safety margin of neuromuscular transmission (see Chapter 2). The EPP amplitudes increased with high-frequency nerve stimulation or bathing in high-calcium solutions. Furthermore, the electrophysiologic abnormalities found in LES patients closely resembled the experimental findings in neuromuscular junctions bathed in low-calcium solutions, suggesting that calcium flux was involved in the pathogenesis of the disorder.

The role of the VGCCs in the disease was elucidated by Fukunaga and colleagues, who described ultrastructural abnormalities of the motor nerve terminal in LES patients (25). They found that the density of the *active zones* on the presynaptic nerve terminal was reduced in LES patients. Recall from Chapter 1 that the *active zones* and active zone particles of the nerve terminal seen on electron microscopy contain the VGCCs. Normally, the active zone particles are arranged in parallel arrays on the presynaptic nerve membrane. In patients with LES, these arrays are disrupted (Fig. 5.2), and the active zones cluster and are reduced in number. These findings indicated that a

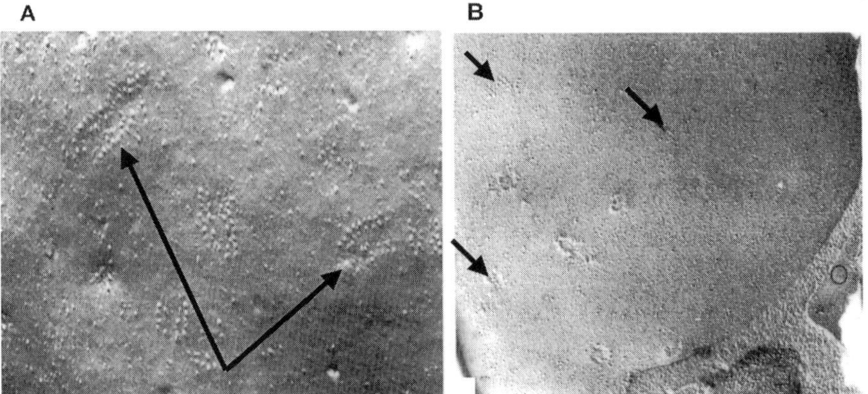

Figure 5.2 Freeze-fracture electron micrographs of presynaptic membrane from normal muscle (A), and from a patient with LES (B). Note the multiple, double parallel rows of membrane particles (arrows) representing the voltage-gated calcium channels in the normal presynaptic membrane. In contrast, the presynaptic membrane from the patient with LES shows scattered clusters of membrane particles without the normal double parallel row arrangement. Reproduced from Ref. 25.

reduction in the number of functional VGCCs was involved in the pathogenesis of LES and that the VGCCs were the likely target of the disease.

The hypothesis that LES was an autoimmune disease preceded Fukunaga's report of the probable autoantigen by more than 10 years (7). This hypothesis was initially based on the association of LES and other autoimmune disorders, such as autoimmune thyroid disease and pernicious anemia. Additional observations in favor of an autoimmune etiology included the disease's favorable response to plasma exchange and other immunosuppressive medications. More direct evidence is the ability to transfer clinical, electrophysiological, and morphological features of the disease to mice using serum from affected patients (26). The finding of autoantibodies binding to the VGCCs in the majority of patients with LES solidified the autoimmune argument. Subsequently, the blocking effect of anti-VGCC antibodies on calcium influx in cells expressing the α_{1A} subunit of the VGCC (as found on P/Q-type VGCCs) suggested that this subunit was the relevant autoantigen in the disease (27).

Since we have seen that there are clear morphological alterations that occur on the presynaptic membrane in LES, the binding of anti-VGCC antibodies must do more than simply block conductance through the channel pore. In fact, the interaction of the anti-VGCC antibodies with their target antigen may set into motion a series of events (perhaps similar to myasthenia gravis in which there is cross-linking and internalization of receptor proteins) that eventually leads to depletion of the number of functional calcium channels. As a consequence, the influx of calcium into the nerve terminal is impaired resulting in a decreased quantal release of acetylcholine. Maneuvers that increase the calcium concentration in the nerve terminal (repetitive nerve stimulation or brief sustained exercise) improve neuromuscular transmission in LES, and underlie the characteristic and often diagnostic electrophysiological findings (see below and Chapter 3).

The prominent autonomic symptoms frequently observed in LES may be understood by examining the role of VGCCs in autonomic neuroeffector transmission. Transmitter release from autonomic neurons is dependent on calcium entry through mainly N-type (but also P/Q- and/or R-type) VGCCs (28). The relevant channel subtype varies according to the transmitter released and the specific tissue involved. Table 5.1 is a partial list of the distribution of VGCC subtypes in the human nervous system. At autonomic synapses, it is believed that LES immunoglobulin impairs transmitter release at sympathetic and parasympathetic neurons through down-regulation of one or more subtypes of VGCCs (P/Q, N, etc.) (29). This down-regulation inhibits autonomic transmission and likely underlies the symptoms of autonomic dysfunction observed in LES. Only a minority of LES patients with autonomic symptoms (31%) are seropositive for antibodies to the N-type VGCCs, arguing against a pathogenic role for these antibodies (30). In contrast, the vast majority of these patients are seropositive for antibodies to the P/Q-type VGCCs, as are the majority of LES patients in general. Neither of these antibodies is correlated with the severity of autonomic dysfunction.

Table 5.1 Distribution of Voltage-Gated Calcium Channel Sub-Types in the Nervous System

Site	L type	N type	P/Q type
Brain	−	+	+
ANS	−	+	+
NMJ	−	−	+
Muscle	+	−	−

NMJ, neuromuscular junction; ANS, autonomic nervous system; +, present; −,absent.

B. LES and Cancer

The association of LES with an underlying cancer (particularly SCLC) was apparent from the initial reports describing the syndrome. Cancer is present at the time of diagnosis of LES or is subsequently found in approximately 40% of cases (Fig. 5.3). In the vast majority of cases, this is SCLC, but other malignancies have been associated with LES including hematologic (31–33), breast (34), prostate (35,36), and neuroendocrine malignancies (37,38), as well as malignant thymoma (39,40). Today LES is the most common and one of the best characterized paraneoplastic syndromes. Paraneoplastic neurological syndromes are believed to be triggered by the presence of a tumor, most often SCLC (41). The tumor is believed to express "onconeural" antigen, which share features with molecules normally expressed in tissues composing the nervous system (neurons, axons, muscle, etc.). In rare instances, it is believed that the immune response initially mounted against the tumor "spills

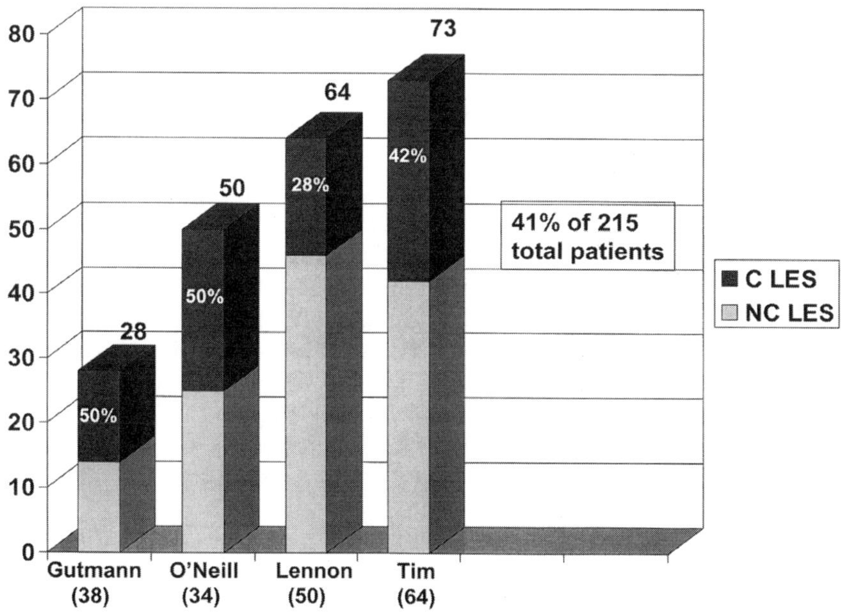

Figure 5.3 Incidence of malignancy associated with LES in four large patient series. C LES = LES with documented malignancy, NC LES = LES without evidence of cancer. Numbers at top of each column indicate total number of patients in each study.

over" to attack tissues of the nervous system expressing similar or related antigens (42).

There are several solid lines of evidence that support the above mechanism in P-LEMS: (a) the P/Q-type VGCCs are the primary mediators of acetylcholine release at the neuromuscular junction (43); (b) functional P/Q-type VGCCs are expressed in SCLC cells (44,45); (c) autoantibodies from LEMS patients immunoprecipitate the same VGCC subtype (46); and (d) imunoglobulin obtained from LEMS patients down-regulates P/Q-type calcium channels in SCLC cells (47). This evidence suggests that SCLC cells (specifically P/Q-type calcium channels) provoke a cross-reactive autoantibody response targeted to the P/Q type VGCCs on the presynaptic nerve terminal. Clinical support for this hypothesis is the observation that patients with LEMS may have striking remission of symptoms of muscle weakness and fatigue with management of the underlying SCLC (48). Interestingly, the prognosis of SCLC appears to be better in patients with LES compared to patients without (49). This may be explained by a more effective immunological response to the cancer, which leads to the development of LES but also improves survival. On the other hand, the presence of LES allows for early detection of an underlying carcinoma, and this may contribute to the more favorable outcome in these patients.

C. LES in the Absence of Malignancy

If this is the mechanistic explanation for P-LES, what is the provoking trigger in NP-LES? One possibility is that patients with NP-LES in fact have an underlying tumor that remains undetected for an extended period. This seems unlikely because there have been patients with LES who have no detectable tumor after many years of follow-up. Both NP-LES and P-LES have an increased association with other autoimmune illnesses, which was the observation that initially led to the hypothesis that LES is an autoimmune disease. O'Neill et al. (34) found a personal or family history of autoimmune disease in 34% of their patients (Fig. 5.4). Lennon and colleagues (50) found that the incidence of detectable organ-specific antibodies (thyroid, gastric, and/or skeletal muscle) in the serum of LES patients was increased in comparison with a matched control population. In patients without detectable cancer, these autoantibodies were found in 52% of patients compared with 28% of patients with a known tumor. An increased association with human leukocyte antigen (HLA) B8 and an increased frequency of IgG heavy chain markers have also been reported in NP-LES patients (51).

These data indicate that there is evidence for immune dysregulation in patients with NP-LES that may predispose them to developing the disease. However, there are no major distinguishing clinical, serological, or patho-

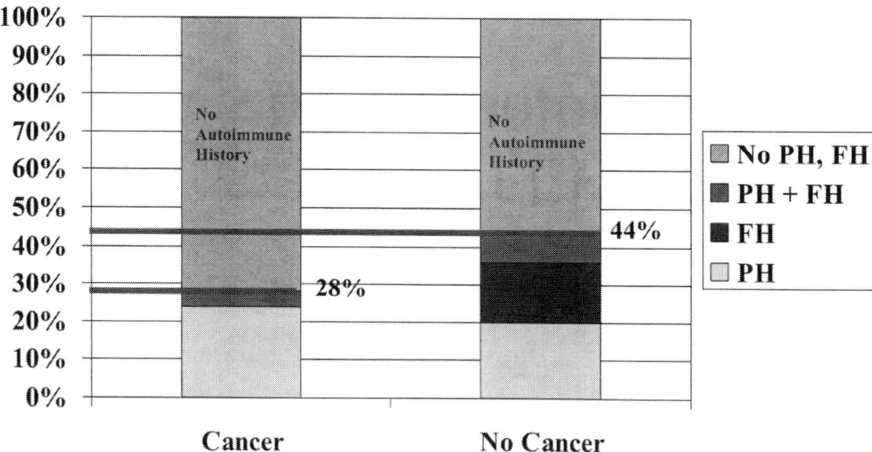

Figure 5.4 Organ specific autoimmune disease in LES. PH = personal history, FH = family history. Data from Ref. 34.

logical differences that separate NP-LES from P-LES, with the exception of the fact that elevated titers of antibodies to the P/Q-type VGCCs are more commonly found in P-LES compared with NP-LES. In addition, there is a male predominance and a higher age at disease onset in patients with P-LES (52). Unfortunately, these are not features that will allow for a clear distinction. As with nonthymomatous myasthenia gravis, the specific provoking factor in NP-LES is simply not known. This argues that there may be more than one trigger that leads to the development of a single autoimmune disease like LES, but once the autoimmune response is initiated the resulting clinical syndromes are virtually indistinguishable.

In general, once a patient with LES has been symptomatic for more than 5 years without discovery of an underlying malignancy, LES is unlikely to be paraneoplastic and is probably caused by a primary (nonparaneoplastic) autoimmune process.

V. CLINICAL PRESENTATION

Patients with LES typically have a characteristic presentation consisting of progressive proximal muscle weakness prominently affecting the hip girdle muscles, diminished or absent muscle stretch reflexes, and autonomic disturbance. Despite this, the diagnosis is frequently missed or delayed, likely due to the fact that symptoms usually begin insidiously and physical examination findings may be minimal (particularly early in the course of the disease). Many patients have symptoms for months or even years before a diagnosis is made.

A. Symptoms

Weakness is the major symptom, with proximal muscles (particularly in the lower extremities) more effected than distal muscles (Table 5.2). Weakness in the hip and proximal leg muscles is most often the presenting symptom (34). Virtually all patients complain of leg weakness at some stage during the illness. The symptoms of weakness often affect the patient's ability to run, walk, climb stairs, or arise from a chair. The affected muscle groups may ache, feel stiff, or be tender to palpation. These painful symptoms may also be worsened by exercise, occasionally leading to the misdiagnosis of neurogenic claudication due to lumbar canal spinal stenosis. Symptoms may be worse in warm weather or after a hot bath.

Upper limb weakness is usually mild in comparison with the lower extremity weakness in LES but is also more prominent in proximal than distal

---

CASE 5.1   A 65-year-old man complained of progressive leg weakness and pain for the past 3 months. He had smoked two packs of cigarettes per day for more than 40 years. Magnetic resonance images of the lumbosacral spine showed degenerative changes at multiple levels. A provisional diagnosis of lumbosacral spinal stenosis (causing neurogenic claudication) was made, but the patient sought a second opinion.

Physical examination revealed mild weakness of shoulder abductors and hip flexors. The patient could not arise from a squat and could not hold his arms above his head for more than 15 seconds. He had a very mild right ptosis with normal extraocular muscle function. Muscle stretch reflexes were absent. The results of repetitive nerve stimulation of the ulnar nerve demonstrated a low compound muscle action potential amplitude, a 20% decrement with 3 Hz stimulation, and postactivation facilitation of 225%. A diagnosis of LES was made. Computed tomography scan of the chest revealed a lung mass which on biopsy was found to be small cell lung cancer. Treatment directed to the cancer resulted in virtual remission of his symptoms of weakness.

Discussion   This man presented with progressive leg weakness and an examination that was classic for LES. The symptoms of exertional leg pain (which may be seen in LES) led to the initial misdiagnosis of lumbosacral spinal stenosis. His age and smoking history strongly suggested that he had an underlying lung cancer. In LES patients with cancer, the initial therapeutic priority is management of the malignancy, which may in certain cases result in significant improvement in the symptoms of muscle weakness as seen in this patient.

muscles. Although less common than leg weakness, upper extremity weakness occurs in the majority of LES patients. Patients may complain of difficulty holding their arms above their heads, a complaint reminiscent of myopathy. However, they may also complain of weakness and stiffness brought on by repetitive use of the hand or arm.

Cranial nerve symptoms are experienced by 70% of patients (34). These symptoms are usually mild and frequently transient. Diplopia and ptosis are the most commonly reported. Occasionally, oropharyngeal muscles are involved, causing dysarthria, dysphagia, difficulty chewing, or even dysphonia. The cranial nerve-innervated muscles are typically not affected to the degree seen in myasthenia gravis. Symptomatic respiratory muscle involvement is uncommon, although it may rarely be the presenting symptom.

Autonomic dysfunction is a very common manifestation of LES. The most common symptoms are dry mouth, which is reported in 77% of patients,

Table 5.2 Symptoms and Signs in 50 LES Patients

Symptoms and Signs	%
Symptoms	
Lower limb weakness	100
Dry mouth	74
Fatigability with exercise	62
Diplopia	50
Ptosis	42
Muscle pain/stiffness	36
Weight loss	24
Signs	
Muscle weakness	92
Lower limbs	90
Upper limbs	82
Depressed/absent reflexes	92
Cranial nerve signs	62

Source: Data from Ref. 34.

and impotence, which is seen in 44% of men (30). Most patients complain of dry mouth often preceding the onset of limb weakness and fatigability. Many patients do not report the symptoms of dry mouth unless specifically questioned. Patients occasionally complain of an unpleasant, metallic taste in the mouth. Other less common autonomic manifestations include dry eyes, orthostatic hypotension, and hyperhidrosis.

Weight loss or other systemic symptoms are occasionally reported. Interestingly, there does not appear to be a significant difference in the incidence of weight loss in patients with P-LES compared with NP-LES (34). A preceding viral illness is reported by a minority of patients.

B. Signs

Muscle weakness is the most common physical examination finding in LES (Table 5.2). Strength is usually reduced in proximal muscle groups, and the lower extremities are usually more prominently involved than the upper limbs. The pattern of weakness is very suggestive of a myopathy, and some patients may even have a waddling, "myopathic" gait. Often, the degree of weakness is mild compared with the severity of the patient's complaints. The ocular and oropharyngeal muscles may be involved in LES but usually not to the degree seen in myasthenia gravis. Ptosis, which is usually mild, may be seen in approximately half of LES patients. Neck weakness is also relatively common. Facial and palatal weakness are less commonly observed. Despite the fact that transient diplopia is a relatively common symptom in LES, clinical evidence of extraocular muscle weakness is rare.

Augmentation of strength during the first few seconds of sustained maximal effort is a feature often described in LES. This effect is observable for such a brief period that it is frequently difficult to demonstrate conclusively on examination. The brief period of increased strength is followed by increasing weakness as sustained contraction produces fatigue due to depletion of the store of readily releasable synaptic vesicles. This phenomenon is the likely explanation for the finding of relatively mild weakness on examination compared to a patient's subjective complaints, i.e., manual muscle testing with brief activation of a muscle during testing, is of sufficient duration to augment strength (but not sufficient to fatigue muscles) in some patients, thus masking the true severity of their weakness. Repeat testing of an individual muscle over several seconds may be more effective in eliciting observable augmentation of muscle strength.

Muscle stretch reflexes are depressed or absent in more than 90% of patients with LES (34), even in muscles with relatively normal clinical strength. The reason for this disparity is not addressed in most monographs discussing the clinical and pathophysiological features of LES. Since the afferent (sensory) limb of the muscle stretch reflex should be intact in LES patients, and the efferent (motor) limb is mildly affected, why are reflexes often absent under these conditions? In myopathies, muscle stretch reflexes are not affected until there is severe atrophic weakness impairing the efferent limb of the reflex. The answer requires a knowledge of the physiology of the muscle stretch reflex. The motor endplates of gamma motor neurons supplying the intrafusal muscle fibers of the muscle spindle have presynaptic VGCCs like those of alpha motor neurons. A presynaptic block affecting these intrafusal fibers would impair the function of these fibers, which is to adjust the sensitivity of the spindle to the length of the muscle. This, in effect, would "desensitize" the spindle producing dysfunction in the afferent limb of the muscle stretch reflex, resulting in areflexia with mild associated extrafusal muscle weakness.

Muscle stretch reflexes in LES can frequently be augmented or provoked by activating the appropriate muscle (sustaining voluntary contraction for 10–15 seconds) or by repeatedly tapping the tendon. This potentiation of hypoactive reflexes is virtually diagnostic of LES. Postexercise potentiation of reflexes in LES was first reported in 1978 (53). Thirty-nine of 50 patients (79%) exhibited this physical finding in O'Neill's series (34), although a more recent study reported a lower rate (31.3%) in 16 patients (54). It is likely that postexercise potentiation of reflexes is more likely to be demonstrated in mild LES where the effects of calcium accumulation (in the presynatic nerve terminal of gamma motor neurons) are sufficient to reverse the presynaptic block. On the other hand, in severe LES the presynaptic defect is so large that brief exercise is not sufficient to enhance the quantal content enough to facilitate the reflex.

As noted, autonomic dysfunction is a very common manifestation of LES, with dry mouth (77%) and impotence (45% of men) representing the most common symptoms. A sluggish pupillary reaction to light is probably the most common physical sign of autonomic dysfunction. The results of autonomic function testing are abnormal in most LES patients, showing evidence of both sympathetic and parasympathetic involvement, even when there are no clear clinical signs of autonomic dysfunction (30). Autonomic failure may be more severe in older patients with an underlying malignancy.

Respiratory muscle weakness may be demonstrated in most patients with LES by tests of respiratory mechanics (46) despite the fact that symptoms of dyspnea are relatively uncommon and, when present, are usually attributable to underlying lung disease. Rarely, severe respiratory weakness causing respiratory failure may be the presenting feature of LES (55,56). LES may be initially discovered when prolonged paralysis and ventilator dependence occurs after neuromuscular blocking agents are used during surgery (57).

The sensory examination is normal in most patients unless a coexistent peripheral neuropathy is present, which may occur in patients with underlying cancer. Likewise, cerebellar function is unaffected in most patients, although a concomitant paraneoplastic cerebellar degeneration may be seen in some patients with P-LES.

C. Distribution of Weakness: LES vs. Myasthenia Gravis

The above discussion points out several clinical differences that distinguish LES from autoimmune myasthenia gravis (MG), such as depression of muscle stretch reflexes and autonomic symptoms and signs. However, MG is frequently listed as an important alternative diagnosis that should be considered in patients with suspected LES. In the majority of cases, LES may be confidently distinguished from MG on clinical grounds. Wirtz and colleagues (58) compared the distribution of muscle weakness at the time of initial presentation in 101 patients with MG and 38 patients with LES. In LES, no patient in their group had initial ocular weakness, 5% had bulbar weakness, and the remaining 95% had limb weakness as their initial symptom. In contrast, 88% of their patients with MG had initial ocular or bulbar weakness, with only 12% presenting with weakness in the limb muscles. Thus, in a patient with suspected LES, initial ocular symptoms essentially exclude the diagnosis.

However, as the disease progresses, most LES patients eventually develop oculobulbar symptoms. In one study, oculobulbar signs or symptoms were present in 18 of 23 (78%) patients (59). Thus, it is the initial distribution of symptoms and subsequent progression that are distinguishing clinical features. In general, the weakness in LES progresses in an ascending pattern, compared to MG which generally spreads in a craniocaudal direction. The severity of ocular symptoms in LES is practically never as functionally significant as it typically is in MG. The physiology of the extraocular muscles may help explain this difference in the degree and severity of their involvement in these two acquired autoimmune neuromuscular junction disorders. The ocular muscles are tonically active and fire at rapid rates, which may predispose them to developing neuromuscular block in a post-synaptic disorder like MG; these same characteristics could potentially protect them from developing synaptic failure in LES because of "autofacilitation," i.e., buildup of calcium in the presynaptic terminal at high firing frequencies (see Chapter 2).

VI. DIAGNOSIS

The diagnosis of LES is based on recognition of the clinical triad of fatigable proximal limb weakness, reduced or absent reflexes, and autonomic dysfunction. Antibodies to the VGCCs are elevated in most patients and essentially confirm the diagnosis in a patient with a suggestive clinical presentation. However, not all patients have antibodies to the VGCCs, and the results are often delayed for days to weeks in those who do. Fortunately, the responses to repetitive nerve stimulation are highly distinctive and are probably the most definitive diagnostic test available.

A. Electrodiagnostic Studies

Repetitive nerve stimulation is the most specific test to confirm the diagnosis in patients with suspected LES (Chapter 3). The repetitive nerve stimulation findings in LES are the diagnostic hallmark of the disease and include low-amplitude compound muscle action potentials (CMAPs) with a decremental response at baseline, and a marked postactivation facilitation (PAF) of greater than 100% (Fig. 5.5). These findings are usually most pronounced in distal hand muscles. Care must be taken not to exercise the muscle too long as this may deplete neurotransmitter release and blunt the facilitory response. In contrast to postsynaptic disorders in which 30 s to 1 min of exercise is best to demonstrate PAE, 10 s is all that is required to best elicit PAF in LES.

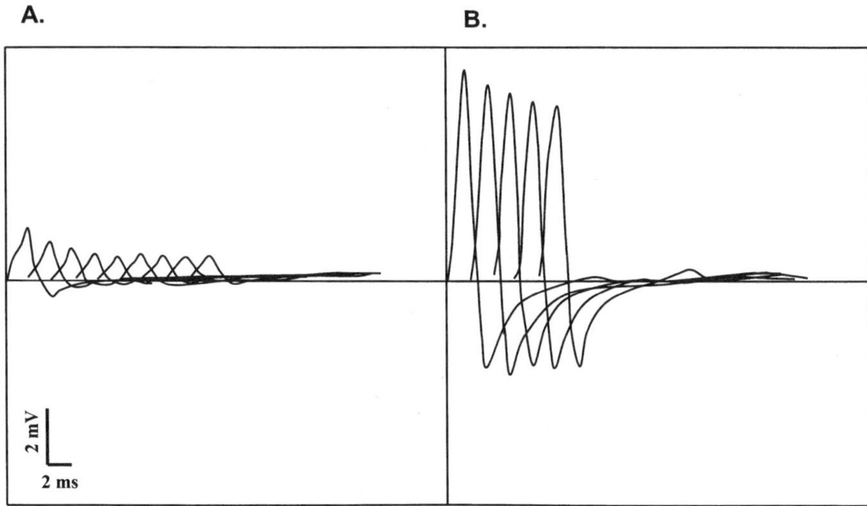

Figure 5.5 Classic electrodiagnostic findings in LES. Repetitive nerve stimulation (RNS) of the ulnar nerve at 3 Hz, recording from the abductor digiti minimi muscle. (A.) RNS of resting muscle. Note low compound muscle action potential (CMAP) amplitude, and decremental response at baseline; (B.) RNS immediately after 10 s of voluntary exercise. Note prominent facilitation of CMAP amplitude (>300%).

One approach to a patient with suspected LES is as follows:

1. Routine nerve conduction studies, including motor studies in at least two distal hand muscles and one foot muscle. Look for low-amplitude CMAPs.
2. Repetitive nerve stimulation (RNS) in two hand muscles and one foot muscle according to the following protocol:

   a. RNS, train of 9 stimuli at 3 Hz in fully rested muscle.
   b. Maximal isometric exercise for 10 s.
   c. RNS, train of 5–9 stimuli at 3 Hz *immediately* after exercise.
   d. RNS, train of 5–9 stimuli at 3 Hz after several minutes of rest.
   e. Repeat a–d for a total of three trials.
   f. Calculate average PAF for three trials.

A rapid screening test for LES (Case 3.2) involves delivering a single supramaximal stimulus to the nerve innervating a fully rested muscle and measuring the amplitude of the obtained CMAP. The patient is then instructed to maximally exercise the muscle for 10 s. Another single supramaximal stimulus is delivered and the amplitude of the CMAP is measured. An increase in CMAP amplitude of greater than 100% is consistent with a presynaptic disorder of neuromuscular transmission.

RNS at a rate of 20–50 Hz may also be used to demonstrate facilitation in LES (Fig. 5.6). In this technique, the maximal amplitude of the CMAPs

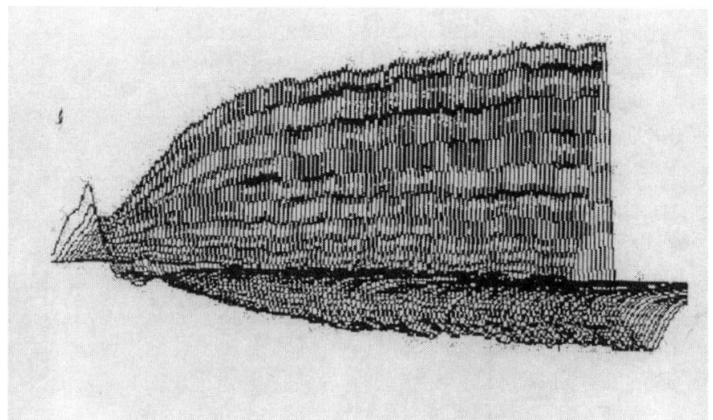

Figure 5.6 High frequency (20 Hz) repetitive stimulation of the ulnar nerve. Note initial decrement (arrow) followed by marked facilitation of CMAP amplitude.

at the end of the stimulation train is compared to the CMAP amplitude at baseline. Potentiation of the CMAP amplitude due to factors other than changes in neuromuscular transmission (i.e., pseudofacilitation; see Chapter 3) may significantly contribute to the observed amplitude changes produced by high-frequency stimulation. Furthermore, high-frequency stimulation is also quite painful and may limit the ability of some patients to fully cooperate with testing. For this reason, it is preferable to assess for the presence of facilitation after sustained voluntary exercise of the muscle rather than after high-frequency RNS, since it is less painful and just as effective for demonstrating PAF (60).

Single-fiber electromyography (EMG) demonstrates abnormal jitter in virtually all patients with LES, usually with prominent impulse blocking. Although this test is highly sensitive, it lacks specificity. Abnormal jitter with blocking is indicative of a defect in neuromuscular transmission but does not allow one to distinguish between pre- and postsynaptic localizations. Jitter

---

CASE 5.2 A 65-year-old man complained of a 6-month history of progressive muscle weakness and fatigue. He had no associated ocular, bulbar, or sensory symptoms. His physical examination was remarkable only for symmetrical hyporeflexia and minimal ptosis. Electrodiagnostic studies showed a decrement of 15% on RNS of the ulnar nerve recording from the abductor digiti minimi (ADM) muscle. Postactivation facilitation of 48% was also demonstrated. Acetylcholine receptor antibodies were negative.

Three months later, he complained of dry mouth, increased weakness, and severe fatigability. His examination now indicated moderate proximal weakness and areflexia. Repeat electrodiagnostic studies revealed a reduced baseline compound muscle potential amplitude in the ADM with a decrement of 28% and postactivation facilitation of 300%. The diagnosis of LES was confirmed by finding elevated serum VGCC antibodies.

Discussion This case illustrates the point that patients with early LES may present with electrodiagnostic findings suggestive of a postsynaptic disorder of the neuromuscular junction, i.e., myasthenia gravis. The distribution of weakness and absence of ocular or bulbar symptoms made the clinical presentation more consistent with LES than myasthenia gravis in this case.

typically decreases with increasing firing rate in LES, although this finding may not be entirely specific and is not seen in all patients (61,62).

Although the predominant clinical feature of LES is proximal lower extremity weakness, the electrophysiological abnormalities are most readily detected in the distal upper extremity muscles. Maddison et al. (63) found that the distal hand muscles were the most sensitive for demonstrating low resting CMAP amplitudes and postexercise facilitation. Tim et al. (64) found that the most sensitive electrophysiological finding in a group of 61 LES patients was a greater than 10% decrement in a distal hand muscle, which was present in all but one of their patients (Fig. 5.7). A reduced CMAP in at least one hand muscle was observed in 97% of patients; 13% of patients failed to demonstrate postexercise facilitation of greater than 100% in any of three tested muscles, despite the fact that this is the criterion used to diagnose LES most often.

B. Voltage-Gated Calcium Channel Antibodies

Antibodies against the P/Q-type VGCC are detectable in significant titers in up to 95% of LES patients (65). In 33% of these patients, elevated titers of antibodies to the N-type VGCC are also found (66). The high frequency of

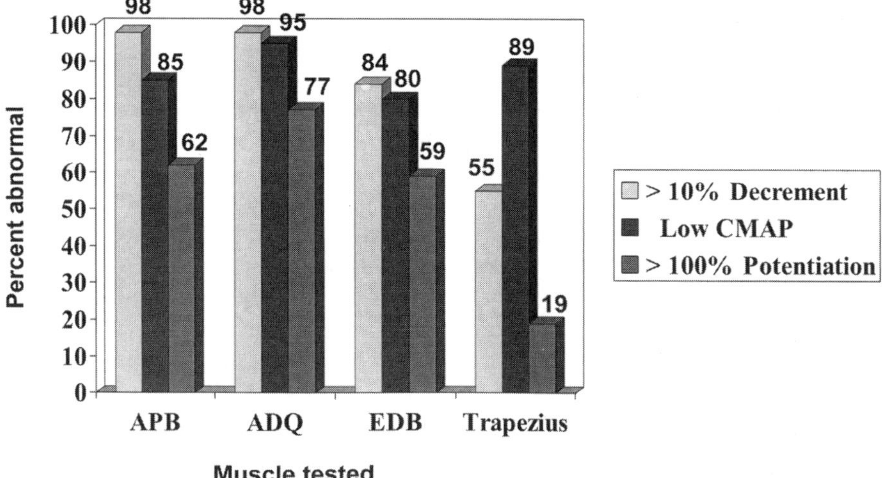

Figure 5.7 Sensitivity of various electrodiagnostic tests in 61 LES patients. CMAP = compound muscle action potential, APB = abductor pollicis brevis, ADM = abductor digiti minimi, EDB = extensor digitorum brevis. Number at top of each column represent percent of patients with abnormal findings for the indicated test. Data from Ref. 64.

anti-P/Q-type VGCC antibodies suggests that it is these antibodies are pathophysiologically important. As previously noted, VGCC antibodies are more frequently detected in LES patients with SCLC, being present in up to 100%, compared to LES patients without underlying cancer in whom elevated titers are found 50–90% of the time.

In general, there is no clear correlation between VGCC antibody titer and disease severity. However, titers decrease in patients as the disease improves, as a result of either immunotherapy or therapy of the underlying cancer. Thus, testing for the presence of VGCC antibodies should be done prior to initiating immunotherapy or cancer therapy, since titers may become undetectable after treatment. Longitudinal studies in individual patients indicate that there is an inverse relationship between the anti-VGCC antibody titer and clinical state as measured by an electrophysiological parameter (CMAP amplitude) (67).

Anti-VGCC antibodies may be detected in 18% of patients with SCLC *without* LES, in 15–40% of patients who have paraneoplastic cerebellar ataxia without LES, regardless of cancer type, and rarely in individuals with autoimmune MG or other autoimmune conditions such as systemic lupus erythematosus and scleroderma (65). The sensitivity and specificity of the VGCC antibody assay are affected by the source of the antigen and the specific laboratory performing the measurements.

The immunological diagnosis of LES is usually straightforward, as long as there is a high index of clinical suspicion. It is important to recognize that the anti-VGCC antibody titers may fall to zero after the initiation of immunotherapy, so that patients referred for fatigable proximal muscle weakness who had previously been misdiagnosed as having autoimmune MG may have misleading antibody profiles. Rarely, these patients may even have binding antibodies to the acetylcholine receptor (as described above) or anti–striated muscle antibodies as their only serological abnormality. The electrophysiological findings may also be misleading in early/mild LES (Case 5.2). In these cases, the initial distribution of weakness may be an important clue in distinguishing LES from MG. An appropriate diagnosis has obvious practical consequences in light of the potential for unnecessary thymectomy or delayed detection of an underlying malignancy.

C. Muscle Biopsy

Muscle biopsy is not required to confirm the diagnosis of LES. A variety of nonspecific changes are usually noted when patients with LES undergo muscle biopsy. However, serial muscle biopsies in one patient showed progressive atrophy and loss of type 1 muscle fibers resulting in a marked type 2 muscle fiber predominance (68). The authors of this report surmised that reduced transmitter release may have deprived type 1 muscle fibers of the low-frequency discharge rate needed to maintain their metabolic properties.

D. Differential Diagnosis

LES patients are frequently misdiagnosed at the time of initial presentation. In one study, more than 50% of patients were initially given an erroneous diagnosis (34). Some of the factors complicating the clinical assessment of patients with possible LES are discussed above. Other diagnoses that should be considered in a patient presenting with progressive proximal weakness and muscle fatigue include polymyositis, polymyalgia rheumatica, MG, and botulism.

In the classic presentatin of LES, the distribution of weakness is "myopathic," with proximal hip girdle greater than shoulder girdle weakness. Like LES, certain inflammatory myopathies may also be associated with an underlying malignancy. Additional confusion may arise when short-duration, polyphasic motor unit action potentials are demonstrated on needle electromyography. While this electrodiagnostic finding is typically observed in myopathy, it may also be seen in LES. The clinical features that distinguish LES from myopathy include absent or depressed reflexes despite relatively mild muscle weakness, the potentiation of these reflexes after brief voluntary contraction of the involved muscle, and the symptom of dysautonomia (dry mouth). The electrodiagnostic findings (particularly the responses to repetitive nerve stimulation) also serve to distinguish LES from myopathy.

Occasionally, patients with LES may present with muscle pain in addition to weakness and fatigability. Generalized muscle pain of subacute onset occurs in the rheumatological disorder polymyalgia rheumatica. Typically, true muscle weakness and fatigability are not a part of this syndrome, but the severity of the pain may make assessment of these signs and symptoms difficult. Unlike LES, polymyalgia rheumatica is associated with an elevated sedimentation rate and has a dramatic response to corticosteroids (69).

Other disorders of neuromuscular transmission may be mistakenly considered in a patient with LES. In the majority of cases, the initial distribution of weakness usually helps to clarify the diagnosis. As we have seen, ocular symptoms at the time of presentation are quite common in MG, whereas presence of initial ocular symptoms virtually rules out the diagnosis of LES. Initial bulbar symptoms are also much less common in LES compared to MG. However, as LES progresses, oculobulbar symptoms become more prevalent. While in most cases the electrodiagnostic and serological findings distinguish the two conditions, there are situations in which this distinction is difficult (see above). Although botulism, like LES, causes progressive weakness and autonomic dysfunction, the more fulminant onset and progression of symptoms often leading to respiratory failure is characteristic of botulism and unusual for LES. The descending pattern of weakness and early pupillary involvement are other potential distinguishing features. The electrodiagnostic features are similar in LES and botulism, although postactivation facilitation is less prominent in the latter (70).

VII. TREATMENT AND MANAGEMENT

Once the diagnosis of LES is confirmed, the first task for the clinician is to determine whether an associated underlying malignancy exists. Next, specific cancer therapy should be initiated in those cases with an underlying cancer. In NP-LES and in P-LES patients who have completed courses of chemotherapy and continue to have symptomatic weakness, treatment considerations may be divided into (a) pharmacological or symptomatic therapy to improve neuromuscular transmission and (b) immunological therapy. Table 5.3 summarizes the treatment and management options of the patient with LES.

A. The Search for an Underlying Malignancy

All adult patients with LES must undergo a thorough investigation for underlying cancer. In general, lung cancer must be the focus of the inves-

Table 5.3 Management of LES

Symptomatic
3,4-Diaminopyridine
Pyridostigmine
Guanidine hydrochloride

Immunotherapy
Severe weakness:
  Plasma exchange
  Intravenous immunoglobulin
Weakness not controlled with symptomatic agents
  Prednisone
  Azathioprine
  Cyclosporine
  Mycophenolate mofetil

tigation, but the possibility of an associated lymphoproliferative disorder should also be considered. Thus, CT of the chest for cancer detection should be performed. A complete blood count, serum chemistries, and serum electrophoresis are obtained to screen for a hematological malignancy. If imaging of the chest is negative in a patient with a substantial risk of having lung cancer (i.e., significant history of tobacco use), bronchoscopy should be performed. Cancer may be found on bronchoscopy even after results of CT and/or magnetic resonance imaging of the chest are normal. If both bronchoscopy and chest imaging are negative, these studies should be repeated at least every 6 months in high-risk individuals. Malignancy surveillance should probably continue for at least 5 years because in most patients with P-LES the cancer is discovered within 5 years after onset of LES symptoms.

The importance of a thorough evaluation for an associated lung cancer cannot be overemphasized. Although SCLCs are rapidly growing and widely disseminating carcinomas with a poor prognosis, outcome is significantly better in limited disease than in extensive disease (71). The majority of these tumors are unresectable at the time of diagnosis, but early detection may increase the chance of resectability. In limited disease, thoracic radiotherapy further improves survival (71)—an option that is not available for tumors with regional or distant metastases. As previously noted, it appears that SCLC patients with LES have an improved survival in comparison with SCLC patients without LES, likely due to an effective immune-mediated attack mounted against the tumor that "spills over" to involve neural "self" tissues.

B. Management of the Underlying Malignancy

The diagnosis of LES should not preclude prompt treatment of the underlying cancer. In fact, antitumor therapy often results in clinical improvement in the signs and symptoms of muscle weakness and fatigability. Chalk et al. (48) reported that 7 of 11 LES patients with SCLC who survived specific treatment for their malignancy (consisting of surgical resection, chemotherapy, and local radiotherapy) experienced progressive improvement in their neurological symptoms. Presumably, resection of the tumor and prevention of recurrence reduces, or even eliminates, the antigenic driving of the autoimmune response. If management of the tumor results in remission of symptoms of weakness, no further intervention is necessary.

In some patients, however, symptoms of weakness persist and are functionally disabling even after successful management of small cell lung cancer. In these patients, other forms of therapy (see below), either symptomatic or immunomodulatory, are required.

C. Specific Symptomatic and Immune Therapy of LES

1. Symptomatic Treatment

Treatment with 3,4-diaminopyridine (3,4-DAP) produces symptomatic improvement in most patients ($\approx$80%) with LES. The mechanism of action of this drug is blockade of voltage-gated potassium channels prolonging the duration of the action potential at nerve terminals and lengthening the open time of the VGCCs (72). This results in increased influx of calcium thereby facilitating the release of transmitter. 3,4-DAP has been used in the management of LES for over 20 years in Europe. Despite this, it has never been approved for clinical use in the United States and therefore is not available for general clinical use.

The efficacy and relative safety of 3,4-DAP in the management of LES has been well documented (73). A randomized trial of 3,4-DAP in LES showed that patients who received 3,4-DAP had a significantly greater improvement in quantitative muscle strength test results and in the summated amplitude of CMAPs recorded from three limb muscles than patients receiving placebo (74). All but one of 26 LES patients who received 3,4-DAP in the subsequent open-label phase of this study showed significant clinical improvement.

The optimal dosing schedule of 3,4-DAP varies considerably between patients and is empirically determined based on the clinical response. The usual starting dose is 5 mg three times daily. This dose is gradually increased by 5 mg/day and titrated to optimize the clinical response. It is usually not necessary to dose more frequently than four times per day. Therapeutic doses may vary from 15 to 100 mg/day. Patients should notice the onset of effect within 30 min after taking a dose, and this beneficial effect typically lasts for 2–4 h. Many patients notice a cumulative effect of repeated fixed doses. The beneficial effect of 3,4-DAP can often be enhanced by concurrent administration of low doses of pyridostigmine (30–60 mg).

In general, 3,4-DAP is very well tolerated when doses between 15 and 60 mg are used. Patients very frequently complain of circumoral paresthesias within several minutes after taking doses greater than 10 mg. These symptoms are transient (typically lasting for 5–10 min) usually do not require any dose change, and are more likely to occur when 3,4-DAP is taken on an empty stomach or when it is taken with pyridostigmine. The use of 3,4-DAP with pyridostigmine may aggravate the latter drug's gastrointestinal side effects leading to abdominal cramping and diarrhea. These symptoms can usually be minimized by reducing the dosage of pyridostigmine. Some patients have insomnia when 3,4-DAP is taken within 2 h of bedtime. Finally, caution is required in patients with asthma because 3,4-DAP may induce asthma attacks.

Since they act on central as well as peripheral synapses, the aminopyridines [3,4-DAP and 4-aminopyridine (4-AP)] may cause seizures. 3,4-DAP has significantly less risk in this regard since it has limited cerebrospinal fluid penetration. Rarely, seizures may be observed in patients taking doses approaching 100 mg/day (75). The risk is obviously greater in patients with brain metastases, a possibility which must be considered given the association with SCLC. In general, doses greater than 100 mg/day should not be used, and doses greater than 60 mg/day should be used with caution particularly in the elderly.

Cholinesterase inhibitors used alone usually do not produce significant improvement in muscle weakness in LES, although some patients may note improvement in their symptoms of dry mouth in response to treatment. Guanidine hydrochloride, which increases the release of acetylcholine from the presynaptic terminal by inhibiting uptake of calcium by subcellular organelles, has been used with some success in patients with LES, but its use is limited by potentially severe side effects. Low-dose guanidine (less than 1000 mg/day) in combination with pyridostigmine is reportedly effective and may have a more favorable safety profile (76). This regimen may be used as an alternative approach to symptomatic treatment when 3,4-diaminopyridine is not readily available.

2. Immunotherapy of LES

Patients whose symptoms are not adequately controlled by the symptomatic agents described above are candidates for immunotherapy. Severe weakness, particularly with bulbar and/or respiratory muscle involvement, requires consideration of plasmapheresis or IVIg. Plasmapheresis may induce a short-term benefit when a course of at least five daily exchanges is given (77). The clinical response to plasmapheresis occurs at about 10 days and lasts for about 6 weeks. The time course of improvement is notably slower than that observed for management of MG. Alternatively, IVIg may be used. In a double-blind crossover trial of IVIg infusion (2 g/kg administered over 2 days) in LES, significant increases in strength were noted in the IVIg-treated patients compared with placebo (78). This clinical effect was accompanied by reductions in anti-VGCC antibody titer. Improvement was first observed at 2 weeks and lasted for 6–8 weeks. Both plasmapheresis and IVIg appear to be comparably effective short-term treatment strategies. Plasmapheresis may be preferable in patients with initial respiratory depression (55). There is no evidence for any cumulative benefit of repeated treatments for either plasma-pheresis or IVIg.

Chronic immunosuppressive treatment with prednisone should be instituted when symptomatic, antitumor, and short-term treatments fail to result in remission of symptoms. Prednisone may induce improvement in LES and is not contraindicated in patients with an active malignancy. Doses of 0.75–1.0 mg/kg/day are typically used, and are gradually tapered as tolerated. As is the case for MG, either daily or alternate-day regimens have been used. Prednisone may be initiated at a high daily dose (60–80 mg/day) and then switched to alternate-day dosing (100–120 mg every other day) when improvement is seen. This dose is then gradually decreased over many months until the minimal dose required to maintain benefit is identified. High-dose alternate-day prednisone treatment may also result in a complete clinical remission of symptoms, although the clinical response is usually slow (77). Azathioprine can produce symptom remission when combined with prednisone and may allow for more successful tapering of the prednisone dose. The efficacy of prednisone combined with azathioprine has been demonstrated in a retrospective study (77), and this regimen may be an appropriate long-term treatment for NP-LES (see below). Azathioprine is started at 50 mg/day and the dose is increased by 50 mg weekly to a total of 2–3 mg/kg/day. Complete blood counts and liver function tests should be performed weekly for the first month, then monthly for the next 6 months, then every 2–3 months thereafter provided a stable dose has been maintained. In patients who cannot tolerate azathioprine, cyclosporine at a dosage of 3–5 mg/kg/day divided into twice-daily administration should be considered (79). The role of mycophenolate mofetil in the management of LEMS has not been investigated.

3. Tailoring Therapy: P-LES vs. NP-LES

The decision to initiate immunotherapy in patients with LES is impacted by the presence/absence of an underlying malignancy. In patients with a known cancer, management of the underlying cancer is the priority. Patients with persistent weakness after cancer therapy should be treated with 3,4-DAP (with or without pyridostigmine) as described above. Prednisone may be safely used in patients with P-LES, although one must be cognizant of the many side effects of this medication. Immunosuppressive medications such as azathioprine and cyclosporine should be avoided because of the theoretical possibility that such treatment will accelerate tumor growth by impairing the immune system's antitumor response. This applies to both patients with a known malignancy and those who are at an increased risk of having a malignancy, i.e., those patients with a smoking history who have had symptoms of LES for less than 5 years. It should be noted that patients with LES who do not respond adequately to symptomatic treatment or high-dose prednisone rarely become functionally normal in response to even highly aggressive immunosuppressive treatment.

In patients without an underlying malignancy, 3,4-DAP with or without pyridostigmine is the first line of treatment. If this results in adequate symptom control, no further therapy is necessary. In those with persistent functionally limiting symptoms, treatment with prednisone alone or prednisone with azathioprine (if symptoms are more than mild) should be commenced. Plasmapheresis or IVIg is used to manage severe symptoms. A management algorithm for LES is shown in Fig. 5.8.

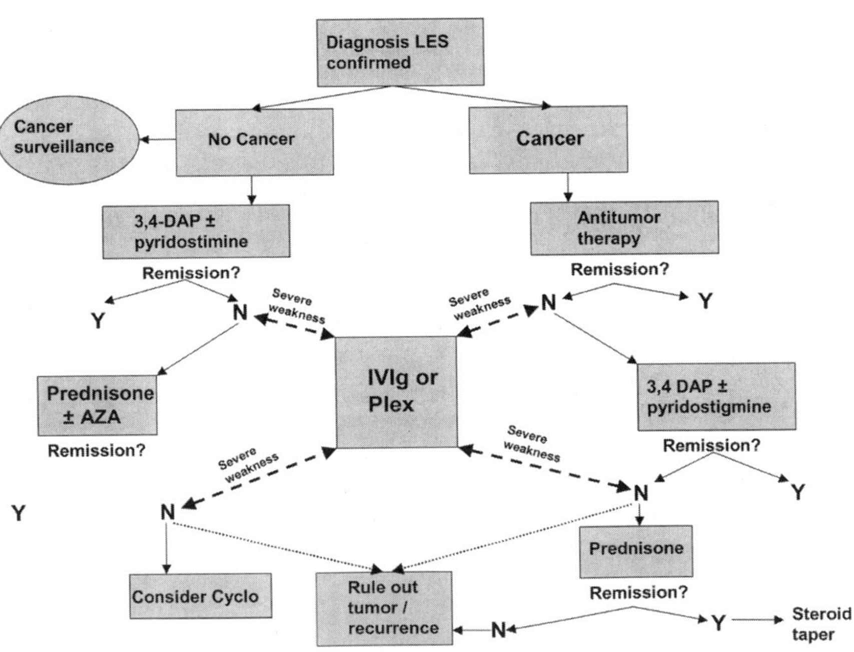

Figure 5.8 Treatment algorithm. The first step is to determine if there is an underlying malignancy. Malignancy surveillance in patients who have no detectable malignancy at the time of diagnosis should continue for five years. Plasma exchange (Plex) and intravenous immune globulin (IVIg) should be used to treat severe symptoms particularly bulbar or respiratory weakness. In patients who are refractory to treatment, it is important to thoroughly investigate for the presence of an undetected malignancy in patients without known cancer, and to consider tumor recurrence in patients with known, treated cancer.

VIII. SPECIAL CIRCUMSTANCES

A. "Overlap Syndromes"

Rare reports of patients presenting with combined features of LES and MG
(80,81) have been published. These reports are primarily based on mixed
electrophysiological and/or immunological features. Newsom-Davis and
colleagues described two patients with clinical features of LES who had
both VGCC antibodies and acetycholine receptor antibodies (82). Lennon
et.al. (65,83) have reported that a small number of patients with clinically
defined LES may have elevated acetylcholine receptor antibodies as their
only serological abnormality. Katz and colleagues (84) reported two such
patients who had clinical and electrodiagnostic findings classic for LES,
with no clinical evidence for MG. Although the presence of acetylcholine
receptor binding antibodies is generally highly specific for MG, as many as 5–
13% of LES patients may have these antibodies (50,65). However, until the
demonstration of a true overlap syndrome based on ultrastructural and
microphysiological techniques is clearly documented, the acetylcholine
receptor antibodies in these cases must be viewed as a nonpathogenic epi-
phenomenon.

B. LES in Children

There are few case reports of LES occurring in patients prior to the age of 18
(85–87). A 10-year-old boy with leukemia was the first child observed with
LES in 1974 (87). A handful of cases with and without underlying cancer
have been subsequently reported. The diagnosis in most of these cases was
determined by the characteristic electrodiagnostic features, but the presence
of antibodies to the VGCCs was not tested. More recently, Tsao et al. (88)
reported two children with LES and positive VGCC antibodies without evidence of underlying malignancy. Both patients responded to immunotherapy.
The presence of VGCC antibodies and the response to immunosuppressive
treatment are important features distinguishing autoimmune LES from congenital LES (see Chapter 6).

C. Medications that May Exacerbate Symptoms in LES

Drugs that compromise neuromuscular transmission may exacerbate weakness in patients with LES. The curare-like agents often have an exaggerated
and/or prolonged effect in these patients. As previously mentioned, it is not
unusual for the initial diagnosis of LES to occur when prolonged weakness or
ventilator dependence follows the use of these agents as part the anesthetic
regimen for surgical procedures. As for MG, the aminoglycosides and certain

of the antiarrhythmics (quinidine and procainamide) should not be used because of their neuromuscular blocking effects. Although the main mechanism of action of calcium channel blocking drugs is inhibition of L-type calcium channels, there are a few reports of severe worsening of weakness in LES patients receiving calcium channel antagonists (89,90). Therefore, drugs like verapamil and diltiazem should probably be used with caution in patients with LES.

IX. OVERVIEW

Lambert-Eaton syndrome is a rare autoimmune disorder in which the autoimmune attack is targeted to the VGCCs on the presynaptic nerve terminals of motor axons. The clinical presentation is usually characterized by progressive proximal muscle weakness, hyporeflexia, and autonomic dysfunction (particularly dry mouth). In roughly 40–50% of patients with LES, an associated malignancy (usually SCLC) either predates the onset of LES or is discovered subsequently (usually within 5 years). Regular surveillance (chest CT every 6 months) for an underlying lung malignancy is an important part of the clinical management of LES.

The diagnosis of LES is readily confirmed by the characteristic electrophysiological findings of reduced CMAP amplitudes, a decremental response at slow stimulation rates, and a prominent facilitation of CMAP amplitudes (>100%) with high-frequency stimulation or immediately after sustained voluntary activation. Roughly 80% of patients will have elevated serum VGCC antibodies, and these antibodies are more likely to be positive in patients with an underlying SCLC.

Management of LES may be divided into (a) symptomatic forms of treatment and (b) immunotherapy. The choice of therapy is influenced on by the presence or absence of an underlying malignancy. 3,4-DAP with or without pyridostigmine is an effective treatment for most patients with LES with or without malignancy. Prednisone, plasmapheresis, or IVIg may likewise be used in P-LES and NP-LES. The latter two choices are used to manage severe muscle weakness. Azathioprine with prednisone is appropriate long-term treatment for NP-LES patients who are not adequately treated with 3,4-DAP alone. Immunosuppressive agents such as azathioprine should be avoided in P-LES.

REFERENCES

1. Anderson HJ, Churchill-Davidson HC, Richardson AT. Bronchial neoplasm with myasthenia: prolonged apnoea after administration of succinylcholine. Lancet 1953; 2:1291–1293.

2. Lambert EH, Eaton LM, Rooke ED. Defect of neuromuscular conduction associated with malignant neoplasms. Am J Physiol 1956; 187:612–613.

3. Eaton LM, Lambert EH. Electromyography and electric stimulation of nerves in diseases of the motor unit: observations on myasthenic syndrome associated with malignant tumors. JAMA 1957; 163:1117–1124.

4. Lambert EH, Rooke ED, Eaton LM, Hodgson CH. Myasthenic syndrome occasionally associated with bronchial neoplasm: neurophysiologic studies. In: Viets HR, ed. Myasthenia Gravis. Springfield, IL: Charles C Thomas, 1961: 362–410.

5. Elmqvist D, Lambert EH. Detailed analysis of neuromuscular transmission in a patient with the myasthenic syndrome sometimes associated with bronchogenic carcinoma. Mayo Clin Proc 1968; 43:689–713.

6. Lambert EH, Elmqvist D. Quantal components of end-plate potentials in the myasthenic syndrome. Ann NY Acad Sci 1971; 183:183–199.

7. Gutmann L, Crosby TW, Takamori M, Martin JD. The Eaton-Lambert syndrome and autoimmune disorders. Am J Med 1972; 53:354–356.

8. Vroom FQ, Engel WK. Non-neoplastic steroid responsive Lambert-Eaton syndrome. Neurology 1969; 19:281.

9. Lundh H, Nillsson O, Rosen I. Effects of 4-aminopyridine in myasthenia gravis. J Neurol Neurosurg Psychiatry 1979; 42:171–175.

10. Lundh H, Nilsson O, Rosen I. Treatment of Lambert-Eaton syndrome: 3,4-diaminopyridine and pyridostigmine. Neurology 1984; 34:1324–1330.

11. McEvoy KM, Windebank AJ, Daube JR, Low PA. 3–4–Diaminopyridine in the treatment of Lambert-Eaton myasthenic syndrome. N Engl J Med 1989; 321:1567–1571.

12. Sanders DB, Howard JF Jr, Massey JM. 3,4-Diaminopyridine in Lambert-Eaton myasthenic syndrome and myasthenia gravis. Ann NY Acad Sci 1993; 681:588–590.

13. Newsom-Davis J, Murray NM. Plasma exchange and immunosuppressive drug treatment in the Lambert-Eaton myasthenic syndrome. Neurology 1984; 34: 480–485.

14. Bird SJ. Clinical and electrophysiological improvement in Lambert-Eaton syndrome with intravenous immunoglobulin therapy. Neurology 1992; 42:1422–1423.

15. Croft PB, Wilkinson M. The incidence of carcinomatous neuromyopathy with special reference to lung and breast carcinoma. In: Brain R, Norris FH, eds. The Remote Effects of Cancer on the Nervous System. New York: Grune and Stratton, 1965: 44–64.

16. Hawley RJ, Cohen MH, Saini N, Armbrustmacher VW. The carcinomatous neuromyopathy of oat cell lung cancer. Ann Neurol 1980; 7:65–72.

17. De la Monte S, Hutchins GM, Moore GW. Paraneoplastic syndromes in prediction of metastatic behaviour of small cell carcinoma of the lung. Am J Med 1984; 77:851–857.

18. Travis WD, Lubin J, Ries L, Devesa S. United States lung carcinoma incidence trends: declining for most histologic types among males, increasing among females. Cancer 1996; 77:2464–2470.

19. Zochbauer-Muller S, Pirker R, Huber H. Treatment of small cell lung cancer patients. Ann Oncol 1999; 10(suppl 6):83–91.

20. Schiller JH. Current standards of care in small-cell and non-small-cell lung cancer. Oncology 2001; 61(suppl 1):3–13.

21. Maddison P, Lang K, Mills K, Newsom-Davis J. Long term outcome in Lambert-Eaton myasthenic syndrome without cancer. J Neurol Neurosurg Psychiatry 2001; 70:212–217.

22. Greenberg DA. Calcium channels in neurological disease. Ann Neurol 1997; 42:275–282.

23. Olivera BM, Miljanich GP, Ramachandran J, Adams ME. Calcium channel diversity and neurotransmitter release: the ω-conotoxins and the ω-agatoxins. Annu Rev Biochem 1994; 63:823–867.

24. Protti DA, Reisin R, Mackinley TA, Uchitel OD. Calcium channel blockers and transmitter release at the normal human neuromuscular junction. Neurology 1996; 46:1391–1396.

25. Fukunaga H, Engel AG, Osame M, et al. Paucity and disorganization of presynaptic membrane active zones in the Lambert-Eaton myasthenic syndrome. Muscle Nerve 1982; 5:686–697.

26. Fukunaga H, Engel AG, Lang B, Newsom-Davis J, Vincent A. Passive transfer of Lambert-Eaton myasthenic syndrome with IgG from man to mouse depletes the presynaptic membrane active zones. Proc Natl Acad Sci USA 1983; 80: 7636–7640.

27. Pinto A, Moss F, Lang B, Boot J, Brust P, Williams M, Staudferman K, Harpold M, Newsom-Davis J. Differential effect of Lambert-Eaton myasthenic syndrome immunoglobulin on cloned neuronal voltage-gated calcium channels. Ann NY Acad Sci 1998; 841:687–690.

28. Waterman SA. Voltage-gated calcium channels in autonomic neuroeffector transmission. Prog Neurobiol 2000; 60:181–210.

29. Waterman SA. Autonomic dysfunction in Lambert-Eaton myasthenic syndrome. Clin Auton Res 2001; 11:145–154.

30. O'Suilleabhain P, Low P, Lennon VA. Autonomic dysfunction in the Lambert-Eaton myasthenic syndrome: serologic and clinical correlates. Neurology 1998; 50:88–93.

31. Argov Z, Shapira Y, Averbuch-Heller L, Wirguin I. Lambert-Eaton myasthenic syndrome (LEMS) in association with lymphoproliferative disorders. Muscle Nerve 1995; 18:715–719.

32. Liveseld JL, Stern A, Rosenthal SN. Myasthenic (Eaton-Lambert) syndrome in association with an indolent non-Hodgkin's lymphoma. NY State J Med 1991; 91:29–30.

33. Morrow JD, Manian FA, Clinton ME, Stein RS. Eaton-Lambert syndrome in a patient with acute T-cell lymphocytic leukemia. South Med J 1988; 81:1578–1579.

34. O'Neill JH, Murray NM, Newsom-Davis J. The Lambert-Eaton myasthenic syndrome: a review of 50 cases. Brain 1988; 111:577–596.

35. Delahunt B, Abernethy DA, Johnson CA, Nacey JN. Prostate carcinoma and the Lambert-Eaton myasthenic syndrome. J Urol 2003; 169:278–279.

36. Agarawal SK, Birch BR, Abercrombie GF. Adenocarcinoma of the prostate and Eaton-Lambert syndrome. A previously unreported association. Scand J Urol Nephrol 1995; 29:351–353.
37. Burns TM, Juel VC, Sanders DB, Phillips LH II. Neuroendocrine lung tumors and disorders of the neuromuscular junction. Neurology 1999; 52:1490–1491.
38. Gutmann L, Phillips LH, Gutmann L. Trends in the association of Lambert-Eaton myasthenic syndrome with carcinoma. Neurology 1992; 42:848–850.
39. Lauritzen M, Smith T, Fischer-Hansen B, Sparup J, Olesen J. Eaton-Lambert syndrome and malignant thymoma. Neurology 1980; 30:634–638.
40. Tabbaa MA, Leshner RT, Campbell WW. Malignant thymoma with dysautonomia and disordered neuromuscular trmansmission. Arch Neurol 1986; 43:955–957.
41. Lang B, Vincent A. Autoimmunity to ion-channels and other proteins in paraneoplastic disorders. Curr Opin Immunol 1996; 8:865–871.
42. Dropcho EJ. Principles of paraneoplastic syndromes. Ann NY Acad Sci 1998; 841:246–251.
43. Uchitel OD, Protti DA, Sanchez V, Cherksey M, Sugimori M, Llinas R. P-type voltage dependent calcium channel mediates presynaptic calcium influx and transmitter release in mammalian synapses. Proc Natl Acad Sci USA 1992; 89:3330–3333.
44. McCann FV, Pettengill OS, Cole JJ, Russell JAG, Sorenson GD. Calcium spike electrogenesis and other electrical activity in continuously cultured small cell carcinoma of the lung. Science 1981; 212:1155–1157.
45. Roberts AS, Perera S, Lang B, Vincent A, Newsom-Davis J. Paraneoplastic myasthenic syndrome IgG inhibits $^{45}Ca^{2+}$ flux in a human small cell carcinoma line. Nature 1985; 317:737–739.
46. Lennon VA, Lambert EH. Autoantibodies bind solubilized calcium channel–omega-conotoxin complexes from small cell lung carcinoma: a diagnostic aid for Lambert-Eaton myasthenic syndrome. Mayo Clin Proc 1989; 64:1498–1504.
47. Viglione MP, O-Shaugnessy TJ, Kim YI. Inhibition of calcium currents and exocytosis by Lambert-Eaton syndrome antibodies in human lung cancer cells. J Physiol 1995; 488:303–317.
48. Chalk CH, Murray NM, Newsom-Davis J, O'Neill JH, Spiro SG. Response of the Lambert-Eaton myasthenic syndrome to treatment of associated small-cell lung carcinoma. Neurology 1990; 40:1552–1556.
49. Maddison P, Newsom-Davis J, Mills KR, Souhami RL. Favourable prognosis in Lambert-Eaton myasthenic syndrome and small cell lung carcinoma. Lancet 1999; 353:117–118.
50. Lennon VA, Lambert EH, Whittingham S, Fairbanks V. Autoimmunity in the Lambert-Eaton myasthenic syndrome. Muscle Nerve 1982; 5:S21–S25.
51. Wilcox N, Demaine AG, Newsom-Davis J, Welsh KI, Robb SA, Spiro SG. Increased frequency of IgG heavy chain marker G1m(2) and of HLA-B8 in Lambert-Eaton myasthenic syndrome with and without associated lung carcinoma. Hum Immunol 1985; 14:29–36.
52. Wirtz PW, Smallegange TM, Wintzen AR, Verschuuren JJ. Differences in the clinical features between the Lambert-Eaton myasthenic syndrome with and

without cancer: an analysis of 227 published cases. Clin Neurol Neurosurg 2002; 104:359–363.

53. Nilsson O, Rosen I. The stretch reflex in the Eaton-Lambert syndrome, myasthenia gravis and myotonic dystrophy. Acta Neurol Scand 1978; 57:350–357.

54. Odabasi Z, Demirci M, Kim DS, Lee DK, Ryan HF, Claussen GC, Tseng A, Oh SJ. Postexercise facilitation of reflexes is not common in Lambert-Eaton myasthenic syndrome. Neurology 2002; 59:1085–1087.

55. Nicolle MW, Stewart DJ, Remtulla H, Chen R, Bolton CF. Lambert-Eaton myasthenic syndrome presenting with severe respiratory failure. Muscle Nerve 1996; 19:1328–1333.

56. Barr CW, Claussen G, Thomas D, Fesenmeier JT, Pearlman RL, Oh SJ. Primary respiratory failure as the presenting symptom in Lambert-Eaton myasthenic syndrome. Muscle Nerve 1993; 16:712–715.

57. Smith AG, Wald J. Acute ventilatory failure in Lambert-Eaton myasthenic syndrome and its response to 3,4 diaminopyridine. Neurology 1996; 46:1143–1145.

58. Wirtz PW, Sotodeh M, Nijnuis M, van Doorn PA, van Engelen BGM, Hintzen RQ, de Kort PLM, Kuks JB, Twijnstra A, de Visser M, Visser LH, Wokke JH, Wintzen AR, Verschuuren JJ. Difference in the distribution of muscle weakness between myasthenia gravis and Lambert-Eaton myasthenic syndrome. J Neurol Neurosurg Psychiatry 2002; 73:766–768.

59. Burns TM, Russell JA, LaChance DH, Jones HR. Oculobulbar involvement is typical with the Lambert-Eaton myasthenic syndrome. Ann Neurol 2003; 53:270–273.

60. Tim RW, Sanders DB. Repetitive nerve stimulation studies in the Lambert-Eaton myasthenic syndrome. Muscle Nerve 1994; 17:995–1001.

61. Trontelj JV, Stalberg E. Single motor end-plates in myasthenia gravis and LEMS at different firing rates. Muscle Nerve 1991; 14:226–232.

62. Sanders DB. The effect of firing rate on neuromuscular jitter in Lambert-Eaton myasthenic syndrome. Muscle Nerve 1992; 15:256–258.

63. Maddison P, Newsom-Davis J, Mills KR. Distribution of electrophysiological abnormality in Lambert-Eaton myasthenic syndrome. J Neurol Neurosurg Psychiatry 1998; 65:213–217.

64. Tim RW, Massey JM, Sanders DB. Lambert-Eaton myasthenic syndrome: electrodiagnostic findings and response to treatment. Neurology 2000; 54:2176–2178.

65. Lennon VA, Kryzer TJ, Griesmann GE, O'Suilleabhain PE, Windebank AJ, Woppman A, Miljanich GP, Lambert EH. Calcium-channel antibodies in the Lambert-Eaton myasthenic syndrome and other paraneoplastic syndromes. N Engl J Med 1995; 332:1467–1474.

66. Motomura M, Lang B, Johnston I, Palace J, Vincent A, Newsom-Davis J. Incidence of serum anti-P/Q-type and anti-N-type calcium channel antibodies in the Lambert-Eaton myasthenic syndrome. J Neurol Sci 1997; 147:35–42.

67. Leys K, Lang B, Johnston I, Newsom-Davis J. Calcium channel autoantibodies in the Lambert-Eaton myasthenic syndrome. Ann Neurol 1991; 29:307–314.

68. Squier M, Chalk C, Hilton-Jones D, Mills KR, Newsom-Davis J. Type 2 fiber predominance in Lambert-Eaton myasthenic syndrome. Muscle Nerve 1991; 14:625–632.

69. Salvarani C, Cantini F, Boiardi L, Hunder GG. Polymyalgia rheumatica and giant cell arteritis. N Engl J Med 2002; 347:261–271.

70. Guttmann L, Pratt L. Pathophysiologic aspects of human botulism. Arch Neurol 1976; 33:175–179.

71. Simon GR, Wagner H. Small cell lung cancer. Chest 2003; 123(1 Suppl):259S–271S.

72. Molgo J, Lundh H, Thesleff S. Potency of 3,4-diaminopyridine and 4-amino-pyridine on mammalian neuromuscular transmission and the effect of pH changes. Eur J Pharmacol 1980; 61:25–34.

73. McEvoy KM, Windebank AJ, Daube JR, Low PA. 3,4-Diaminopyridine in the treatment of Lambert-Eaton myasthenic syndrome. N Engl J Med 1989; 321:1567–1571.

74. Sanders DB, Massey JM, Sanders LL, Edwards LJ. A randomized trial of 3,4-diaminopyridine in Lambert-Eaton myasthenic syndrome. Neurology 2000; 54:603–607.

75. Sanders DB. 3,4-Diaminopyridine in the treatment of Lambert-Eaton myasthenic syndrome. Ann NY Acad Sci 1998; 841:811–816.

76. Oh SJ, Kim DS, Head TC, Claussen GC. Low-dose guanidine and pyridostigmine: relatively safe and effective long-term symptomatic therapy in Lambert-Eaton myasthenic syndrome. Muscle Nerve 1997; 20:1146–1152.

77. Newsom-Davis J, Murray NMF. Plasma exchange and immunosuppressive drug treatment in the Lambert-Eaton myasthenic syndrome. Neurology 1984; 34:480–485.

78. Bain PG, Motomura M, Newsom-Davis J, Misbah SA, Chapel HM, Lee ML, Vincent A, Lang B. Effects of intravenous immunoglobulin in Lambert-Eaton myasthenic syndrome. Neurology 1996; 47:678–683.

79. Sanders DB. Lambert-Eaton myasthenic syndrome: clinical diagnosis, immune-mediated mechanisms, and update on therapies. Ann Neurol 1995; 37(S1):S63–S73.

80. Oh SJ, Dwyer DS, Bradley RJ. Overlap myasthenic syndrome: combined myasthenia gravis and Eaton-Lambert syndrome. Neurology 1987; 37:1411–1414.

81. Taphoorn MJB, Van Duijn H, Wolters ECH. A neuromuscular transmission disorder: combined myasthenia gravis and Lambert-Eaton syndrome in one patient. J Neurol Neurosurg Psychiatry 1988; 51:880–882.

82. Newsom-Davis J, Leys K, Ferguson I, Modi G, Mills K. Immunological evidence for the co-existence of the Lambert-Eaton myasthenic syndrome and myasthenia gravis in two patients. J Neurol Neurosurg Psychiatry 1991; 54:452–453.

83. Lennon VA. Serological diagnosis of myasthenia gravis and the Lambert-Eaton

myasthenic syndrome. In: Lisak R, ed. Handbook of Myasthenia Gravis and Myasthenic Syndromes. New York: Marcel Dekker, 1994: 147–164.

84.   Katz JS, Wolfe GI, Bryan WW, Tintner R, Barohn RJ. Acetylcholine receptor antibodies in the Lambert-Eaton myasthenic syndrome. Neurology 1998; 50:470–475.

85.   Chelmicka E, Bernstein LP, Zurbrugg EB, Huttenlocher PR. Eaton-Lambert syndrome in a 9-year-old girl. Arch Neurol 1979; 36:572–574.

86.   Dahl DS, Sato S. Unusual myasthenic state in a teen-age boy. Neurology 1974; 24:897–901.

87.   Shapira Y, Cividalli G, Szabo G, Rozin R, Russell A. A myasthenic syndrome in childhood leukemia. Dev Med Child Neurol 1974; 16:668–671.

88.   Tsao CY, Mendell JR, Friemer ML, Kissel JT. Lambert-Eaton myasthenic syndrome in children. J Child Neurol 2002; 17:74–76.

89.   Krendel DA, Hopkins LC. Adverse effect of verapamil in a patient with the Lambert-Eaton myasthenic syndrome. Muscle Nerve 1986; 9:519–522.

90.   Ueno S, Hara Y. Lambert-Eaton myasthenic syndrome without anti–calcium channel antibody: adverse effect of calcium antagonist diltiazem. J Neurol Neurosurg Psychiatry 1992; 55:409–410.

6

Congenital Myasthenic Syndromes

I. INTRODUCTION

Congenital myasthenic syndromes (CMSs) are inherited disorders of neuromuscular transmission that do not involve immunologic mechanisms. The mutations that produce CMSs alter the expression and function of ion channels, receptors, enzymes, or other accessory molecules that are needed to maintain the safety margin of neuromuscular transmission. In addition to a neuromuscular transmission defect, some CMSs are associated with secondary degenerative changes of muscle (i.e., endplate myopathy). Most CMSs are autosomal recessive disorders although at least one subtype, the slow-channel syndrome (SCCMS), is typically autosomal dominant. Ultrastructural, physiologic, and molecular genetic techniques have been used to define and classify the various CMSs (Table 6.1) and to design treatment strategies. Although these highly specialized studies are often necessary to make a specific diagnosis, correlation of these data with clinical manifestations and findings on electrodiagnostic studies, as well as increasing availability of genetic probes for specific mutations, has made it possible to diagnose and accurately classify many patients with CMS without the need for intercostal or anconeus muscle biopsy.

Table 6.1 Classification of Congenital Myasthenic Syndromes

Presynaptic defects
  CMS with episodic apnea (endplate choline acetyltransferase)
  Paucity of synaptic vesicles
  Lambert-Eaton syndrome–like CMS
Synaptic defects
  Endplate acetylcholinesterase deficiency
Postsynaptic defects
  Primary AChR kinetic abnormality with or without AChR deficiency
    Slow-channel CMS
    Fast-channel CMS
  Primary AChR deficiency with or without kinetic abnormality
    Reduced AChR expression due to AChR mutations
    Reduce AChR expression due to rapsyn mutations
    Reduced AChR expression with plectin deficiency
  Sodium channel CMS (mutations of perijunctional sodium channels)

CMS, congenital myasthenic syndrome; AChR, acetylcholine receptor.

II. MOLECULAR BASIS OF NEUROMUSCULAR TRANSMISSION

A brief overview of concepts that are important to the understanding of CMS is presented below. The reader is referred to Chapter 1 for a more comprehensive review of the anatomy of the neuromuscular junction (NMJ) and the physiology of neuromuscular transmission. The NMJ is a specialized cholinergic synapse that is designed for efficient and reliable generation of a muscle fiber action potential each time a nerve action potential invades the motor nerve terminal. The direct coupling between the nerve and muscle action potential is maintained even at high discharge rates by the safety margin of neuromuscular transmission. The size of the safety margin depends on presynaptic, synaptic, and postsynaptic factors (Table 6.2, Fig. 6.1).

The major source for acetylcholine (ACh) synthesis is the nerve terminal where choline acetyltransferase (ChAT) is the rate-limiting enzyme responsible for synthesis of ACh from recycled choline and acetyl-CoA (Fig. 6.1). Storage and mobilization of ACh rely on energy-dependent vesicle uptake and transport mechanisms that involve a number of cytoskeletal proteins and other molecules (e.g., synapsin-1, calcium calmodulin-dependent kinase-2). Release of ACh vesicles from the active zone of the nerve terminal also depends on a variety of vesicle membrane–, cytoplasmic, and nerve terminal membrane–associated proteins (e.g., synaptobrevin, synaptotagmin, synaptophysin, synaptosome-associated protein of 25,000 daltons (SNAP-25), N-ethylmaleimide-sensitive ATPasePage (NSF), rab-3, etc). This

Table 6.2 Factors That Determine the Safety Margin of Neuromuscular Transmission

Presynaptic
1. Synthesis, storage, and mobilization of ACh
2. Concentration of ACh vesicles (quanta) in active zones of the nerve terminal
3. Probability of ACh release primarily dependent on the number and function of P/Q-type voltage-gated calcium channels (Cav2.1) (1)

Synaptic/Postsynaptic
1. Anatomic integrity of the synaptic cleft including postsynaptic folds of muscle fiber
2. Concentration and function of AChE
3. Expression and function of AChR
4. Expression and function of perijunctional voltage-gated sodium channels (Nav1.4)

ACh, acetylcholine; AChE, acetylcholinesterase; AChR, acetylcholine receptor.

complicated process of ACh release relies on the influx of calcium into the nerve terminal through PQ-type voltage-gated calcium channels (Cav2.1) (1). The anatomic configuration of the synaptic cleft concentrates ACh receptor (AChR) at the site of ACh release and provides for rapid diffusion and metabolism of ACh after detachment from the receptor. The acetylcholinesterase (AChE) molecule is concentrated in the synaptic clefts, where the globular catalytic subunits are anchored into the basal lamina by a collagen-like tail (Fig. 6.1). The adult isoform of the nicotinic AChR is a ligand-gated ion channel consisting of five subunits 2α, 1β, 1δ, 1ε (Fig. 6.2). The ε subunit is replaced with the γ subunit in the fetal isoform. Each subunit is encoded by different genes on one of two chromosomes (Table 6.3).

The structure of the AChR is homologous. Each subunit consists of four transmembrane domains (M1–M4) with a large extracellular amino terminal segment and a smaller extracellular carboxy terminal segment (Fig. 6.3). When folded in three dimensions, the subunit associate to form a globular glycoprotein transmembrane pore containing two binding sites for ACh on the α subunit (C192-193 of the amino terminal segment). The M2 segment lines the pore of the channel and is important for channel gating. The intracellular segment linking M3 and M4 stabilizes the gating mechanism, contains phosphorylation sites that are important for desensitization, and serves to attach the AChR to cytoskeletal proteins such as utrophin. Postsynaptic AChRs undergo regular turnover, a process that is under the influence of the motor nerve terminal. Rapsyn, a 43-kDa postsynaptic protein, plays an essential role in clustering of AChR in the postsynaptic membrane. Other nerve-derived factors, such as agrin and muscle-specific kinase (MuSK), are involved in clustering and linking AChR to cytoskeletal proteins (2). Activation of the AChR requires binding of ACh in two locations, one

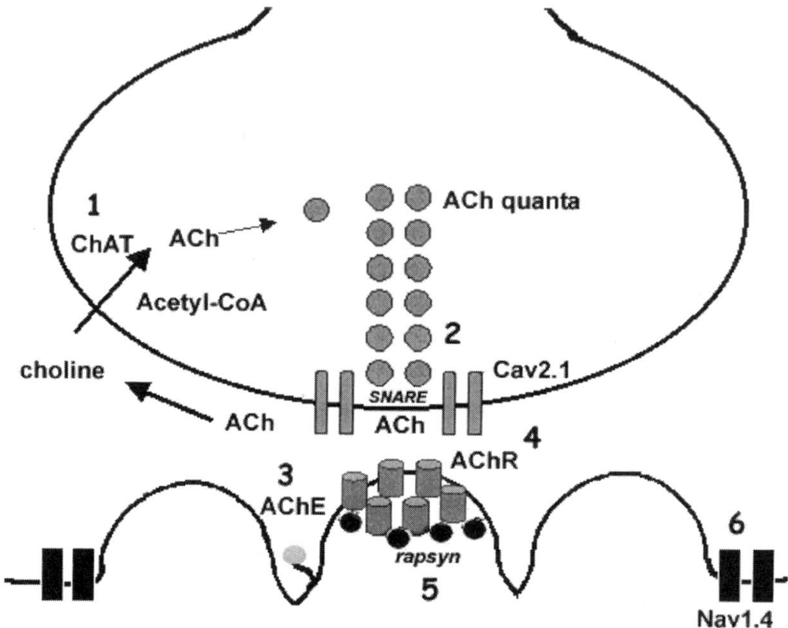

Figure 6.1 Overview of neuromuscular transmission. The numbers represent documented mechanisms affecting neuromuscular transmission in various subtypes of congenital myasthenic syndromes (CMSs). 1, Reduced synthesis of acetylcholine (ACh) caused by congenital choline acetyltransferase (ChAT) deficiency (CMS with episodic apnea); 2, congenital Lambert-Eaton–like syndrome; 3, congenital endplate acetylcholinesterase (AChE) deficiency; 4, primary ACh receptor (AChR) deficiency due to mutations that affect expression or kinetics of AChR; 5, AChR deficiency secondary to rapsyn mutations (failure of proper AChR aggregation); 6, sodium channel myasthenia (mutations of voltage-gated perijunctional sodium channels; Nav1.4); SNARE, complex of vesicle, cytoplasmic, and neuronal membrane–associated proteins that lead to docking, fusion, and release of ACh-containing vesicles.

at the interface between the α and ε subunit (γ in the fetal isoform) and one at the α–δ interface. Thus, amino acid residues in this region of the α, ε, γ, and δ subunits often affect the binding affinity and activation of the AChR.

Binding of two ACh molecules opens the AChR channel allowing conductance of sodium and other cations into the muscle fiber. A single open episode or burst actually consists of one or more openings due to oscillation of the receptor between the open and closed state. The amplitude and duration of single AChR currents correlate directly with the amplitude and dura-

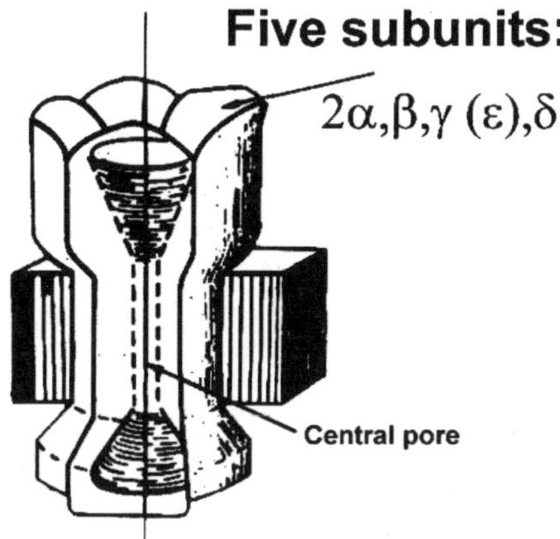

Figure 6.2 Nicotinic acetylcholine receptor. Glycoprotein with molecular weight of 250 kD made of five subunits [2α, β, γ (fetal isoform), ε (adult isoform), δ]. The subunits are arranged like staves of a barrel around the central pore.

tion of the miniature endplate current (MEPC) generated by spontaneous release of individual quanta of ACh from the nerve terminal. With the exception of the number of ACh molecules per vesicle (i.e., quantal size), the amplitude and duration of the MEPC (as well as the miniature endplate potential, MEPP) primarily depend on synaptic/postsynaptic factors. These include the anatomic configuration of the synapse, as well as the expression and function of the AChR and AChE molecules. The endplate current (EPC) or potential (EPP) is the graded receptor response attributable to the release of quanta generated by a single motor nerve action potential. The amplitude and duration of the EPC (and EPP) depend on all of the synaptic/postsynaptic factors that determine the MEPC (or MEPP), as well as two important

Table 6.3 Genes Encoding Subunits of the Acetylcholine Receptor

Subunit	Gene	Locus (OMIM ref.)
α	*CHRNA1*	C2q24-23 (100690)
β	*CHRNB*	C17p12-11 (100710)
δ	*CHRND*	C2q33-34 (100720)
γ	*CHRNG*	C2q33-34 (100730)
ε	*CHRNE*	C17p13-12 (100725)

OMIM, Online Mendelian Inheritance of Man.

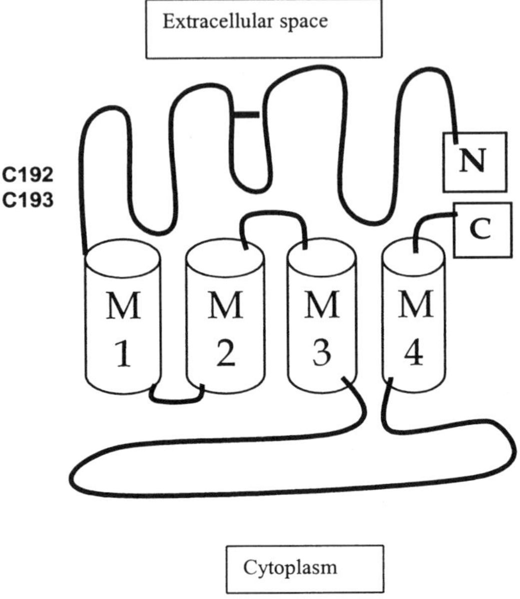

Figure 6.3 Schematic of AChR α subunit with binding site of ACh at C192-193 of the extracellular N-terminal segment. The M2 segment lines the channel pore. The cytoplasmic loop between M3 and M4 links the AChR to cytoskeletal proteins and participates in desensitization.

presynaptic factors: the immediately available stores of ACh in the active zones and the probability of release (primarily determined by the Cav2.1).

III. DIAGNOSTIC METHODS

A. Clinical Manifestations

Like autoimmune myasthenia gravis, the CMSs are typically associated with a combination of static and exertional weakness. Involvement of ocular, bulbar, axial, and limb muscles is common, with some subtypes having a fairly characteristic distribution of weakness (e.g., neck and digit extensors in SCCMS, pupillary involvement in AChE deficiency). Manifestations that raise suspicion of CMS are a history of myasthenic symptoms from birth or early childhood, siblings or other family members with similar symptoms, a family history of sudden infant death syndrome (SIDS) skeletal deformities (e.g., high-arched palate, scoliosis or exaggerated lumbar lordosis when standing, pectus deformities), and small underdeveloped muscles. In some

CMSs static weakness is prominent, making it difficult to differentiate CMS from a congenital myopathy, muscular dystrophy, or metabolic myopathy. Most CMSs respond to cholinesterase inhibitors, but no response or worsening of myasthenic symptoms occurs in congenital endplate AChE deficiency or in SCCMS. Atypical cases that make diagnosis difficult include those that occur sporadically and those that present later in life. These cases are often misdiagnosed as seronegative autoimmune myasthenia gravis or a myopathy, and a high index of suspicion is required to make the correct diagnosis of congenital myasthenia in these situations.

B. Laboratory

By definition, all CMSs have negative tests for AChRs, other ion channels (e.g., Cav2.1, potassium channels), or other recently defined endplate targets for autoimmunity (e.g., MuSK). Serum levels of creatine kinase and other muscle enzymes are normal in congenital myasthenia. Additional laboratory studies that are performed in all suspected cases include electrodiagnostic studies (nerve conduction study, NCS; and needle electromyography, EMG) and standard muscle biopsy. In some cases, the diagnosis of a specific subtype of congenital myasthenia can be established on the basis of clinical, electrodiagnostic, and standard muscle biopsy data. In others, additional morphologic, histochemical, electrophysiologic, and molecular genetic studies are required to make a specific diagnosis. These studies require special expertise and are only performed at a few academic centers.

1. Electrodiagnostic Studies

Since many patients with suspected CMS are children, the electrodiagnostic studies are best performed under conscious sedation, particular under the age of 10–12 years. A variety of sedatives (midazolam, ketamine) and anesthetics (propofol, nitrous oxide) are administered by a nurse anesthetist or anesthesiologist with appropriate cardiorespiratory monitoring. In many cases it is best to perform the standard concentric needle examination first when the patient is able to voluntarily activate muscles, and then perform NCS and if needed single-fiber EMG under deeper levels of sedation.

Standard NCS are usually normal in CMS. The compound muscle action potential (CMAP) is reduced in size in some cases, particularly when there is static weakness due to poor muscle development (hypotrophy), an endplate myopathy, or an associated muscular dystrophy. In CMSs associated with prolonged open time of the AChR (AChE deficiency or SCCMS), there is typically one or more repetitive compound muscle action potential (R-CMAPs) that follows the main CMAP after delivery of a single supramaximal stimulus (Fig. 6.4). The R-CMAP results from persistent elevation of the EPP

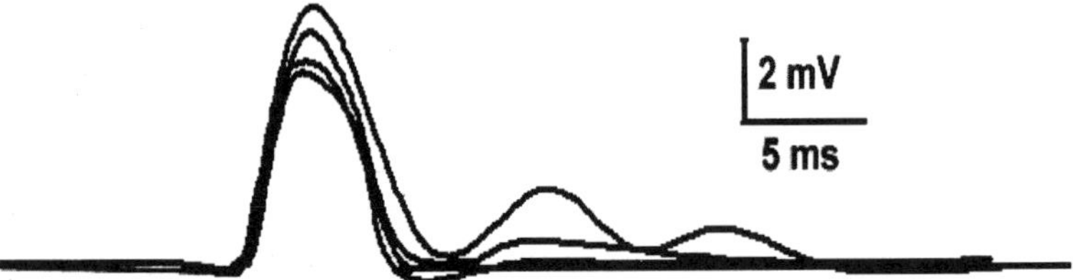

Figure 6.4 Repetitive stimulation of ulnar nerve at 2 Hz recording from surface electrodes over the abductor digiti minimi muscle in a patient with slow-channel congenital myasthenic syndrome (SCCMS). Note the repetitive compound muscle action potentials (R-CMAPs) that follow the main CMAP by about 6 ms. The R-CMAPs are smaller and decrement to a greater degree than the main CMAP. Sensitivity is in millivolts (mV).

above threshold in some muscle fibers beyond the refractory period of the initial action potential. The persistent elevation of the EPP is produced by its prolonged duration. This can be induced pharmacologically in normals with cholinesterase inhibitors, where R-CMAPs are also observed. The R-CMAP is smaller than the main CMAP because the EPP remains just above threshold in a limited number of muscle fibers. This creates a tenuous situation and accounts for the observation that R-CMAPs decrement faster than the main CMAP with slow rates of repetitive stimulation and disappear completely at faster stimulation rates or with exercise.

Repetitive stimulation is a very useful diagnostic tool in the evaluation of suspected CMS. Although a few cases of CMS with normal repetitive stimulation studies have been observed, the vast majority have abnormal studies, particularly when performed in areas of clinical weakness. When multiple nerves are tested using slow and fast rates of stimulation (and exercise when feasible), the absence of a decrement on repetitive stimulation studies does not exclude but rather raises doubt about the diagnosis of CMS. The pattern of CMAP decrement observed with slow rates (2–5 Hz) in CMS is nonspecific and in most cases is indistinguishable from the pattern observed in autoimmune myasthenia gravis. The initial CMAP is normal and is followed by a tapering decrement affecting the subsequent three or four potentials, which is then followed by a gradual repair of the decrement if the train of potentials is carried out beyond four or five stimuli. Following exercise or brief periods of tetanic stimulation there is partial or complete repair of the decrement, which then worsens 1–3 min afterward due to postactivation exhaustion. With higher rates of repetitive stimulation (10–50 Hz), most types of CMS are associated with a progressive CMAP decrement, which increases with the rate of stimulation (Fig. 6.5). This rate-dependent pattern of

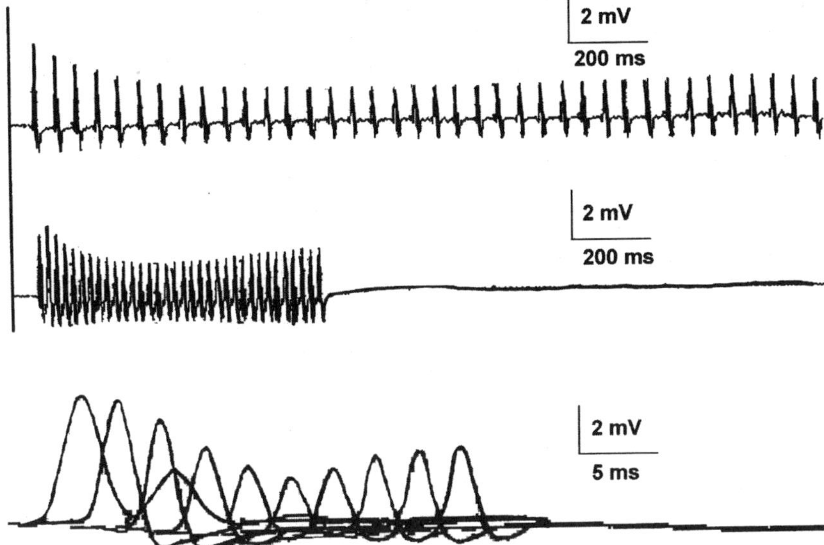

Figure 6.5 Rate-dependent decrement observed in congenital endplate acetyl-cholinesterase (AChE) deficiency and the slow-channel congenital myasthenic syndrome (SCCMS). Repetitive stimulation is applied at frequencies of 20 and 50 Hz to the ulnar nerve, recording over the abductor digiti minimi (ADM) muscle in a patient with AChE deficiency (top two traces). Repetitive stimulation is applied at a frequency of 20 Hz to the median nerve recording over the abductor pollucis brevis muscle in a patient with SCCMS (bottom trace).

decrement differs from the typical pattern of repair or mild facilitation observed in autoimmune myasthenia gravis, and can help distinguish CMS from immune-mediated myasthenia gravis.

Severe "postsynaptic" cases of CMS (e.g., AChR deficiency) can have a "presynaptic" pattern on repetitive stimulation studies. These cases as well as some forms of presynaptic CMS (e.g., Lambert-Eaton–like syndrome) are associated with a low amplitude baseline CMAP that exhibits facilitation with higher frequency repetitive stimulation. Likewise some presynaptic disorders (e.g., CMS with paucity of synaptic vesicles) are associated with a "post-synaptic" pattern on repetitive stimulation studies with a CMAP decrement at low rates that is partially repaired but does not display facilitation at higher rates or following exercise. Other presynaptic CMSs (i.e., ChAT deficiency) may exhibit a decrement only after prolonged repetitive stimulation at intermediate rates (10 15 Hz). It is clear from these observations that the pattern of findings on repetitive stimulation does not always predict the site of the neuromuscular transmission defect in CMS.

Standard concentric needle examination is useful in assessing patients with suspected CMS. Since they are so rare in CMS, the observation of fibrillation potentials and other forms of spontaneous activity suggests an alternative diagnosis such as muscular dystrophy, an acquired myopathy, or a neurogenic disorder. Motor unit potentials are small, relatively simple in configuration, and display prominent variation in amplitude on consecutive discharges. Highly polyphasic motor unit potentials are rare but may be observed in CMSs associated with a muscular dystrophy, e.g., plectin deficiency (3), or an endplate myopathy, e.g., SCCMS or AChE deficiency.

Single-fiber EMG is a very sensitive but nonspecific indicator of a defect of neuromuscular transmission. It is useful as a diagnostic tool when standard NCS, repetitive stimulation studies, and standard concentric needle examination are normal. Mild abnormalities on single-fiber EMG should be interpreted with caution in suspected cases of CMS, as they may also occur in conditions such as congenital myopathies in the setting of a normal standard electromyograms. Most CMSs are associated with prominent abnormalities on single-fiber EMG with increased jitter and blocking. Some cases of AChE deficiency have displayed a fairly unique pattern with greatly increased jitter but very little blocking (4). Voluntary single-fiber EMG can be performed in older children or adults, while in younger children stimulated single fiber is done along with other electrodiagnostic studies under sedation. Measuring the effect of stimulation rate on jitter and blocking can sometimes help distinguish between presynaptic and postsynaptic defects of neuromuscular transmission.

When abnormalities are noted on standard electrodiagnostic studies, administration of pharmacologic agents can assist in the diagnosis and determine potential effectiveness of therapy in various subtypes of CMS. Administration of edrophonium is frequently associated with an increase in the number and amplitude of R-CMAP in SCCMS but has no effect in AChE deficiency. Repair of the CMAP decrement with cholinesterase inhibitors and/or 3,4-diaminopyridine suggests that these medications will provide clinical benefit in individual subtypes of CMS.

2. Muscle Biopsy

The abnormalities on standard muscle biopsy in all subtypes of CMS are minimal and typically confined to type 2 muscle fiber atrophy. If endplates are identified, then qualitative histochemical or immunofluorescence analysis can be performed to assess the presence and abundance of AChR, AChE, agrin, utrophin, rapsyn, and components of complement at the endplate. The presence of C3 and C5b9 complement proteins suggests the diagnosis of sero-

Table 6.4 Information Obtained from Microelectrode Studies in Congenital Myasthenic Syndromes

Technique/modality	Interpretation
Conventional microelectrode studies	
MEPP/MEPC	
Frequency	Reduced in some presynaptic disorders (e.g., LES)
Amplitude	Reduced in most synaptic/postsynaptic disorders[a]
Duration (decay time constant)	Increased with prolonged AChR open time[b]
EPP/EPC	
Amplitude	Reduced in presynaptic, synaptic/postsynaptic disorders[c]
Duration	Increased with prolonged AChR open time[b]
Quantal release per impulse (m)	Reduced in presynaptic disorders
Number of readily releasable quanta (n)	Reduced in some presynaptic disorders (e.g., ChAT deficiency)
Probability of quantal release (p)	Reduced in presynaptic disorders affecting Cav2.1[d]
Single-channel patch-clamp studies	
Amplitude, duration channel openings	Increased in SCCMS, AChE deficiency, fetal AChR expression Decreased in FCCMS
Stability of open/closed states	Increased/decreased in SCCMS Decreased/increased in FCCMS

[a] Can also be reduced in disorders that reduce the number of ACh per vesicle (quanta).
[b] Can occur with SCCMS, congenital or acquired AChE deficiency, overexpression of fetal AChR.
[c] EPP amplitude defines the safety margin of NMT. Reduction of the EPP with preservation of the MEPP amplitude suggests a presynaptic disorder. Reduction of both the EPP and MEPP suggests a postsynaptic or mixed disorder.
[d] Disorders of other components of vesicle release mechanism will also reduce the probability of release.
CMS, congenital myasthenic syndromes; MEPP, miniature endplate potential; MEPC, miniature endplate current; EPP, endplate potential; EPC, endplate current; LES, Lambert-Eaton syndrome; AChR, acetylcholine receptor; Cav2.1, P/Q-type voltage-gated calcium channel; ChAT, choline acetyltransferase; SCCMS, slow-channel congenital myasthenic syndrome; FCCMS, fast-channel congenital myasthenic syndrome; NMT, neuromuscular transmission.

negative autoimmune myasthenia gravis. Electron microscopy of the NMJ may provide useful information in selected cases. Degenerative changes in endplate region of the muscle are seen in the endplate myopathy that occurs in SCCMS and some cases of AChE deficiency. Ultrastructural studies may reveal changes in size of nerve terminal, density and size of synaptic vesicles, size of the synaptic cleft, and other compensatory changes in endplate morphology.

Intercostal or anconeus muscle biopsy is performed when in vitro electrophysiologic studies are required to confirm the diagnosis and define the mechanism of neuromuscular transmission defect in suspected cases of congenital myasthenia. Since endplates are abundant, this type of specimen is also ideal for ultrastructural and histochemical studies including quantitative analysis of AChR density using ^{125}I-α-bungarotoxin. The types and utility of information obtained from microelectrode studies are listed in Table 6.4.

3. Molecular Genetic Studies

More than 100 mutations in various structural proteins, enzymes, and other regulatory molecules have been reported to cause CMS. The majority of reported mutations involve the AChR molecule causing reduced expression of the adult receptor and/or abnormal receptor kinetics by alteration of the adult AChR or overexpression of the fetal receptor. Mutations in AChE, ChAT, rapsyn, and in perijunctional sodium channels have also been reported to cause various subtypes of CMS.

Most CMS mutations have been discovered after morphologic and electrophysiologic studies suggest a defect in a particular gene product or gene. Once potential candidate genes are identified, then expression of the genetically engineered mutant allele in human cell lines can be done to study the pathogenicity of the mutation and to test the effect of candidate drugs for potential management of the condition.

Molecular genetic screening for diagnosis is available for some CMS syndromes with a restricted number of mutations. However, genetic heterogeneity, particularly in the case of AChR mutations, continues to limit the utility of genetic testing as an initial diagnostic tool.

IV. CONGENITAL MYASTHENIC SYNDROME SUBTYPES

A. CMS with Episodic Apnea (Endplate Choline Acetyltransferase Deficiency)

1. Definition and Genetics

CMS with episodic apnea (CMS-EA) is an autosomal recessive disorder associated with deficiency of endplate ChAT, in which the early course is dominated by recurrent episodes of severe generalized, respiratory, and bulbar weakness that may produce sudden death or require hospitalization for airway protection and respiratory support. All reported cases of CMS-EA with molecular genetic studies have been associated with mutations in the *CHAT* gene (C10q11.2), which codes for ChAT, the rate-limiting enzyme in the synthesis of ACh from recycled choline and acetyl-CoA (5). These mutations produce a defect in synthesis of ACh within the motor nerve terminal. The syndrome could theoretically result from other defects of synthesis and vesicular uptake of ACh, but none of these other mechanisms have been documented.

CMS-EA was initially reported by Greer and Schotland in 1960 (6) and later given the name "familial infantile myasthenia" by Conomy et al. (7). In 2001, Ohno et al. proposed the name "congenital myasthenic syndrome with episodic apnea" (CMS-EA) and reported the association with mutations in the *CHAT* gene (5). CMS-EA emphasizes the important clinical feature of episodic crises of generalized weakness often associated with respiratory insufficiency, whereas "ChAT deficiency" refers to the only known cause of CMS-EA that has been documented to date.

2. Clinical Manifestations

The onset of CMS-EA is typically in the infantile or early childhood period with generalized hypotonia and weakness involving bulbar, limb, and respiratory muscles. The baseline weakness is punctuated by acute crises precipitated by excitement or infection. A history of SIDS in siblings is a common and important diagnostic clue (8). In patients who survive the infantile period or in those cases where the onset is delayed to later childhood, there is often gradual improvement of the generalized weakness. Patients may present as adolescents or young adults with symptoms and signs of mild ptosis, bulbar and limb weakness. In these cases, CMS-EA is often incorrectly diagnosed as seronegative autoimmune myasthenia gravis. Again, a history of crises early in life or a family history of SIDS in cases of seronegative myasthenia should raise suspicion of CMS-EA. At all stages of the illness the symptoms are responsive to cholinesterase inhibitors, but as expected no benefit is observed with immunomodulation therapy.

3. Laboratory

Serologic tests for AChR antibodies and serum creatine kinase are normal. In patients with generalized weakness, electrodiagnostic studies show normal or slight reduction in the size of the baseline CMAP and a mild to moderate CMAP decrement with 2- to 5-Hz repetitive stimulation. Exercise or a higher rate of repetitive stimulation produces transient repair of the decrement followed by pronounced postactivation exhaustion. These findings are similar to those in autoimmune myasthenia gravis, except that in CMS-EA, post-activation exhaustion is severe and prolonged especially when exercise is extended for 5–10 min as opposed to the typical 30- to 60-s period. In CMS-EA, the CMAP amplitude remains depressed and 2- to 5-Hz repetitive stimulation produces a prominent decrement for 5–10 min or longer after exercise, while in autoimmune myasthenia the period of postactivation exhaustion is usually under 5 min duration (Harper, Engel, unpublished observation). In older patients with CMS-EA who are mildly affected, standard repetitive stimulation studies may be normal. In these cases, prolonged exercise (5–10 min) or continuous repetitive stimulation at 10 Hz for 5–10 min elicits a fall in the baseline CMAP amplitude and an increase in the decrement in response to 2-Hz repetitive stimulation (Fig. 6.6). Similar findings may occur

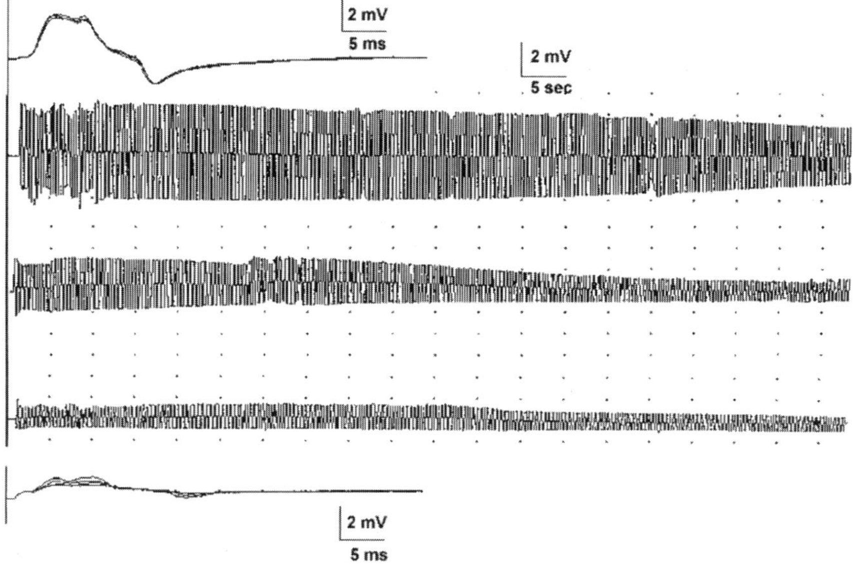

Figure 6.6 Prolonged repetitive stimulation of the peroneal nerve, recording the compound muscle action potential (CMAP) with surface electrodes over the tibialis anterior muscle in a patient with congenital myasthenic syndrome with episodic apnea (CMS-EA) caused by a deficiency of choline acetyltransferase (ChAT). The procedure was performed under sedation with intravenous midazolam and ketamine. The top trace shows repetitive stimulation at 2 Hz (train of 4 superimposed) prior to the start of prolonged repetitive stimulation (no decrement). The middle three traces illustrate a gradual decline in the CMAP amplitude with continuous stimulation at 10 Hz for 5 min. The bottom trace shows repetitive stimulation at 2 Hz (train of 4 superimposed) 1 min after prolonged stimulation was discontinued (50% decrement).

in autoimmune myasthenia gravis or other forms of CMS, but the extended period of recovery from postactivation exhaustion strongly suggests the diagnosis of CMS-EA. Standard concentric needle EMG in CMS-EA reveals normal insertional activity and small varying motor unit potentials of simple configuration. Single-fiber EMG demonstrates increased jitter and blocking commensurate with the degree of motor unit variation of standard EMG.

The routine muscle biopsy is normal or shows only type 2 fiber atrophy. Morphologic and histochemical analysis of the endplate is normal. Micro-electrode studies show a normal MEPP amplitude and quantal content of the EPP (m) at rest but a steady decrease in both with prolonged repetitive stimulation at 10 Hz (5,9). This pattern mimics the effect of hemicholinium in vitro (9) and is associated with a gradual reduction in the number of quanta available for ready release (n). This pattern confirms the presynaptic origin of the neuromuscular transmission defect and could be produced by "an alteration of choline reuptake or resynthesis, or by packaging or mobilization of ACh stores."

4. Treatment

Cholinesterase inhibitors produce a modest benefit in CMS-EA by prolonging the presence and effect of ACh within the synaptic cleft. Drug-induced desensitization is uncommon because of the progressive reduction in quantal content associated with CMS-EA secondary to ChAT deficiency. 3,4-Diaminopyridine has been tried in CMS-EA but, as expected, the benefit is transient because the drug tends to rapidly worsen the already depleted stores of ACh.

CASE 6.1   This female patient was the product of a normal pregnancy and delivery. Immediately after birth she experienced respiratory difficulty and required apnea monitoring during the neonatal and early childhood period. At age 15 months, in the setting of acute otitis media, she developed severe generalized weakness, feeding difficulties, and respiratory insufficiency requiring intubation. She recovered after 1 week. Tests for AChR antibodies were negative and a EMG, including repetitive stimulation studies on multiple nerve, produced normal results. Two of six siblings died of SIDS during childhood infections. Examination of the patient at age 5 years showed mild ptosis but no clear weakness. She complained of being "tired" after 5 min of "playing," which included a mixture of walking, running, and climbing activities.

Routine motor and sensory nerve conduction studies were normal. Repetitive stimulation of the ulnar peroneal and facial nerves at 2 Hz was normal. Routine needle examination was normal. Under conscious sedation with medazolam and nitrous oxide, continuous repetitive stimulation of the peroneal nerve at 10 Hz for 5 min revealed a gradual decrement of the tibialis anterior CMAP, which eventually reached 40% of the baseline amplitude. Repetitive stimulation at 2 Hz performed after the period of prolonged repetitive stimulation at 10 Hz revealed a decrement of 25% between the first and fourth response. The CMAP amplitude returned to normal and the decrement disappeared gradually over the ensuing 15–20 min.

An intercostal muscle biopsy was performed. Microelectrode studies showed normal MEPP amplitude and quantal release per nerve impulse at 1 Hz. Repetitive stimulation at 10 Hz for 5 min showed a progressive 90% decrease of the EPP amplitude followed by a slow return to baseline over the next 7 min. The MEPP amplitude recorded over 5 min after stimulation was reduced to about 50% of normal. Patch-clamp recordings from endplates showed no kinetic abnormality of the AChR channel. Electron microscopy showed a normal concentration of AChR at the endplate and normal endplate morphology. Mutational analysis revealed two mutations in the *CHAT* gene (L210P and S498L). Both mutations markedly reduce the catalytic efficiency of ChAT.

The patient was treated with pyridostigmine with subsequent improvement in physical endurance and no recurrence of respiratory "crises" to date.

B. Paucity of Synaptic Vesicles

1. Definition and Genetics

CMS secondary to a paucity of synaptic vesicles and reduced quantal release is a rare disorder with only one well-defined case described in the literature (10). Since the case was isolated, an autosomal recessive pattern of inheritance is most likely, but confirmation awaits better understanding of the molecular origin of the disorder. The disorder is named after the characteristic findings of reduced density of synaptic vesicles on ultrastructural studies of the endplate.

2. Clinical Manifestations

In the only well-described case of CMS secondary to a paucity of synaptic vesicles, the onset of symptoms was in the infantile period with generalized hypotonia and feeding difficulties (10). Ptosis, bulbar and limb weakness developed by early childhood, and by the time the patient was studied at 23 years of age the pattern of clinical involvement resembled typical seronegative autoimmune myasthenia gravis. There was no history of myasthenic crises and the symptoms were moderately responsive to cholinesterase inhibitors.

3. Laboratory and Treatment

Serum assays for AChR antibodies are negative. Electrodiagnostic studies reveal a pattern indistinguishable from moderately severe seronegative autoimmune myasthenia gravis with a normal baseline CMAP, a decrement with slow rates of repetitive stimulation, and partial repair of the decrement with exercise or high-frequency stimulation (10). Edrophonium produces partial repair of the decrement as well. Needle examination reveals small, rapidly recruited motor unit potentials that are simple in configuration and display prominent amplitude variation on consecutive discharges. Single-fiber EMG findings have not been reported. Ultrastructural studies are normal except for an 80% reduction in the density of synaptic vesicles in the motor nerve terminal (10). Microelectrode studies show a commensurate 80% decrease in the quantal content (m) of the EPP and the number of readily releasable quanta (n), with normal probability of release (p). The presumed pathogenesis of this disorder lies in impaired synthesis or recycling of synaptic vesicles. The only patient described reported a moderate clinical benefit from pyridostigmine (10). No other medications have been tried.

C. Lambert-Eaton Syndrome–Like CMS

1. Definition and Genetics

This is an ill-defined group of rare autosomal recessive or sporadic disorders that share a common pattern on electrophysiologic studies with autoimmune Lambert-Eaton syndrome. The first case reported by Albers et al. in 1984 (11) and all cases reported since have presented in the infantile period (12,13).

2. Clinical Manifestations, Laboratory, and Treatment

Manifestations include hypotonia and severe generalized weakness with poor motor development. Respiratory muscle weakness can be severe enough to require mechanical ventilation. Electrodiagnostic studies show a low-amplitude baseline CMAP, a decrement of the CMAP with low rates of repetitive stimulation, and facilitation of 200% or more with high-frequency stimulation. Needle examination shows small varying motor unit potentials with increased jitter and blocking that may improve at higher rates on stimulated single-fiber EMG. Morphologic studies have been essentially normal and microelectrode studies mimic the results observed in autoimmune Lambert-Eaton syndrome. The MEPP amplitude is normal and the quantal content of the EPP is reduced because of a decreased probability of quantal release (p). In three cases of presynaptic CMS, attempts to identify a mutation in the

Cav2.1 were unsuccessful (14). Defects in other components of the synaptic vesicle release complex could produce the same type of defect as a calcium channel mutation. Cholinesterase inhibitors, guanidine, and 3,4-diaminopyridine have been used for treatment with variable improvement.

D.　Endplate Acetylcholine Esterase Deficiency

1.　Definition and Genetics

Endplate AChE deficiency is an autosomal recessive CMS caused by a deficiency in the asymmetric heteromeric AChE molecule at the motor endplate. Complete deficiency produces a more severe phenotype than partial deficiency. Clinical characteristics that suggest AChE deficiency include generalized weakness, muscle hypotrophy, a slow pupillary response to light, and no response or worsening with cholinesterase inhibitors. The AChE deficiency is caused by mutations in the gene for ColQ, a triple-stranded protein that anchors the globular catalytic subunit of AChE to the basal lamina of the postsynaptic membrane (15–17).

Endplate AChE deficiency was originally described by Engel et al. in 1997 (18). Hutchinson et al. defined the clinical spectrum of endplate AChE deficiency in 1993 (19). In 1998 the molecular pathogenesis was defined when recessive mutations in the *COLQ* gene were identified in patients with AChE deficiency (15). Twenty mutations in 24 kinships have been described since (15–17).

2.　Clinical Manifestations

When the AChE deficiency is complete, the patient presents as an infant with hypotonia, skeletal deformities, and muscle hypotrophy. Severe generalized weakness, feeding difficulties, weak cry, and respiratory insufficiency are also observed. When AChE deficiency is partial, the onset tends to be later in life and manifestations are less severe. Older children and adults have fatigable ptosis, weakness of extraocular muscles, a delayed and incomplete pupillary light reflex, dysarthria, dysphagia, and generalized muscle weakness. Scoliosis and lumbar lordosis are common and often worsen after several minutes of standing. Cholinesterase inhibitors either produce no benefit or cause the symptoms to worsen.

3.　Laboratory and Treatment

Tests for AChR antibodies are negative and the serum creatine kinase is normal. Nerve conduction studies reveal one or more (R-CMAPs) that follow the main CMAP by 3–6 ms, decrement faster than the main CMAP on repetitive stimulation, disappear complete after exercise or higher frequency repetitive stimulation, and are unchanged by administration of cholinesterase inhibitors (Fig. 6.7). The R-CMAP is produced by a prolonged

EPP, which remains above threshold beyond the action potential refractory period in a portion of muscle fibers. The R-CMAP is most readily observed in small hand and foot muscles because of their relatively short CMAP duration. Repetitive stimulation studies show a rate-dependent decrement (i.e., increase in magnitude as the rate of repetitive stimulation is increased; Fig. 5, which is caused by desensitization of AChR and depolarization block

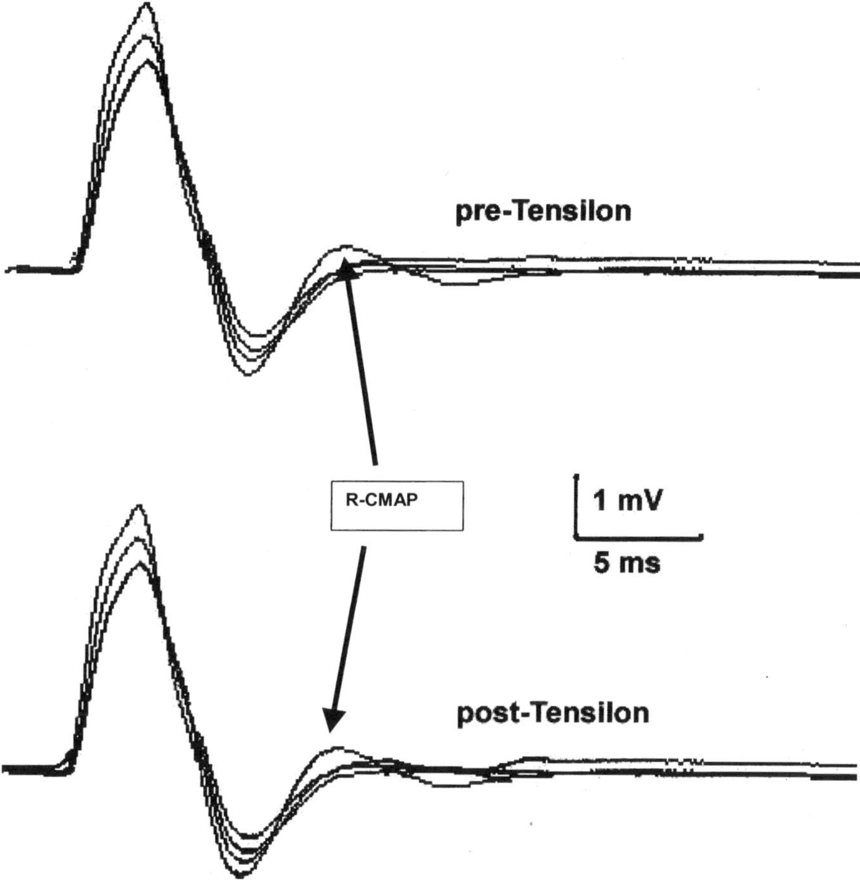

Figure 6.7 Repetitive stimulation of the ulnar nerve recording over the abductor digiti minimi muscle in a patient with congenital endplate acetylcholinesterase (AChE) deficiency. Stimulation rate is 2 Hz with four superimposed consecutive sweeps. Top and bottom groups were obtained before and 30 s after administration of 1 mg of tensilon intravenously. Notice that there is no change in the amplitude or number of repetitive compound muscle action potentials (R-CMAP) after Tensilon administration.

of the muscle membrane (secondary to the long EPP). Standard needle examination shows abundant small, polyphasic, varying motor unit potentials with rapid recruitment and normal insertional activity. The motor unit potentials are smaller and more polyphasic than in other CMS (with the exception of SCCMS) because of the associated endplate myopathy. Single-fiber EMG demonstrates increased jitter with blocking, although the block may be less than expected, presumably because the rise time of the EPP is affected more than the overall amplitude (4).

Ultrastructural studies show small nerve terminals, encroachment of Schwann cells over the nerve terminals, and degeneration of the postsynaptic folds and associated cytoplasm (19). The changes in the nerve terminal are thought to be compensatory and result in a secondary decrease in quantal content. The changes in the muscle are in response to excess flow of calcium through AChR into the muscle and constitute the "endplate" myopathy that is responsible for the static weakness observed in AChE deficiency. Histochemical studies show reduced concentration of AChE at the endplate. Microelectrode studies show MEPPs and EPPs of reduced size and prolonged duration. Patch-clamp studies confirm the prolonged AChR open episodes (19).

Genetic heterogeneity has made the use of molecular genetic testing as a diagnostic tool difficult. The characteristic clinical and electrodiagnostic features along with histochemical studies confirming the reduction in AChE concentrations at the endplate are usually sufficient to confirm the diagnosis of the CMS secondary to endplate AChE deficiency.

Unfortunately, no highly effective treatments have been described for this CMS subtype. Cholinesterase inhibitors do not help and may make symptoms worse. Ephedrine produces subjective benefit in some patients. In one severe case, counteracting desensitization of the AChR by intermittent administration of a controlled infusion of a short-acting neuromuscular blocking agent produced temporary benefit (20).

CASE 6.2   This male patient was a product of a normal pregnancy and delivery. At age 3 months he was noted to have restricted eye movements. He sat and walked on time but was slow and behind his peers in all motor activities. His sister of 5 years younger age was noted to have similar symptoms. No family members were affected in other generations. He complained of generalized weakness that worsened on exertion. On examination at age 13 years there was mild ophthalmoparesis without ptosis, slowed pupillary light reflexes, and normal speech. Manual muscle testing demonstrated diffuse moderately severe weakness of neck muscles and of proximal upper and lower limb muscles. Deep tendon reflexes and sensation were normal. Forward arm elevation was limited to 30 s and he was unable to perform a deep knee bend.

Nerve conduction studies showed clear R-CMAPs in the median and ulnar motor studies. The R-CMAPs disappeared following brief exercise or at repetitive stimulation rates of 1–5 Hz. At 2 Hz, there was a 25–35% decrement of the main CMAP, which increased up to 75% with 50-Hz repetitive stimulation. There was no repair of the decrement and no change in the number or size of the R-CMAP after the administration of intravenous Tensilon. Needle examination showed small varying motor unit potentials with no fibrillation potentials.

An intercostal muscle biopsy was performed. Microelectrode studies showed slight reduction in the amplitude of the MEPP and MEPC, with a twofold prolongation of the MEPC decay time constant. The number of quanta released was markedly reduced (due to compensatory reduction in the size of the motor nerve terminals). Histochemistry confirmed the absence of AChE at the endplate and electron microscopy showed small nerve terminals encased in Schwann cells as well as degeneration of the postsynaptic folds indicating an endplate myopathy. Mutational analysis confirmed a missense mutation in the proline-rich domain of the ColQ gene, which prevents the attachment of the catalytic subunits of AChE to the ColQ tail that anchors the enzyme to the basal lamina.

Attempts to treat the patient with cholinesterase inhibitors, mexiletine, and quinidine have been unsuccessful.

E. Slow-Channel CMS

1. Definition and Genetics

SCCMS is an autosomal dominant disorder with variable expression that is caused by gain of function mutations in the AChR. It is the only CMS to date that has been shown to follow an autosomal dominant pattern of inheritance. The disorder was initially described and characterized both clinically and electrophysiologically by Engel et al. in 1982 (21). Subsequently mutationsin the AChR that produce SCCMS have been found in the α, β, and ε subunits of the AChR (22–29). Most slow-channel mutations are found in the M2 pore-lining segment of the receptor. Mutations produce their effect by either stabilizing the open state of the receptor or increasing the affinity of AChR for ACh. It has been shown that open-channel blockers such as quinidine sulfate and fluoxetine benefit SCCMS clinically (30–32).

2. Clinical Manifestations

The clinical presentation of SCCMS is highly variable. Some patients are asymptomatic but have abnormal electrodiagnostic studies. Severe cases tend to present earlier in life and develop severe disability by the end of the first decade. Others are mildly affected and may not present until the seventh or eighth decade of life. The distribution of weakness in SCCMS is fairly characteristic with prominent weakness involving neck extensors, wrist and digit extensors, and intrinsic hand muscles. There is often atrophy of the intrinsic hand muscles. Other manifestations that are common include variable ptosis, ophthalmoparesis, dysarthria, dysphagia, proximal limb weakness, and respiratory insufficiency. Respiratory involvement can be clinically occult until the first episode of decompensation is triggered by a respiratory infection or some other illness. Nocturnal hypoxemia may contribute to the fatigue and weakness associated with SCCMS and other forms of congenital myasthenia. Asymmetric weakness is common in SCCMS. In severe cases and as the disease progresses, static weakness and muscle atrophy become more prominent due to progression of the endplate myopathy associated with SCCMS. All symptoms characteristically become more severe when patients with SCCMS are given cholinesterase inhibitors.

3. Laboratory

Tests for AChR antibodies are negative and serum creatine kinase is normal in SCCMS. Like AChE deficiency, routine NCS reveals the presence of R-CMAPs in the majority of cases. The characteristics of the R-CMAP in SCCMS and AChE deficiency are identical (see "Laboratory" section under AChE deficiency), except that cholinesterase inhibitors increase the number and size of R-CMAPs in the SCCMS but have no effect on the R-CMAPs in AChE deficiency (Fig. 6.7 and 6.8). Like AChE deficiency, a rate-dependent decrement of the main CMAP is also observed in SCCMS (Fig. 6.9). The R-CMAPs in SCCMS result from a prolonged EPP whereas the rate-dependent decrement is caused by depolarization block. Needle examination in SCCMS shows normal insertional activity and short-duration, polyphasic, varying motor unit potentials with rapid recruitment. The severity of needle examination findings correlates with the severity of the endplate myopathy.

Ultrastructural studies show degeneration of the postsynaptic folds and subsarcoplasmic regions of the muscle fiber in the endplate region (33). The endplate myopathy is often associated with a secondary decrease in the concentration of the postsynaptic AChR. Microelectrode studies show prolonged endplate currents secondary to prolonged opening events of individual AChRs (33). The prolonged opening events are caused by increased affinity of AChRs for ACh, stabilization of the open state, or destabilization of the closed state of the receptor.

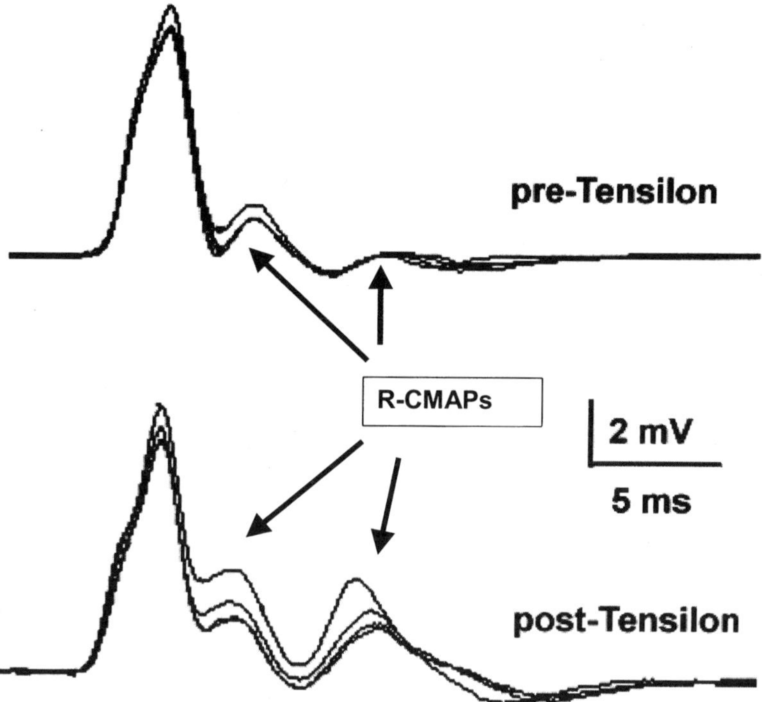

Figure 6.8 Repetitive stimulation of the ulnar nerve recording over the abductor digiti minimi muscle in a patient with congenital slow channel myasthenic syndrome (SCCMS). Stimulation rate is 2 Hz with 4 superimposed consecutive sweeps. Top and bottom groups were obtained before and 30 seconds after administration of 1 mg of Tensilon intravenously. Notice that there the amplitude and number of repetitive compound muscle action potentials (R-CMAP) is increased after Tensilon administration.

4. Treatment

SCCMS gets worse with cholinesterase inhibitors as they enhance the pro-longed openings and promote desensitization and depolarization block of the AChR. Prolonged treatment with cholinesterase inhibitors may worsen the endplate myopathy by promoting the influx of calcium to the muscle fiber. Long-lived open-channel blockers such as quinidine sulfate and fluoxetine have been shown to reduce the channel open time in vitro (30) and improve objective clinical as well as electrophysiologic measures of function in SCCMS (31,32).

CASE 6.3 This female patient was a product of a normal pregnancy and delivery. Shortly after birth she was noted to have mild hypotonia and weakness. In childhood she experienced moderate generalized weakness as well as mild diplopia, ptosis, dysarthria, and dysphagia. Multiple family members in multiple generations were noted to have a similar disorder. At 23 years of age her examination revealed mild weakness of proximal limb muscles as well as extraocular, facial, masseter, and tongue muscles. There was moderately severe weakness of the neck flexors and extensors, as well as finger extensors and intrinsic hand muscles. Cholinesterase inhibitors caused her weakness to worsen, and calcium channel blockers as well as ephedrine produced minimal subjective benefit.

Nerve conduction studies showed clear R-CMAPs on the median, ulnar, and radial motor studies. There was no R-CMAP observed on the facial motor conduction study. Repetitive stimulation at 2 Hz produced decrements of the main CMAP ranging from 5% to 15%, with the greatest decrement in facial muscles. Increasing the stimulation rate to 50% increased the decrement in the ulnar CMAP from 12% to 38%. The number and amplitude of R-CMAPs was increased following the administration of intravenous Tensilon. Needle examination showed small varying motor unit potentials in proximal muscles.

An intercostal muscle biopsy was performed for morphologic and electrophysiologic assessment. Microelectrode studies showed significant prolongation of the MEPC decay time constant but preservation of the MEPC amplitude. Single-channel recording documented a receptor population with four times the normal channel opening time, confirming the diagnosis of "slow-channel" syndrome. Electron microscopy showed simplification and degeneration of the postsynaptic folds indicating an endplate myopathy. Mutational analysis showed a mutation in the extracellular domain of the α subunit (αG153S) near the binding site for ACh.

The patient was placed on quinidine sulfate with significant improvement in muscle strength and reduction in the decrement on repetitive stimulation studies. She continues to improve gradually after 4 years of continuous quinidine therapy.

F. Fast-Channel CMS

1. Definition and Genetics

Fast-channel CMS (FCCMS) is the "mirror" image of SCCMS. FCCMS is an autosomal recessive disorder caused by mutations in the AChR that

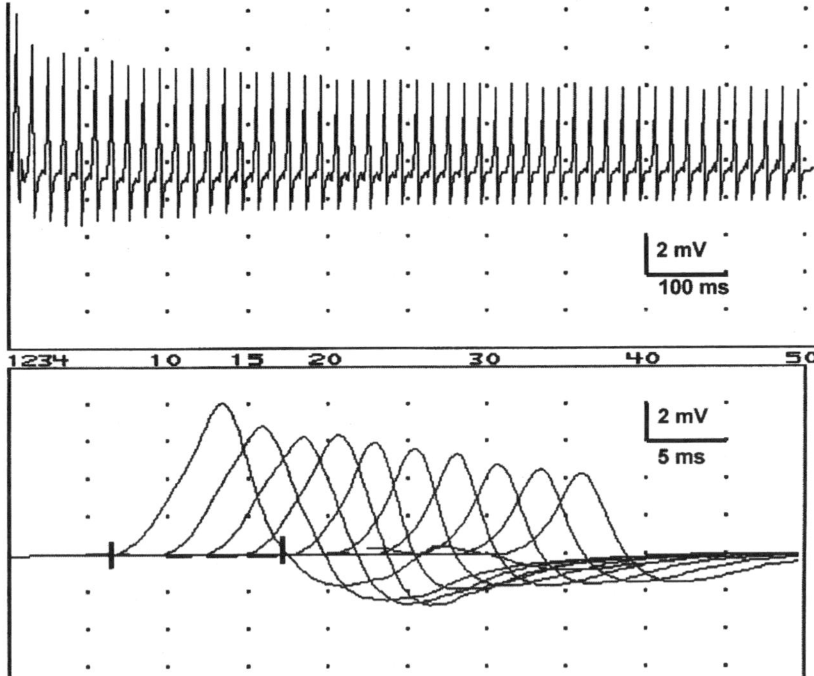

Figure 6.9 Repetitive stimulation of the ulnar nerve recording over the abductor digiti minimi muscle in a patient with slow-channel congenital myasthenic syndrome (SCCMS). Stimulation rate is 50 Hz. The CMAP amplitude and area both decrement by 50%. The decrement with 2 Hz stimulation was 15% (not shown).

shorten the opening episodes of the receptor by decreasing its affinity for ACh, destabilizing the open state or stabilizing the closed state of the receptor (34–36). The first mutation associated with FCCMS was discovered in the extracellular domain of the ε subunit of AChR by Ohno et al. in 1996 (34). Subsequently, two additional mutations that act by different mechanisms to produce FCCMS have been described (33,35–37).

2. Clinical Manifestations, Laboratory, and Treatment

Patients with FCCMS typically present in infancy or early childhood with generalized weakness, fatigue, dysphagia, dysarthria, ptosis, and ophthalmoparesis (33). The picture is indistinguishable from autoimmune myasthenia gravis or many other subtypes of AChR. The symptoms respond to cholinesterase inhibitors. The findings on electrodiagnostic studies are also indistinguishable from mild to moderate autoimmune myasthenia gravis. On NCS, there are no R-CMAPs with single stimuli, and with repetitive stimulation there is a decrement of the main CMAP at low rates that shows postactivation repair and exhaustion following exercise or fast rates of repetitive stimulation. No rate-dependent decrement has been reported in FCCMS. Needle examination is nonspecific with small varying motor unit potentials on standard EMG and increased jitter and blocking on single-fiber EMG. Ultrastructural studies are typically normal or show a reduction in the density of AChR on the postsynaptic membrane.

Microelectrode studies show a small MEPP with short duration MEPP and EPP. Single-channel studies and molecular genetic analysis have defined three separate mutations and mechanisms underlying the FCCMS phenotype. In cases with the εP121L mutation in the extracellular domain of AChR, the symptoms are moderate to severe and single-channel kinetics show decreased affinity of AChR for ACh (33,34). The αV285I mutation in the M3 segment of the AChR reduces the AChR expression and alters the gaiting mechanism (manifested as a decrease in the opening rate and an increase in the closing rate of the AChR) (33,37). Symptoms are relatively mild in this form of FCCMS. The third subtype of FCCMS is caused by mutations that alter the mode-switching kinetics of AChR, causing it to open and close rapidly and inefficiently (35).

In addition to cholinesterase inhibitors, the FCCMS responds to 3,4-diaminopyridine, either alone or in combination with cholinesterase inhibition (38).

CASE 6.4 This female patient had good health until late childhood when she began to complain of intermittent diplopia and generalized fatigue. She was noted to have severe restriction of her extraocular movements. She developed fluctuating generalized weakness and dyspnea on exertion, difficulty chewing, and dysphagia. She experienced intermittent exacerbation of symptoms lasting several days to weeks. During these periods she experienced increased generalized weakness, dyspnea on exertion, orthopnea, and dysphagia. Her symptoms were partially responsive to pyridostigmine. On examination at 29 years of age, there was near-complete ophthalmoplegia, mild ptosis and facial weakness, and mild-moderate generalized weakness.

Routine motor and sensory nerve conduction studies were normal. No R-CMAPs were observed. Repetitive stimulation of the ulnar, median, spinal accessory, and facial nerves revealed decrements ranging from 15% to 28%, which repaired to <10% with brief exercise or separate administration of either Tensilon or 3,4-diaminopyridine.

Needle examination showed small varying motor unit potentials in proximal muscles.

An intercostal muscle biopsy was performed for morphologic and electrophysiologic assessment. Microelectrode studies showed a 20% reduction in the amplitude of the MEPP and MEPC. The MEPC time constant showed a biexponential decay with one normal component shorter than normal. The number of acetylcholine receptors per endplate, as determined by ^{125}I-α-bungarotoxin binding, was reduced to 5% of normal. Electron microscopy showed mild simplification of the postsynaptic folds and reduced expression of AChR on the junctional folds. Mutational analysis revealed two mutations: (a) a frame-shifting mutation in the extracellular domain of the epsilon AChR subunit (ε553del7), and (b) a point mutation (εR311W) in the N-terminal region of the long cytoplasmic loop of the ε subunit. Expression studies and patch-clamp analysis showed that these mutations produced "fast-channel" properties (short open times). The patient was treated with a combination of 3,4-diaminopyridine and pyridostigmine with significant improvement in muscle strength and decrement on repetitive stimulation studies.

G. Primary AChR Deficiency

1. Definition and Genetics

This is a heterogeneous group of autosomal recessive disorders that result in reduced expression of the AChR at the motor endplate. Some mutations exclusively reduce AChR expression while others have minor effects on AChR kinetics as well (33). AChR kinetics can also be altered when mutations in the ε subunit lead to compensatory expression of the fetal γ subunit. The AChR deficiency is caused by homozygous and heterozygous autosomal recessive mutations. More than 50 different mutations have been shown to cause the CMS secondary to primary AChR deficiency (33,39–55). The mutations are of many types including null, frameshift, and missense mutations in structural or regulatory portions of the gene. The majority of mutations affect the ε subunit, but mutations causing AChR deficiency have also been described in the α, β, and δ subunit genes and in the gene which codes for rapsyn (55), a molecule that regulates aggregation and expression of AChR at the muscle endplate.

2. Clinical Manifestations

The onset and severity of symptoms varies greatly in primary AChR deficiency (33). Some patients present in infancy with severe hypotonia and generalized weakness, which includes bulbar and respiratory muscles. Others present in childhood with manifestations that are indistinguishable from autoimmune myasthenia gravis. Common cranial manifestations include variable ptosis, ophthalmoparesis, dysphagia, dysarthria, and chewing difficulties. Weakness also typically affects neck, proximal limb, and respiratory muscles. As with autoimmune myasthenia gravis the weakness is variable and worsens with exertion; in addition, most patients with CMS have some static weakness and their muscles are generally smaller than those of normal subjects of similar age. Clinical clues to the diagnosis of AChR deficiency CMS include the presence of symptoms in early childhood or infancy, association with skeletal anomalies such as high arched palate and scoliosis, history of a similar disorder in siblings, and a beneficial response to cholinesterase inhibitors. AChR deficiency has been observed in association with muscular dystrophy secondary to plectin deficiency (3).

3. Laboratory

Tests for AChR antibodies are negative and creatine kinase levels are normal [except in rare cases associated with plectin deficiency (3)]. The findings on clinical electrodiagnostic studies are variable and depend primarily on the severity and distribution of weakness. There are no R-CMAPs with single stimuli. In severe cases the baseline CMAP is reduced in size and may facilitate more than 200% with exercise or high frequency stimulation (Fig. 6.10). This pattern demonstrates that the severity of the neuromuscular transmission defect is a greater determinant of the pattern of findings on repetitive stimulation studies than is the site or mechanism of the defect. Milder cases produce findings on repetitive stimulation studies that are identical to autoimmune myasthenia gravis. The CMAP amplitude is normal at baseline but displays a decrement of 10–50% with low-frequency stimulation. The decrement is repaired with exercise or high-frequency stimulation and then worsens for several minutes due to postactivation exhaustion. The decrement is frequently repaired with either cholinesterase inhibitors or 3,4-diaminopyridine (Fig. 6.11). In mutations that are associated with a kinetic abnormality of the AChR, the CMAP may decrement rather than repair with higher frequency stimulation. In mild cases the abnormalities on repetitive stimulation may be confined to facial muscles or be seen only in the phase of postactivation exhaustion, even when there is mild generalized muscle weakness. Standard needle EMG shows small varying motor unit potentials. In cases associated with plectin deficiency, fibrillation potentials and other forms of abnormal spontaneous activity can be observed. Single-fiber EMG shows increased jitter and blocking.

Routine muscle biopsy is normal except for atrophy of type 2 fibers. Ultrastructural studies show faint staining for AChR, increased number of

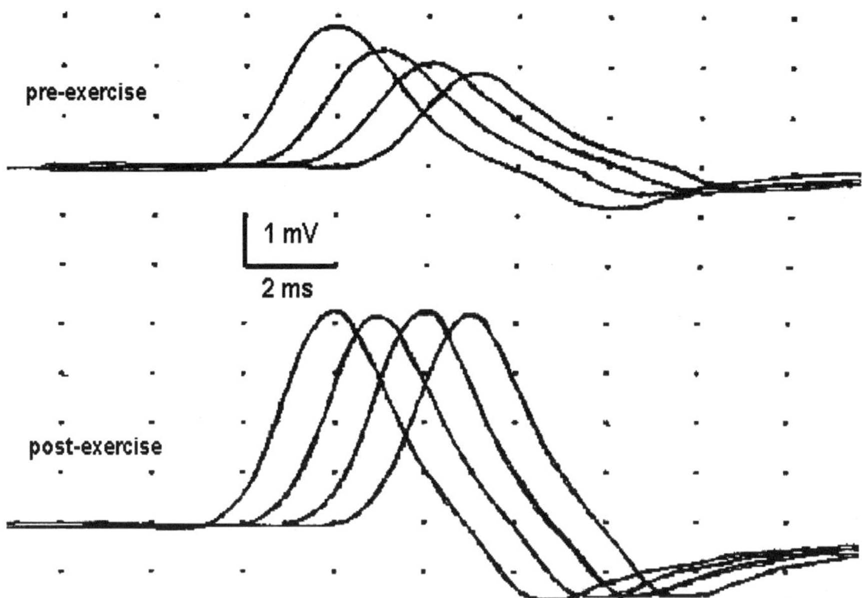

Figure 6.10 Repetitive stimulation of the ulnar nerve at 2 Hz before and immediately after 10 s of isometric exercise in a patient with severe congenital acetylcholine receptor (AChR) deficiency. Microelectrode studies in this patient showed reduced miniature endplate potential amplitudes with normal quantal release, and mild prolongation of the AChR open time consistent with expression of the fetal receptor (γ subunit). Note that the amplitude of the initial compound muscle action potential (CMAP; top group of traces) is below normal. After exercise there (bottom group of traces) there is facilitation of the CMAP amplitude and repair of the decrement.

endplates per muscle fiber, and simplification of the postsynaptic membrane (33). Quantitative staining for AChR with α-bungarotoxin confirms reduced expression of AChR. Microelectrode studies show reduced MEPP and EPP amplitudes with normal quantal content. The duration of endplate currents and single-channel openings is sometimes prolonged, but this is less prominent than in SCCMS. The abnormal kinetics result directly from mutations that alter AChR activation or from overexpression of the γ subunit in cases of severe loss of the ε subunit.

4. Treatment

The response to treatment in cases of primary AChR deficiency is highly variable. Almost all cases improve somewhat with cholinesterase inhibitors.

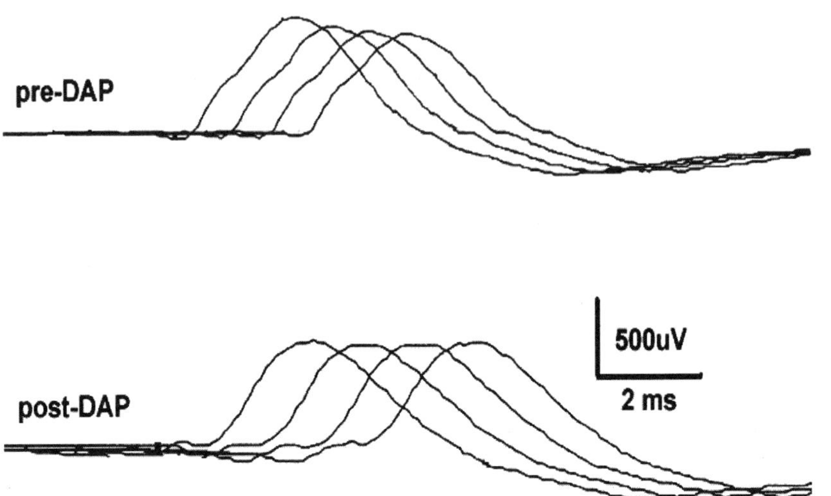

Figure 6.11   Repetitive stimulation of the facial nerve at 2 Hz before and 1 h after administration of 15 mg of 3,4-diaminopyridine (DAP) in a patient with mild congenital AChR deficiency. The compound muscle action potential is recorded over the nasalis muscle. The facial nerve was the only nerve to exhibit a decrement in this patient. Note repair of the decrement following administration of DAP.

Addition of 3,4-diaminopyridine also benefits some patients (38). Medications that increase the availability of ACh to the AChR (i.e., cholinesterase inhibitors or 3,4-diaminopyridine may produce desensitization and worsening of symptoms in cases of severe AChR deficiency. Thus, the effect of cholinesterase inhibitors and 3,4-diaminopyridine effect is sometimes short lived and is followed by subjective worsening of symptoms. As a result, patients should be started on low doses with gradual titration and close monitoring for signs of worsening myasthenic symptoms. For the same reason, some patients with primary AChR deficiency benefit from an intermittent "drug holiday," which may minimize receptor desensitization. Ephedrine also produces subjective benefit in AChR deficiency CMS; however, the mechanism of action is unknown.

H. Sodium Channel CMS (Mutations of Perijunctional Sodium Channels)

Sodium channel CMS is a new syndrome that was recently described as a single case studied by Tsujino et al. in 2002 (56). The patient presented in early adulthood with mental retardation and a history of recurrent acute episodes of respiratory insufficiency and weakness of bulbar muscles since birth. The episodes typically lasted several minutes but no longer than 30 min and recurred several times per month. Nerve conduction studies were normal including brief trains of repetitive stimulation at 2 and 50 Hz. No change was noted after brief exercise. When 10- or 50-Hz repetitive stimulation was continued for 1 min or more, the CMAP amplitude fell dramatically by up to 85% of baseline, and subsequent brief trains of 2-Hz repetitive stimulation elicited a significant decrement. These changes in the CMAP repaired rapidly within several minutes.

An intercostal muscle biopsy was performed and revealed normal ultrastructure of the endplate. Microelectrode studies showed no abnormalities of the MEPP or EPP, or AChR kinetics. However, the muscle fibers were electrically unexcitable. Subsequent genetic studies revealed two mutations in the skeletal muscle sodium channel gene *SCN4A*, S246L in the cytoplasmic linker between S4 and S5, and V1442E in the S3-S4 extracellular linking segment. Expression of the latter mutation in human embryonic kidney cells showed enhancement of fast inactivation of the sodium channel very close to the resting membrane potential and inactivation of the channel with high-frequency stimulation. This defect in perijunctional sodium channels was felt to explain the clinical and electrodiagnostic findings in this novel case.

REFERENCES

1. Ertel EA, Campbell KP, Harpold MM. Nomenclature of voltage-gated calcium channels. Letter to the Editor. Neuron 2000; 25:533–535.
2. Burden SJ. The formation of neuromuscular synapses. Genes Dev 1998; 12:133–148.
3. Banwell BL, Russel J, Fukudome T, Shen X-M, Stilling G, Engel AG. Myopathy, myasthenic syndrome, and epidermolysis bullosa simplex due to plectin deficiency. J Neuropathol Exp Neurol 1999; 58:832–846.
4. Kohara N, Lin TS, Fukudome T, Kimura J, Sakamoto T, Kaji R, Shibasaki H. Pathophysiology of weakness in a patient with congenital end-plate acetylcholinesterase deficiency. Muscle Nerve 2002; 25:585–592.
5. Ohno K, Tsujino A, Brengman J, Harper CM, Bajzer Z, Udd B, Beyring R, Robb S, Kirkham F, Engel AG. Choline acetyltransferase mutations cause myasthenic syndrome associated with episodic apnea in humans. PNAS 2001; 98:2017–2022.
6. Greer M, Schotland M. Myasthenia gravis in the newborn. Pediatrics 1960; 26:101–108.
7. Conomy JP, Levisohn M, Farnoff A. Familial infantile myasthenia gravis: a cause of sudden death in young children. J Pediatr 1975; 87:428–429.
8. Byring RF, Pihko H, Tsujino A, Shen XM, Gustafsson B, Hackman P, Ohno K, Engel AG, Udd B. Congenital myasthenic syndrome associated with episodic apnea and sudden infant death. Neuromusc Disord 2002; 12:548–553.

9. Mora M, Lambert EH, Engel AG. Synaptic vesicle abnormality in familial infantile myasthenia. Neurology 1987; 37:206–214.

10. Walls TJ, Engel AG, Nagel AS, Harper CM, Trastek VF. Congenital myasthenic syndrome associated with paucity of synaptic vesicles and reduced quantal release. Ann N Y Acad Sci 1993; 681:461–468.

11. Albers JW, Faulkner JA, Dorovini-Zis K. Abnormal neuromuscular transmission in an infantile myasthenic syndrome. Ann Neurol 1984; 16:28–34.

12. Bady B, Chauplannaz G, Carrier H. Congenital Lambert-Eaton myasthenic syndrome. J Neurol Neurosurg Psychiaty 1987; 50:476–478.

13. Harper CM. Congenital myasthenic syndromes. In: Brown WF, Bolton CR, Aminoff MJ, eds. Neuromuscular Function and Disease. Philadelphia: WB Saunders, 2002:1687–1696.

14. Maselli RA, Kong DZ, Bowe CM, McDonald CM, Ellis WG, Agius MA, Gomez CM, Richman DP, Wollmann RL. Presynaptic congenital myasthenic syndrome due to quantal release deficiency. Neurology 2001; 57:279–289.

15. Ohno K, Brengman J, Tsujino A, Engel AG. Human endplate acetylcholinesterase deficiency caused by mutations in the collagen-like tail subunit (ColQ) of the asymmetric enzyme. Proc Natl Acad Sci USA 1998; 95:9654–9659.

16. Ohno K, Brengman JM, Felice KJ, Cornblath DR, Engel AG. Congenital endplate acetylcholinesterase deficiency caused by a nonsense mutation and an A→G splice-donor-site mutation at position +3 of the collagen like-tail-subunit gene (COLQ): how does G at position +3 result in aberrant splicing? Am J Hum Genet 1999; 65:635–644.

17. Shapira YA, Sadeh ME, Bergtraum MP, Tsujino A, Ohno K, Shen XM, Brengman J, Edwardson S, Matoth I, Engel AG. Three novel COLQ mutations and variation of phenotypic expressivity due to G240X. Neurology 2002; 58:603–609.

18. Engel AG, Lambert EH, Gomez MR. A new myasthenic syndrome with endplate acetylcholinesterase deficiency, small nerve terminals, and reduced acetylcholine release. Ann Neurol 1977; 1:315–330.

19. Hutchinson DO, Engel AG, Walls TJ, Kakano S, Camp S, Taylor P, Harper CM, Brengman JM. The spectrum of congenital end-plate acetylcholine receptor deficiency. Ann N Y Acad Sci 1993; 681:469–486.

20. Breningstall GN, Kurachek SC, Fugate JH, Engel AG. Treatment of congenital endplate acetylcholinesterase deficiency by neuromuscular blockade. J Child Neurol 1996; 11:345–346.

21. Engel AG, Lambert EH, Mulder DM. A newly recognized congenital myasthenic syndrome attributed to a prolonged open time of the acetylcholine-induced ion channel. Ann Neurol 1982; 11:553–569.

22. Sine SM, Ohno K, Bouzat C, Auerbach A, Milone M, Pruitt JN, Engel AG. Mutation of the acetylcholine receptor α subunit causes a slow-channel myasthenic syndrome by enhancing agonist binding affinity. Neuron 1995; 15:229–239.

23. Engel AG, Ohno K, Milone M, Wang H-L, Nakano S, Bouzat C, Pruitt JN, Hutchinson DO, Brengman JM, Bren N, Sieb JP, Sine SM. New mutations in

acetylcholine receptor subunit genes reveal heterogeneity in the slow-channel congenital myasthenic syndrome. Hum Mol Genet 1996; 5:1217–1227.

24. Gomez CM, Maselli R, Gammack J, Lasalde J, Tamamizu S, Cornblath DR, Lehar M, McNamee M, Kuncl RW. A beta-subunit mutation in the acetylcholine receptor gate causes severe slow-channel syndrome. Ann Neurol 1996; 39:712–723.

25. Milone M, Wang H-L, Ohno K, Fukudome T, Pruitt JN, Bren N, Sine SM, Engel AG. Slow-channel syndrome caused by enhanced activation, desensitization, and agonist binding affinity due to mutation in the M2 domain of the acetylcholine receptor alpha subunit. J Neurosci 1997; 17:5651–5665.

26. Ohno K, Milone M, Brengman JM, Lo Monaco M, Evoli A, Tonali P, Engel AG. Slow-channel congenital myasthenic syndrome caused by a novel mutation in the acetylcholine receptor ε subunit. Neurology 1998; 50:A432.

27. Ohno K, Wang H-L, Shen X-M, Milone M, Bernasconi L, Sine SM, Engel AG. Slow-channel mutations in the center of the M1 transmembrane domain of the acetylcholine receptor α subunit. Neurology 2000; 54(suppl 3):A183.

28. Zeevaert B, Hansen I, Crielaard JM, Wang FC. Slow channel syndrome due to an autosomal translocation at 2q31-9p27. Rev Neurol (Paris) 2002; 158:605–608.

29. Gomez CM, Maselli RA, Vohra BP, Navedo M, Stiles JR, Charnet P, Schott K, Rojas L, Keesey J, Verity A, Wollmann RW, Lasalde-Dominicci J. Novel delta subunit mutation in slow-channel syndrome causes severe weakness by novel mechanisms. Ann Neurol 2002; 51:102–112.

30. Fukudome T, Ohno K, Brengman JM, Engel AG. Quinidine normalizes the open duration of slow-channel mutants of the acetylcholine receptor. Neuroreport 1998; 9:1907–1911.

31. Harper CM, Engel AG. Quinidine sulfate therapy for the slow-channel congenital myasthenic syndrome. Ann Neurol 1998; 43:480–484.

32. Harper CM, Engel AG, Fukodome T, Zochodne DW, Freidli WG. Treatment of slow channel congenital myasthenic syndrome with fluoxetine. Neurology 2002; 58:A329.

33. Engel AG, Ohno K. Congenital myasthenic syndromes. Adv Neurol 2002; 88: 203–215.

34. Ohno K, Wang HL, Milone M, Bren N, Brengman JM, Nakano S, Quiram P, Pruitt JN, Sine SM, Engel AG. Congenital myasthenic syndrome caused by decreased agonist binding affinity due to a mutation in the acetylcholine receptor epsilon subunit. Neuron 1996; 17:157–170.

35. Milone M, Wang HL, Ohno K, Prince R, Fukudome T, Shen XM, Brengman JM, Griggs RC, Sine SM, Engel AG. Mode switching kinetics produced by a naturally occurring mutation in the cytoplasmic loop of the human acetylcholine receptor epsilon subunit. Neuron 1998; 20:575–588.

36. Wang HL, Milone M, Ohno K, Shen XM, Tsujino A, Batocchi AP, Tonali P, Brengman J, Engel AG, Sine SM. Acetylcholine receptor M3 domain: stereochemical and volume contributions to channel gating. Nat Neurosci 1999; 2:226–233.

37. Wang HL, Ohno K, Milone M, Brengman JM, Evoli A, Batocchi AP,

Middleton LT, Christodoulou K, Engel AG, Sine SM. Fundamental gating mechanism of nicotinic receptor channel revealed by mutation causing a congenital myasthenic syndrome. J Gen Physiol 2000; 116:449–462.

38. Harper CM, Engel AG. Treatment of 31 congenital myasthenic syndrome patients with 3,4-diaminopyridine. Neurology 200;54 (suppl 3):A395.

39. Akabas MH, Karlin A. Identification of acetylcholine receptor channel-lining residues in the M1 segment of the α subunit. Biochemistry 1995; 34:12496–12500.

40. Ohno K, Engel AG, Milone M, Brengman JM, Sieb JP, Iannaccone S. A congenital myasthenic syndrome with severe acetylcholine receptor deficiency caused by heteroallelic frameshifting mutations in the epsilon subunit. Neurology 1995; 45(suppl 4):A283.

41. Ohno K, Fukudome T, Nakano S, Milone M, Feasby TE, Tyce GM, Engel AG. Mutational analysis in a congenital myasthenic syndrome reveals a novel acetylcholine receptor epsilon subunit mutation. Soc Neurosci Abstr 1996; 22:234–234.

42. Milone M, Ohno K, Pruitt JN, Brengman JM, Sine SM, Engel AG. Congenital myasthenic syndrome due to frameshifting acetylcholine receptor epsilon subunit mutation. Soc Neurosci Abstr 1996; 22:1942.

43. Ohno K, Quiram P, Milone M, Wang H-L, Harper CM, Pruitt JN, Brengman JM, Pao L, Fischbeck KH, Crawford TO, Sine SM, Engel AG. Congenital myasthenic syndromes due to heteroallelic nonsense/missense mutations in the acetylcholine receptor ε subunit gene: identification and functional characterization of six new mutations. Hum Mol Genet 1997; 6:753–766.

44. Ohno K, Anlar B, Özdirim E, Brengman JM, De Bleecker J, Engel AG. Myasthenic syndromes in Turkish kinships due to mutations in the acetylcholine receptor. Ann Neurol 1998; 44:234–241.

45. Brengman JM, Ohno K, Shen X-M, Engel AG. Congenital myasthenic syndrome due to two novel mutations in the acetylcholine receptor ε subunit gene. Muscle Nerve 1998; 21(suppl 7):S120.

46. Abicht A, Stucka R, Karcagi V, Hercegfalvi A, Horváth R, Mortier W, Schara U, Ramaekers V, Jost W, Brunner J, Janssen G, Seidel U, Schlotter B, Muller-Felber W, Pongratz D, Rudel R, Lochmuller H. A common mutation (ε1267 delG) in congenital myasthenic patients of Gipsy ethnic origin. Neurology 1999; 53:1564–1569.

47. Banwell BL, Russel J, Fukudome T, Shen X-M, Stilling G, Engel AG. Myopathy, myasthenic syndrome, and epidermolysis bullosa simplex due to plectin deficiency. J Neuropathol Exp Neurol 1999; 58:832–846.

48. Croxen R, Newland C, Betty M, Vincent A, Newsom-Davis J, Beeson D. Novel functional ε-subunit polypeptide generated by a single nucleotide deletion in acetylcholine receptor deficiency congenital myasthenic syndrome. Ann Neurol 1999; 46:639–647.

49. Middleton L, Ohno K, Christodoulou K, Brengman JM, Milone M, Neocleous V, Serdaroglu P, Deymeer F, Ozdemir C, Mubaidin A, Horany K, Al-Shehab A, Mavromatis I, Mylonas I, Tsingis M, Zamba E, Pantzaris M, Kyriallis K, Engel AG. Congenital myasthenic syndromes linked to chromosome 17p are

caused by defects in acetylcholine receptor ϵ subunit gene. Neurology 1999; 53:1076–1082.

50. Nichols P, Croxen R, Vincent A, Rutter R, Hutchinson M, Newsom-Davis J, Beeson D. Mutation of the acetylcholine receptor ϵ-subunit promoter in congenital myasthenic syndrome. Ann Neurol 1999; 45:439–443.
51. Ohno K, Anlar B, Engel AG. Congenital myasthenic syndrome caused by a mutation in the Ets-binding site of the promoter region of the acetylcholine receptor ϵ subunit gene. Neuromuscul Disord 1999; 9:131–135.
52. Brengman JM, Ohno K, Milone M, Friedman RL, Feldman RG, Engel AG. Identification and functional characterization of eight novel acetylcholine receptor mutations in six congenital myasthenic syndrome kinships. Neurology 2000; 54(suppl 3):A182–A183.
53. Croxen R, Vincent A, Newsom-Davis J, Beeson D. Myasthenia gravis in a woman with congenital AChR deficiency due to epsilon-subunit mutations. Neurology 2002; 28(58):1563–1565.
54. Abicht A, Stucka R, Schmidt C, Briguet A, Hopfner S, Song IH, Pongratz D, Muller-Felber W, Ruegg MA, Lochmuller H. A newly identified chromosomal microdeletion and an N-box mutation of the AChR epsilon gene cause a congenital myasthenic syndrome. Brain 2002; 125:1005–1013.
55. Ohno K, Engel AG, Shen XM, Selcen D, Brengman J, Harper CM, Tsujino A, Milone M. Rapsyn mutations in humans cause endplate acetylcholine-receptor deficiency and myasthenic syndrome. Am J Hum Genet 2002; 70:875–885.
56. Tsujino A, Harper CM, Engel AG. Unpublished observations.

7

Neurotoxicology of the Neuromuscular Junction

I. INTRODUCTION

The neuromuscular junction (NMJ) is uniquely sensitive to the effects of neurotoxins. Unlike the blood–brain barrier that protects the brain and spinal cord and the blood–nerve barrier that protects peripheral nerve, there are no barriers to protect the NMJ from the deleterious effects of these agents. Worldwide, the most common neurotoxicity of the neuromuscular junction results from envenomation. All forms of NMJ neurotoxicity are characterized by progressive, typically symmetric muscle weakness. Muscles of eye movement or the eyelids are most often involved as are muscles of neck flexion and the pectoral and pelvic girdles. In more severe situations there may be involvement of bulbar and/or respiratory musculature. Cognition and sensation are usually spared unless other elements of the nervous system are simultaneously involved. Muscle stretch reflexes are often preserved or only minimally diminished particularly during the early phases of the illness but may be lost if muscle weakness is severe.

II. CLOSTRIDIAL NEUROTOXINS

The clostridial neurotoxins are gram-positive, anaerobic, spore-forming bacteria found ubiquitously in the environment. The neurotoxins of clostridial organisms produce botulism and tetanus by the inhibition of neurotransmitter release, although the site of action and subsequent clinical picture of each is quite different (1). The clostridial neurotoxins are the most toxic substances known to mankind. The neurotoxins produced from *Clostridium botulinum* are the result of food poisoning, although there are rare incidents of wound botulism and a colonizing infection of neonates. Humans are usually exposed to the neurotoxin produced by *Clostridium tetani* as a result of wounds, and this remains a serious public health problem in developing countries around the world. However, nearly everyone reared in the Western world is protected from tetanus toxin as a result of the ordinary course of childhood immunizations.

A. Botulism

Historically, Justinus Kerner of Germany reported in 1820 cases of what we now know as botulism from ingestion of improperly smoked sausage and later found that ingestion of an extract from the sausage reproduced clinical botulism (2). However, it was Emile van Ermengen of Ghent who identified the bacterial toxin to be the cause of botulism after isolating an anaerobic bacterium from ham and reproducing the disease in laboratory animals following injection of the toxin produced by the bacteria (3). The term *botulism* is derived from the Latin word *botulus*, meaning sausage.

1. Pathogenesis

Botulinum toxin is ubiquitously found in soil and survives under anaerobic and alkaline conditions. The toxin itself is heat labile, but its spores are capable of surviving extreme weather conditions, are very heat resistant, and may survive for decades (4–6). Eight immunlogically distinct serotypes of the toxin exist (A, B, C_α, C_β, D, E, F, and G). Type A is distributed worldwide and predominates in the western part of the United States, Russia Asia, and South America. Type B is also distributed worldwide but is most common in the eastern part of the United States, Europe, and Russia. Types C and D are responsible for outbreaks in animals only. Type C botulism occurs principally in waterfowl and other birds living in an aquatic environment, but other species of mammals have been infected. Type E has been associated with outbreaks in northern Europe, Scandinavia, Canada, Alaska, Japan, and Russia, usually in association with the consumption of fish (7). Type F is very uncommon and has been associated with two outbreaks: one in Denmark and the other in the United States (8). Type G was found in Argentina, but no outbreaks have been recognized (9).

All forms of the toxin block ACh release at the presynaptic motor nerve terminal, parasympathetic and sympathetic ganglia as initially described in

1949 (10). The intracellular target of botulinum toxin appears to be a protein of the ACh vesicle membrane. Like tetanus toxin, botulinum toxin is introduced inside the nerve terminal through a receptor-mediated endocytosis process (11). There is internalization, membrane translocation, and subsequent cytosolic targeting (1). The toxin is a zinc-dependent protease that cleaves protein components of the neuroexocytosis apparatus, thus impairing the docking and fusion of synaptic vesicles to the terminal membrane (12). Different toxin isoforms exert their effects on different proteins (13–16). Type A and E toxins hydrolyze synaptosomal-associated protein-25 (SNAP-25), type B, D, F, and G toxins cleave synaptobrevin, and type C toxin cleaves both SNAP-25 and syntaxin (see Chapter 1). Considered the most potent of neurotoxins, lethality may be seen following exposure doses of 0.05–0.10 ps.

2. Clinical Features

Clinical botulism occurs as five entities: classic or food-borne botulism, infantile botulism, wound botulism, hidden botulism, and iatrogenic botulism. The classic form of botulism occurs after the ingestion of food contaminated by a preformed neurotoxin of *C. botulinum*. Most cases are caused by type A, B, or E. All three forms may cause death. Type E botulism is associated with the ingestion of contaminated seafood. Clinical presentations of type A, B, and E are similar. Type A poisoning is often more severe and longer lasting than type B or E poisoning (17). Infrequent cases of human botulism are caused by type F toxin, and type G organisms have been recovered from human tissues at autopsy (18). Toxin types C and D cause disease in animals (19). The clinical pattern of weakness is stereotypical to all categories, i.e., beginning with cranial nerve dysfunction followed by a descending pattern of weakness. However, the pathogenesis of weakness differs for the various forms. Classic botulism is caused by the ingestion of preformed toxin. In contrast, infant, hidden, and wound botulism are infectious forms of botulism. In the infant and hidden forms, ingested organisms colonize the digestive tract and produce toxin, whereas in wound botulism, bacteria generate toxin following proliferation in the wounds. The iatrogenic form is observed among patients who receive botulinum toxin for therapeutic purposes.

Classic (Food-Borne) Botulism Within hours (usually 2–36) of ingestion of contaminated food, most patients develop signs and symptoms of ocular and bulbar muscle weakness: blurred vision, diplopia, ptosis, ophthalmoplegia, dysarthria, and dysphagia. These symptoms are quickly followed by a descending pattern of muscle weakness affecting the upper limbs, then lower limbs and, in severe cases (most), respiratory muscle weakness. Weakness is usually bilateral but can be asymmetric. Sensation and cognition are typically preserved. Because botulinum toxin inhibits ACh release at cholinergic motor nerve terminals, parasympathetic and sympathetic ganglia signs and symptoms include constipation (most commonly), dry mouth, postural hypotension, urinary retention, and pupillary abnormalities.

Advances in critical care management have reduced the fatality rates to less than 10% (19). Death usually results from the complication of long-term ventilatory support. Recovery from botulism is prolonged and usually complete, but symptoms of general fatigue and autonomic dysfunction can persist for months after normal muscle strength is regained (20). The long recovery process (many months) results from the necessity for nerve terminal sprouting at motor endplates and axonal reinnervation.

Infantile Botulism First identified in the mid-1970s, infantile botulism has become the most frequently reported form of botulism (21). Spores of *C. botulinum* are ingested and germinate in the intestinal tract in infantile botulism. The source of toxin is not identified in most cases. The toxin subsequently is absorbed and carried by the bloodstream to peripheral cholinergic synapses. In contrast to adults, the infant's intestinal tract lacks the protective bacterial flora and the clostridium-inhibiting bile acids. Consequently, the infant intestinal tract is more susceptible to colonization by toxin-producing *C. botulinum*. Most cases occur before the age of 6 months. Typically constipation is the initial symptom, and often the infant has listlessness, lethargy, a weak cry, difficulty feeding or sucking, and weakness of bulbar and limb muscles. Epidemiologic studies implicate honey consumption as a significant risk factor for infant botulism (22). Microbiological analysis of honey products indicates the presence of clostridial spores (mostly type B) in up to 25% of products (23,24). For these reasons, the American Academy of Pediatrics suggests that honey should not be fed to children younger than 1 year.

Wound Botulism Wound botulism, initially reported in 1943, has previously been a rare disorder occurring in patients with traumatic wound complications. However, it has increased dramatically in frequency since the early 1990s in intravenous drug users (25–29). *C. botulinum* has been recovered from abscesses forming at injection sites in drug abusers and has also been recovered from the nasal passages of cocaine sniffers (30). The clinical features of wound botulism are identical to those of the classic form of the disease. Similarly, treatment is the same along with the appropriate management of the specific wound (31).

Hidden Botulism A small number of patients with clinical botulism show no obvious source of toxin. In these cases, there is no known food contamination, no wound, and no history of drug abuse (32,33). For this reason, such patients stated to have the hidden form of botulism. They are felt to represent adult variations of infant botulism, i.e., adults who accommodate toxin-producing clostridial bacteria in their intestinal tract. Epidemiologically there is an abnormality of the gastrointestinal tract, such as prior diverting surgery, achlorhydria, Crohn's disease, or recent antibiotic treatment (34).

Iatrogenic Botulism There is potential for symptomatic complications from excess botulinum toxin as this toxin has become increasingly utilized for focal dystonia, spasticity, and, most recently, cosmetic purposes. Its effect is both local at the site of injection in muscle and (to a lesser degree) remote from the site of injection (35). Dysphagia is a common side effect of botulinum injection for laryngeal dysphonia, typically lasting for about 2 weeks. On occasion the dysphagia is severe, especially when patients report some degree of pretreatment dysphagia or when both sternocleidomastoid muscles are injected with large doses of toxin (36,37). A prospective study of botulinum toxin injection complications for cervical dystonia showed that prior to treatment 11% of patients had symptoms of dysphagia while 22% had radiologic evidence for abnormal peristalsis. After injections of botulinum toxin new symptoms of dysphagia developed in an additional 33% of patients, and 50% developed new peristaltic abnormalities by radiographic study (37). Single-fiber EMG (SFEMG), the most sensitive marker of disturbed synaptic transmission, of the forearm muscle following treatment of cervical dystonia and hemifacial spasm shows abnormal increase in mean jitter. Studies performed 6 weeks after treatment noted an increased fiber density indicating reinnervation (38). In addition, mild abnormalities of cardiovascular reflexes suggest distant effects on autonomic function. Lambert-Eaton syndrome (LES) has been unmasked in a patient following therapeutic botulinum toxin injection (39). Myasthenic crisis has been reported following injections of botulinum toxin (40).

Bioterrorism The potential for intentional poisoning with botulinum toxin has become a major concern in the 21st century. In 1996 at least 17 countries were suspected to include or to be developing biological agents in their offensive weapons programs (41). This number has more than doubled since the initial ratification in 1972 of the *Convention on the Prohibition of the Development, Production and Stockpiling of Bacteriological (Biological) and Toxin Weapons and on Their Destruction* treaty (42). Four of the countries listed by the U.S. government as "state sponsors of terrorism" (Iran, Iraq, North Korea, and Syria) have developed, or are believed to be developing, botulinum toxin as a weapon of mass destruction (43). With the economic difficulties in Russia after the demise of the Soviet Union, some of the thousands of scientists formerly employed by its bioweapons program have been recruited by nations attempting to develop biological weapons (44). The increased interest in botulism as a weapon of terror is in part due to the relative ease in which the toxin can be produced, and because of its high lethality in small quantities. The LD50 is estimated to be 0.001 µg/kg (45). The ability to disseminate large quantities of the toxin by aerosols can produce mass casualties.

Development and use of botulinum toxin as a biological weapon began in the 1940s (46). The head of the Japanese biological warfare group admitted to feeding cultures of *C. botulinum* to prisoners with lethal effect during that country's occupation of Manchuria in the 1930s (47). The U.S. biological weapons program first produced botulinum toxin during World War II due to concerns that Germany had weaponized botulinum toxin (48). RISE, a terrorist group of the early 1970s, reportedly planned to introduce botulinum toxin into the Chicago water supply (49). Iraq revealed to the United Nations that during the Persian Gulf War 19,000 L of concentrated botulinum toxin was prepared of which 11,200 L was loaded into specially designed SCUD missile warheads (50,51). This total amount is more than three times what is necessary to annihilate the entire human race. Furthermore, Aum Shinrikyo, the apocalyptic cult that used sarin in the 1995 terrorist attack on the Tokyo subway system, had produced and stockpiled quantities of botulinum toxin and other biological agents (52). Despite being one of the signatories of the 1972 *Biological and Toxin Weapons Convention*, the then–Soviet Union subsequently produced botulinum toxin for use as a weapon. Botulinum toxin was one of several agents tested at the Soviet site Aralsk-7 on Vozrozhdeniye Island in the Aral Sea (53).

3. Differential Diagnosis

The differential diagnosis of botulism includes other disorders of neuro-muscular transmission, e.g., myasthenia gravis and LES (Table 7.1). It is suggested by the combination of a descending pattern of weakness in association with autonomic dysfunction. The diurnal variability in symptoms and findings will often distinguish these disorders from botulism. Landry-Guillain-Barré (LGB) syndrome, tick paralysis, Miller-Fisher variant of LGB syndrome (MFV), and diphtheritic neuropathy are also considerations. The latter two entities are often the most difficult to distiguish from botulism. The pattern of descending weakness is a clinical feature of botulism that distin-guishes it from the classical form of LGB, which usually presents with ascending weakness. The MFV of LGB syndrome, with ocular and bulbar abnormalities, may present a more difficult diagnostic challenge. The preser-vation of deep tendon reflexes would be more in keeping with botulism than with LGB and MFV. The pharyngeal-cervical-brachial variant of LGB has clinical features similar to botulism. In contrast to botulism, however,

Table 7.1   Differential Diagnosis of Botulism

Disease entity	Characteristic features
Botulism	Initial oculobulbar then rapid descending pattern of weakness, autonomic involvement
Landry-Guillain-Barré syndrome	Rapid ascending pattern of weakness; loss of muscle stretch reflexes, elevated CSF protein
Myasthenia gravis	Variable weakness of ocular, limb and bulbar muscle groups; preserved reflexes
Lambert-Eaton syndrome	Variable weakness (often less than MG); absent or diminished reflexes, autonomic involvement
Tick paralysis	Ascending pattern of weakness; typically children
Diptheritic neuropathy	Tonsilar exudates; peripheral neuropathy (late)
Poliomyelitis	Acute, rapid, asymmetric weakness, CSF pleocytosis with elevated protein
Miller-Fisher variant of LGB	See Landry-Guillain-Barré syndrome; ataxia

patients with the pharyngeal-cervical-brachial variant of LGB have serum antiganglioside antibodies. Infants with suspected botulism must be assessed for the myriad of other causes of hypotonia as well as poliomyelitis and spinal muscular atrophy. In many instances, the rapidity of the course of illness will be the defining feature. The diagnosis of wound botulism should be considered whenever a patient with a wound develops bulbar signs and a rapidly evolving descending pattern of weakness.

4.   Laboratory Diagnosis

A diagnosis of botulism can be established with the detection of *C. botulinum* organism in the stool or of botulinum toxin in the patient's serum, stool, or wound. *C. botulinum* is found in the stool of 60% of patients with botulism but virtually never in the stools of healthy adults (33). Rarely *C. botulinum* can be isolated from the stool of normal infants (54). The toxin type can be identified using mouse bioassay studies with antitoxin neutralization. The suspected food, if available, should also be tested for toxin and bacteria at the Centers for Disease Control (CDC) or appropriate state health facility (19). Laboratory studies are not confirmatory in all instances. This is especially true when the collection of the specimens is deferred for days after the onset of symptoms. If the delay in securing serum samples is more than 2 days after ingestion of the toxin, the chances of obtaining a positive test are less than 30%. Only 36% of stool cultures are positive after 3 days (55).

Electrodiagnostic studies may provide presumptive evidence of botulism in patients with suspected botulism in whom bioassay studies for botulinum toxin and stool cultures or when test results are pending during the early phase of the illness (56–58). The typical electrophysiologic abnormality is a reduced compound muscle action potential (CMAP) amplitude in response to single supramaximal nerve stimulation in clinically affected muscles. Motor conduction velocities are preserved and sensory studies are normal. A decremental response may be seen with slow rates (2 Hz, 3 Hz) of repetitive nerve stimulation. A modest facilitatory response is seen with following brief (10 s), vigorous volitional exercise or following rapid rates (>40 Hz) of stimulation. The degree of facilitation in botulism is usually between 30% and 100% and is often less than that seen in LES (58,57). Needle EMG examination demonstrates an increased number of fibrillation potentials and short-duration, polyphasic motor unit potentials. SFEMG studies reveal increased neuromuscular jitter and impulse blocking, which become less marked after activation (59–61).

5. Management

The primary treatment for severe botulism is high quality intensive care with special attention to respiratory function and, subsequently, an aggressive rehabilitation program. Careful observation of patients for progression of limb and respiratory muscle weakness is mandatory. Recovery in severe cases may take many months because regrowth of nerve and regeneration of new motor endplates is required (62). Other treatments are less effective or speculative. The role of antitoxin administration is controversial. Lack of efficacy has been demonstrated in many cases. Numerous complications have followed including allergic reactions (63,64). Serious side effects occur in as many as 20% of patients (19). A 2% rate of anaphylaxis has been reported, which is high compared to most other equine products (63). Most commercially available botulinum antitoxins are of equine origin, and allergic responses are attributed to antibody products of nonhuman origin. Beneficial effects are more likely with treatment for type E botulism than with types A or B. Efficacy is diminished in many cases because of the time lag in administration of the antitoxin. To be of benefit, antitoxin must be given early, before the toxin is bound to and translocated into the nerve terminal. Administration after the onset of clinical symptoms is not protective (65).

Because the incidence of botulinum poisoning is so low in the United States, vaccination of the general public is unwarranted. Because of the possible use of botulinum toxin as a biological warfare agent, the U.S. Army has developed vaccine and antiserum to botulinum toxin and nearly all stocks of these products are presently held by the military. The vaccine, developed in the 1950s by the military at Fort Detrick, Maryland, protects from serotypes A–E (66).

Guanidine and the aminopyridines (4-AP, 3,4-diaminopyridine) are reported to improve ocular and limb muscle strength in some patients (67–74). Unfortunately, the aminopyridines have little or no effect in reversing respiratory muscle weakness (75). Similarly, the aminopyridines were ineffective in treating mice exposed to botulinum toxin and their use only prolonged the time to death (76,77). Both drugs facilitate the release of ACh from nerve terminals. The aminopyridines are potassium channel–blocking agents that increase calcium influx through presynaptic voltage-gated membrane channels. Aminopyridine therapy can be complicated by the development of seizures and insomnia (78,79). The serious side effects of guanidine (bone marrow suppression and nephritis) are dose and time related, thus limiting the use of this drug (69,80).

B. Tetanus

The word tetanus is derived from the Greek *tetanos*, which is derived from the term *teinein*, meaning "to stretch." Tetanus has been recognized since the 5th century B.C. when discovered by Hippocrates but the modern era of understanding tetanus begins in 1884 (81). Carle and Rattone first produced tetanus in animals by injecting them with pus from a deceased human tetanus patient in 1884. During the same year, Nicolaier produced tetanus in animals by injecting them with samples of soil. In 1889, Kitasato isolated the organism from a human victim, showed that it produced disease when injected into animals, and reported that the toxin could be neutralized by specific antibodies. In 1897, Nocard demonstrated the protective effect of passively transferred antitoxin, and passive immunization in humans was used during World War I. Tetanus toxoid was developed by Descombey in 1924, and the effectiveness of active immunization was demonstrated in World War II (81).

Tetanus is caused by the neurotoxin tetanospasmin that is produced by *C. tetani*, a gram-positive, spore-forming, motile, obligate anaerobic organism. The organism has a distinctive drumstick-like appearance due to the terminal formation of the spore. Tetanospasmin abolishes the inhibitory spinal reflex arcs, allowing excitatory reflexes to predominate (1). This results in increased muscle tone and spasms that are the cardinal manifestations of the disease. Tetanus is predominantly seen in neonates and children in developing countries where immunization programs remain inadequate (82–85). In the Western world, tetanus is most often encountered in patients older than 50 years, often after a minor injury acquired outdoors, and in drug addicts (86–88). Tetanus occurs in three clinical forms: localized, generalized, and cephalic.

1.   Pathogenesis

Clostridium tetani is a worldwide ubiquitous organism. The spores are relatively resistant to drying and various disinfectants (e.g., phenol, formaldehyde, and chloramine) require more than 15 h to kill the spores. Autoclaving, aqueous iodine and 2% glutaraldehyde at pH 7.5–8.5 are destructive. However, the spores of *C. tetani* may survive for decades, especially in manure-rich soil. Spores may also be found in animal and human feces and in domestic dust. Spores germinate into the vegetative form under appropriate anaerobic conditions, particularly in wounds associated with necrosis. Two exotoxins, tetanolysin and tetanospasmin, are elaborated by the vegetative form.

Tetanolysin is not thought to be involved in the pathogenesis of tetanus. Tetanospasmin, a zinc metalloprotease, is formed under plasmid control as a single 1315- amino-acid polypeptide chain that is cleaved by bacterial protease to form a heterodimer consisting of a 100-kD heavy chain and a 50-kD light chain joined by a disulfide bond (89). Biophysical studies indicate that the toxin is similar to other three-dimensional toxins (e.g., diphtheria toxin) and is folded into three functionally distinct domains that have importance in the role of cell intoxication (90). The carboxyl terminal of the H chain in primarily responsible for neurospecific binding, the amino terminal of the same chair is responsible for cell penetration and the L domain is responsible for the blockade of neurotransmitter exocytosis (1).

Cell intoxication occurs in four steps: cell binding, internalization, membrane translocation, and targeted cell dysfunction (91). When tetanospasmin is released in infected wounds, the C fragment binds to specific axonal membrane gangliosides (GDIb and GT) predominantly at the terminals of α motor and, to a lesser extent, autonomic neurons. The toxin is then internalized inside the lumen of synaptic vesicles after vesicle reuptake. It is translocated from the endosomes to the cytosol where it is then transported by retrograde transsynaptic axonal transport to the cell bodies of inhibitory interneurons in the spinal cord and brainstem. The light-chain fragment causes proteolytic cleavage of the synaptosomal-associated protein complexes, particularly the synaptobrevin vesicle-associated membrane protein, and prevents neurotransmitter release [glycine in the spinal cord and γ-aminobutyric acid (GABA) in the brain]. This disinhibition results in uncontrolled excessive efferent discharge of motor and autonomic neurons resulting in muscle rigidity, spasms, and autonomic dysfunction characteristic of tetanus. The amino acid structures of botulinum toxin and tetanospasmin, are partially homologous. The estimated human lethal dose of tetanospasmin is less than 2.5 ng/kg.

2. Clinical Features

Three clinical forms of tetanus exist: localized, generalized, and cephalic. The incubation period for tetanus is usually 7 days after injury but varies from 3 to 21 days although the syndrome may appear as early as 24 h or may be delayed for several months (92). The incubation period is directly related to the distance of the injury from the central nervous system. Injuries to the head and neck are likely to be associated with significantly shorter incubation periods than injuries to the lower extremities. Incubation time is a prognosticator of ultimate outcome. The shorter the incubation period, the greater the likelihood of death. In Western society, tetanus is a disease of older individuals and typically due to a small puncture wound. It is a disease of infants and children in developing countries primarily due to the lack of immunization programs.

Localized Tetanus Localized tetanus is uncommon in humans and is generally mild in severity (93). It accounts for 13% of cases in one reported series but has not been well characterized in the literature (86). Localized tetanus produces painful muscle spasms in a restricted area in proximity to the site of injury. Death occurs in less than 1% of cases. The muscle spasms may persist for several weeks to a few months before spontaneously subsiding. In some instances, they may be the first manifestation of generalized tetanus.

Generalized Tetanus Generalized tetanus is the most common form. Typically the illness starts with spasms of the muscles of mastication, producing trismus or "lockjaw." This is quickly followed by involvement of other muscles of the head and neck causing dysphagia, and proceeding to involvement of the axial muscles, shoulders, hips, and limbs. Symptoms abate in reverse order. Abdominal involvement produces a rigid abdomen and sustained contraction of the facial muscles produces the classic grimace called *risus sardonicus*. The sustained contraction of paraspinal musculature produces the characteristic opisthotonus position, a finding that occurs early in the disease perhaps due to the short length of the nerve innervating these muscles. Death as the result of asphyxia due to laryngospasm may occur. Auditory or tactile stimuli often produce paroxysmal, generalized, repetitive spasms (tentanospasms) that become exhausting to the patient.

Autonomic dysfunction may occur, particularly in severe cases. Cardiac and vasomotor instability and thermoregulatory disturbances are common.

Labile or sustained hypertension, hyperpyrexia, excessive sweating, tachycardia, and other arrhythmias may occur. Severe cardiac instability may lead to cardiac arrest and death.

Cephalic Tetanus Cephalic tetanus is rare (94). It occurs following localized infections about the head and neck, typically in the distribution of the facial nerve. It is characterized by unilateral facial paralysis, trismus, nuchal rigidity, pharyngeal spasms causing dysphagia, frequent laryngeal spasms, and facial stiffness on the unaffected side. There is a risk of death from asphyxia. There may be associated involvement of other cranial nerves: glossopharyngeal, vagus, and rarely, the oculomotor nerves. The incubation period is short and may progress to generalized tetanus.

3. Differential Diagnosis

Tetanus should not be confused with other disorders so long as the clinician has thought of it. The differential diagnosis of tetanus depends on the clinical pattern of presentation (Table 7.2). Those patients presenting with trismus should also be evaluated for the presence of dental caries, peritonsilar and retropharyngeal abscesses, tonsillitis, parotid gland abnormalities, and tem-

Table 7.2 Differential Diagnosis of Tetanus

Disease entity	Characteristic features
Tetanus	Initial oculobulbar then rapid descending pattern of weakness, autonomic involvement
Retropharyngeal or dental abscess	Pseudotrismus, localized findings to the jaw; fever
Meningitis	CSF pleocytosis with elevated protein
Encephalitis	Sensorial clouding; CSF pleocytosis with elevated protein
Rabies	Trismus is not present; usually incubation period is longer. CSF pleocytosis
Hypocalcemic tetany	
Phenothiazine-induced dystonia	Known exposure to drug; multifocal dystonic posturing
Epilepsy	Witnessed seizure, incontinence, postictal state
Strychnine poisoning	Trismus appears late; low serum calcium

promandibular dysfunction (95–102). Less commonly, trismus may be seen with meningitis and encephalitis (103–105). Trismus is not associated with hypocalcemic tetany and in this disorder, the trunk is often spared and the patient will exhibit Trousseau and Chvostek signs. Syndromes of continuous muscle fiber activity (stiff-person syndrome) evolve more insidiously and typically only rarely involve the muscles of the face. However, other elements of the disorder are similar with axial stiffness and spasms provoked by a variety of stimuli (106–108). Antibodies to glutamic acid decarboxylase may be present. Electrodiagnostic features also help to differentiate between the two.

4. Laboratory Diagnosis

There are no laboratory findings characteristic of tetanus. The diagnosis is entirely clinical and does not depend on bacteriologic confirmation. Clues to the diagnosis include a wound or recent history of a wound, no clear history of tetanus toxoid immunization, headache, low-grade fever, irritability, and restlessness. However, the absence of a wound should not preclude a diagnosis of tetanus, and the illness has been reported in those who have been previously immunized (109). *Clostridium tetani* is recovered from the wound in only 30% of cases and, not infrequently, is isolated from patients who do not have tetanus. Routine blood work is typically normal as is the cerebrospinal fluid. Electrodiagnostic studies demonstrate bursts of motor unit potentials, similar to voluntary contraction, during tetanospasim. Characteristically, there is a shortening or absence of the silent period after supramaximal nerve stimulation (110–113).

5. Management

The primary treatment for tetanus is directed at the elimination of the source of toxin; the cleansing and thorough debridement of the wound; the use of appropriate antibiotics; the neutralization of circulating unbound toxins and adequate immunization to prevent infection. Modern critical care units has decreased the fatality rates significantly in developed countries (114–117). Human tetanus immunoglobulin should be given immediately at the time of diagnosis to prevent further spread of the toxin. Tetanus antitoxin does not cross the blood–brain barrier and has no effect on toxin already bound to neurons. Intrathecal antitoxin administration has yet to be of proven benefit.

Tracheostomy and ventilatory support are often necessary when there is laryngeal spasm. Sedatives, muscle relaxants, and a quiet environment are used to reduce rigidity and control tetanospasms. Typically, diazepam is given at a dosage of 0.5–1.0 mg/kg per day either by infusion or in divided doses. An alternative is the intravenous infusion of midazolam (118). Larger doses run the risk of respiratory depression. Baclofen, intravenously, has the advantage of managing spasms and preserving voluntary movement and respiration

(119–121). Dantrolene and propofol have been used in small series with variable results (120). Neuromuscular blockade may be necessary when spasms are refractory to other measures.

The management of the autonomic disturbances may be very problematic (122–125). Hypotension can be managed with fluid load and, if needed, inotropic support. Hypertensive episodes can be treated with short-acting β-blockers, such as an intravenous infusion of esmolol or with labetalol (126). However, the use of β-blockers is not without risk particularly in those patients whose blood pressure and heart rate vary widely and are likely to become either hypotensive or bradycardic (120).

The key to the management of tetanus is prevention. Tetanus immunization, usually combined with diphtheria and pertussis, is recommended for all children older than 6 who have no contraindication to vaccination. Three of the doses are administered usually at 6- to 8-week intervals while the last is delayed for at least 6 months after the third injection. Booster injection should be administered upon entry to school (age 5–6) and at 10-year intervals thereafter. Individuals who have simple wounds should receive tetanus vaccine if they have not been previously in the past 10 years or if the vaccination history is not known. If the wound is severe the same recommendations are employed except that the interval since last immunization is shortened to 5 years.

C. Envenomation

Most biological toxins of animal origin affect the cholinergic system and either facilitates the release of neurotransmitter from the presynaptic nerve terminal or block the AChR. In general, bites from snakes, scorpions, and ticks are more common during summer months when they are inadvertently encountered. In contrast, exposure to marine toxins may occur at any time as they are acquired through ingestion and less rarely by injection or penetration. Specific geographic loci can be demonstrated for each of these vectors. For example, tick envenomation predominates in states west of the Rocky Mountains, the western provinces of Canada, and Australia. The geography of snake envenomation is species specific. The cobras are found in Asia and Africa, the kraits in Southeast Asia, the mambas in Africa, the coral snake in North America, and the sea snakes in the waters of the Pacific near Australia and New Guinea.

1. Arthropods

The venoms of the phylum *Arthropod* have been known since antiquity and are used to incapacitate prey for feeding or as a defense against predators (127). Few of the arthropods, however, produce toxicity at the NMJ. The toxicity at the NMJ occurs by three mechanisms (Table 7.3). In the first there is an initial augmentation of ACh release followed by presynaptic depletion of neurotransmitter. The second causes a facilitation of ACh release without a subsequent presynaptic depletion of neurotransmitter. The third mechanism causes a depletion of ACh release without a subsequent presynaptic depletion of neurotransmitter. Where once these envenomation carried a 12–25% mortality; in the last few decades these intoxications are rarely fatal with the improvement of critical care facilities (128,129).

Spider Bites Only a few spider venoms affect the NMJ. The funnel web spider and the redback spider of Australia are the most dangerous spiders in this group. In North America, only the bite of the black widow spider (*Lactrodectus*) is of concern. The most common victims of a black widow spider bite are small boys, perhaps because of their inquisitiveness around nooks and crannies.

Lathrotoxins found in the venoms from *Latrodectus* cause systemic lathrodectism. These toxins produce a marked facilitation in neurotransmitter release by depolarization of the presynaptic nerve terminal and increasing Ca^{2+} influx into the nerve terminal at all neurosecretory synapses including the NMJ (130–132). There is subsequent depletion of neurotransmitter from the nerve terminal resulting in a blockade of synaptic transmission. It has been demonstrated that this toxin exerts its effects on the presynaptic nerve terminal by several mechanisms. The toxin binds to neurexin and thereby activates the presynaptic protein complex of neurexin, syntaxin, synaptotagmin, and the N-type calcium channel to massively facilitate ACh release (133). Neurotransmitter release in nerve–muscle preparations, as measured by MEPP frequency, increases several hundred fold within a few minutes (134). There is a subsequent depletion of synaptic vesicles, disruption of the highly organized active zone region of the presynaptic nerve terminal thus inhibiting the docking of synaptic vesicles to the terminal membrane, and effective recycling of vesicular membrane (135–140).

Symptoms from a black widow spider bite begin within minutes of the bite and reflect the massive release of neurotransmitter from peripheral, autonomic, and central synapses (141). Severe muscle rigidity and cramps precedes generalized muscle weakness due to the depolarizing neuromuscular blockade. A black widow spider bite is rarely fatal but cardiovascular collapse

Table 7.3 Mechanisms of Arthropod Blockade of Synaptic Transmission

1. Facilitation of ACh release with subsequent exhaustion of neurotransmitter
2. Facilitation of ACh release without subsequent exhaustion of neurotransmitter
3. Depletion of ACh release with subsequent exhaustion of neurotransmitter

may occur in elderly persons or in young children. Treatment is primarily supportive. The administration of calcium gluconate may be helpful in alleviating the severe muscle cramps and rigidity (142). Magnesium salts may be beneficial by reducing neurotransmitter release (141). The administration of a horse serum antivenom is very effective in rapidly reversing the neurotoxic effects (143).

Tick Paralysis   Tick paralysis is a worldwide disorder that was first described at the turn of the 20th century in North America and Australia, although there is vague reference to an earlier case in 1824 (129,144–146). It is one of several kinds of neuromuscular disorders that may result from tick venom exposure. Tick paralysis results from the introduction of a neurotoxin from one of more than 60 tick species (147,148). In North America, the *Dermacentor andersoni, D. variabilis, D. occidentalis, Amblyomma americanum, and A. maculatum* are toxic. The vectors in Europe and the Pacific are *Ixodes ricinus* and *I. cornuatus* and in Australia it is *I. holocyclus.* Geographically, tick paralysis is more common in states west of the Rocky Mountains and in British Columbia and Alberta (149).

The symptoms are stereotypical. Within 5–6 days of attachment, there is a prodrome of paresthesiae, headache, malaise, nausea, and vomiting. The prodromal period parallels the feeding pattern of the tick. Over the next 24–48 h an ascending paralysis occurs. It begins symmetrically in the lower extremities and progresses to involve the trunk and arms. In most instances when a tick is found, it is fully engorged. In contrast to the vectors found most commonly in North America (*Dermacentor* and *Amblyomma species*), the weakness of the Australian tick is more severe and much slower to resolve. In these patients there is often a worsening of symptoms 24–48 h following the removal of the tick (150). Sensation is preserved, but muscle stretch reflexes are often diminished or not present suggesting the LGB Syndrome (Table 7.4),

Table 7.4   Comparative Features of Ascending Paralysis

Clinical and laboratory features	Tick paralysis	Landry-Guillain-Barré syndrome
Rate of progression	Hours to days	Days to 1–2 weeks
Sensory loss	Absent	Mild
Muscle stretch reflexes	Diminished or absent	Diminished or absent
Time to recovery	< 24 h after tick removal	Weeks to months
CSF WBC count	< 10 per mm^2	< 10 per mm^2
CSF protein	Normal	Elevated

a common misdiagnosis (151). There is no demonstrable response to cholinesterase inhibitors (152,153). There is some indication of an association between the proximity of the site of attachment to the brain and the severity of the disease. Resolution of symptoms is dependent in part on how quickly the tick is removed, suggesting that the amount of muscle weakness is a dose-dependent process. Often improvement begins within hours of removing those paralyses due to the *Dermacentor* species and continues over several days. Antitoxin may be of benefit in some situation, but the high frequency of acute allergic reactions makes their widespread use less feasible (154). However, prolonged weakness has been reported (155). Death may occur due to respiratory failure from severe bulbar and respiratory muscle weakness, and the clinical picture may be clouded by the presences of CNS findings (156,149).

The improvement in critical care facilities over the last few decades make envenomation intoxications rarely fatal; previously they carried a 12–25% mortality (128,129). Children are more prone to the disorder than adults. This may be due in part to their play habits or their lower body mass relative to the amount of toxin acquired. The head and neck is the most common site for tick attachment, although any part of the body may be the site of attachment. Some studies suggest that girls are more often affected because their long hair allows the tick to remain hidden for longer periods and therefore allows prolonged feeding (151,157). The identification of the presence of a tick bite is often delayed. This results in the misdiagnosis of the problem and has been confused with LGB syndrome, myasthenia gravis, spinal cord disease, periodic paralysis, diphtheria, heavy-metal intoxication, insecticide poisoning, porphyria, and hysteria (151,158). In many instances, the tick is located by the nurse, the house officer, the mortician, or at the time of autopsy (128, 151,159). Careful, systematic inspection of the scalp, neck, and perineum, often with a fine-toothed comb, is necessary to locate the tick.

In most instances, the characteristics of the toxin from various species are not known. Radiolabeling studies with monoclonal antibodies have demonstrated the presence of toxin in salivary glands (160). The most potent toxin is from the Australian tick, *Ixodus holocyclus*. The mechanism by which weakness occurs following tick envenomation remains controversial. Holocyclotoxin, isolated from the salivary glands of female ticks, causes a temperature-dependent blockade of neurally evoked release of ACh from the nerve terminal (161). Others also have suggested a block of neuromuscular transmission (162). The tick paralysis of the *Dermacentor* species is understood less well. Some authors feel that there is no direct abnormality of synaptic transmission; rather, they postulate an abnormality due to impaired depolarization of the nerve terminal with secondary impairment of ACh release (163,164). There are variable reports of prolonged distal motor latencies, slowed nerve conduction velocities, and reduced CMAP amplitudes (6,148, 165–167).

Scorpion Bites The peptides contained in scorpion neurotoxins may cause a variety of neurologic effects, the most significant of which are those that modulate Na^+ and K^+ channel function. However, some affect the neuromuscular junction and produce an enhanced presynaptic depolarization resulting in release of neurotransmitter from synaptic vesicles (168). Increased excretion of catecholamines has been demonstrated after scorpion sting and may relate to the primary effect of the venom or to a secondary sympathetic adrenergic surge. Treatment is nonspecific and focuses on maintaining respiratory and cardiac as well as coagulation function. Antivenom does not appear to have any efficacy (169,170).

2. Snakebites

Envenomation by snakebite occurs from four major groups; Viperidae (true vipers) *Crotalidae* (rattlesnakes and pit vipers), *Elapidae* (American coral snake, cobras, kraits, mambas), and *Hydrophiodae* (sea snakes). Neuromuscular blockade occurs primarily from the *Elapidae* and *Hydrophiodae* species (171–173). One *Crotalidae* species, *Croatulus durissus terrificus*, a South American rattlesnake, has a very potent neuromuscular blocking venom. Other rattlesnakes and pit vipers act through hematologic and cardiovascular mechanisms. Venom is produced and stored in salivary glands, and inoculation occurs through fangs or modified premaxillary teeth (171).

An in-depth discussion of the pharmacology of snake toxins is beyond the scope of this chapter. These may act either presynaptically or postsynaptically. Presynaptic toxins, β-neurotoxins (β-bungarotoxin, notexin, and taipoxin), act to inhibit the normal release of ACh from the presynaptic cell of the NMJ. Often, there is an initial augmentation of ACh release followed by presynaptic depletion of neurotransmitter. They tend to be more potent than postsynaptic toxins. Postsynaptic neurotoxins, α-neurotoxins, produce a curare-mimetic, nondepolarizing neuromuscular block but vary in the degree to which the block is reversible in the laboratory. Most venoms are chemically an admixture of both types of neurotoxins, although one type may predominate in a given venom. For example, the venom of the Thai cobra is composed primarily of a single postsynaptic neurotoxin (174). In contrast, the venom of *Bungarus multicintus* contains β-bungarotoxin, four other presynaptic toxins, α-bungarotoxin, and two other postsynaptic toxins (175). The venoms of *Hydrophiodae* species is more toxic than land snakes although the amount of toxin injected by sea snakes is smaller than that injected by land-based snakes (176,177). The α-neurotoxins (postsynaptic), like curare, bind to the nicotinic AChR of muscle. They have a slower onset of action, a longer duration of effect, and are 15–40 times more potent than *d*-tubocurarine (178). There are numerous subforms of β-neurotoxins (presynaptic). Most have a phospholipase component that is essential for the presynaptic effects of the toxin. All suppress the release of ACh from the nerve terminal although there is some variability in the precise mechanism by which this occurs. In experimental preparations, toxins from different species will potentiate each other, suggesting different binding sites at the NMJ (179). Taipoxin from the Australian and Papua New Guinean taipan snake is unique. In addition to its potent presynaptic blockade of synaptic transmission, it also has a direct myotoxic component. This produces rapid muscle necrosis and degeneration. There is species variation in the susceptibility to toxin exposure. The venom of the Australian mulga snake is fatal in humans, will produce ptosis in monkeys, and does not appear to produce a neuromuscular block in the rabbit (180,181).

The clinical course of snake envenomation follows a specific pattern. After the bite of a pit viper or cobra, there is local pain. Pain is often absent following the bite of other *Elapidae and Hydrophiodae* organisms. Swelling typically occurs within 1 h following bites from *Viperidae, Crotalidae,* or the cobra but is not seen following bites from other *Elapidae* (mambas, kraits, coral snakes) and *Hydrophiodae.* This is followed by a preparalytic stage whose signs and symptoms include headache, vomiting, loss of consciousness, parasthesiae, hematuria, or hemoptysis (182). These symptoms are not common after envenomation by cobras or mambas. The time period between snakebite and the development of paralytic signs and symptoms may vary from 0.5 to 19 h (183). The first signs of neuromuscular toxicity are usually ptosis and ophthalmoparesis though these are absent following the bite of the South American rattlesnake. Facial and bulbar weakness develops over hours following the development of ocular and periocular muscle weakness (184). Limb, diaphragmatic, and intercostal weakness follows and may continue to evolve for up to 2–3 days (171,185). Cardiovascular collapse, seizures, and coma ensue without appropriate treatment. There is no sensory abnormality other than that which occurs around the bite itself. Other systemic effects of neurologic importance relate to coagulation deficits. Cerebral and subarachnoid hemorrhage have been reported after bites from many species of these snakes and is the leading cause of death following viper bites in several regions of the world (186,187).

Treatment consists of the use of antivenoms, and these are most effective in bites that do not contain significant amounts of phospholipase, a component of presynaptic neurotoxins (184,188,189). If the type of snake is known, a high-titer monovalent type is administered. However, often the type of snake is not known and polyvalent antivenom is necessary. The goal of antivenom is to shorten the duration of weakness. Other respiratory, cardiovascular, and hematologic support measures may be required. Supportive measures are the mainstay of care for most victims of coral snake bite. Intensive care treatment and airway maintenance is similar to patients with myasthenia gravis. Some authors recommend treatment with cholinesterase inhibitors in those cases that are predominantly caused by a postsynaptic abnormality and suggest that electrodiagnostic testing may be useful in determining whether they will be effective (190,191).

3.   Marine Toxins

The rapid rise in marine pollution has spurred a renewed interest in marine toxins. Previously they were only of interest to physiologists and pharmacologists who used them as tools for the investigation of biological systems. Examples of marine neurotoxicology are scattered throughout the literature dating to biblical times (Exodus 7:20-21). The reader is referred to Southcott's paper for an excellent review of the subject (192). Marine neurotoxins affecting the neuromuscular junction are rare and come primarily from poisonous fish, a few mollusks, and perhaps dinoflagellates. Unlike the poisoning from arthropods and snakes, the majority of marine intoxications occur as the result of ingestion. Unique to some marine toxins is the fact that there is an increase in the concentration of toxin though successive predatory transvection up the food chain.

Dinoflagellates are single-celled, biflagellated, algae-like organisms. Diatoms, similar to dinoflagellates, are not flagellated and are encased by a silica shell. The toxins produced by these organisms cause a variety of systemic and neurologic effects. Those that affect the NMJ are rare and indirect. They include paralytic shellfish poisoning (PSP) which results from neurotoxins produced by less than 1% of the 2000–3000 species of known dinoflagellates and diatoms (193). The toxin is rapidly absorbed through the gastrointestinal tract and symptoms begin within 30 min of ingestion. Characteristically, there is an initial burning or paresthesia of the face and mouth, spreading quickly to involve the neck and limbs. Slowly, these sensory symptoms abate and are replaced with numbness, some ataxia, and, in severe cases, progressive generalized weakness and respiratory failure. Overall, the mortality approaches 10%. Most neurotoxins from dinoflagellates and diatoms are sodium channel blockers (e.g., saxitoxin and tetrodotoxin). Brevetoxin, a milder neurotoxin that causes nonlethal neurotoxic shellfish poisoning, depolarizes cholinergic systems by opening sodium channels to a lesser extent. Neuromuscular transmission is altered indirectly as a result.

Conontoxins are a diverse group of toxins from predatory cone snails that inject their venom via a small harpoon-like dart (194). It is only the fish-predatory species (*Conus geographus, C. textile, C. marmoreus, and C. omaria*) of this mollusk that appears dangerous to man (195–197). The effects of these toxins are variable among and within species. Several have direct effects on the NMJ. The α-conotoxins block the binding of ACh to the ligand binding site (198–200). These venoms function similarly to the snake α-neurotoxins described earlier. The ω-conotoxins block the voltage-gated calcium channel of the presynaptic nerve terminal (201). The latter toxin has played an important role in our understanding of LES and serves as the basis for the currently used antibody assay (202,203). Following the injection of toxin there is intense local pain quickly followed by malaise, headache, and within 30 min a progressive generalized weakness. Respiratory failure often occurs within 1–2 h. Most cone shell bites are preventable. These shells should be handled carefully with forceps and thick gloves. The proboscis protrudes from the small end of the shell, but it is flexible and long enough to sting the holder at the other end. The live shells should never be placed in one's pocket because the dart may penetrate cloth (192). Treatment is directed to respiratory and cardiovascular support. There is no antivenom available. There is no literature discussing the potential efficacy of cholinesterase inhibitors. More than 60% of stings have been fatal (197,204).

The most venomous fish is the stonefish (*Synanceja horrida, S. traachynis, S. verrucosa*) found in the Indo-Pacific oceans and Red Sea and the genus *Inimicus* found off the coast of Japan (205). The toxin stonustoxin is inflicted by injection through the 13 dorsal spines when the victim steps on the small fish that is buried in the sand. Neuromuscular blockade occurs as the result of the induced neurotransmitter release with depletion of ACh stores, similar to that of other presynaptic toxins (206,207). Envenomation results in immediate, excruciating pain that may last for 1–2 days. Severe edema occurs due to the actions of hyaluronidase, which promotes the rapid spread of venom through the tissue, and tissue necrosis may occur (192). In addition to gastrointestinal, autonomic, and cognitive difficulties, the victim may experience generalized muscle weakness due to the mechanism noted above. Death results from cardiotoxicity. Treatment is supportive and in some cases the use of a specific antitoxin may be helpful.

4. Plant Toxins

There are very rare instances in which plant neurotoxins affect the NMJ of humans. They are more likely to affect animals. Their neurotoxicity is dependent on the potency, concentration, and interaction with other toxins or substrates in the victim. Many are alkaloids. Coniine, the neurotoxin from the herb *Conium maculatum* (poison hemlock), produces a rapidly ascending paralysis that often results in death. Sensory abnormalities are common and prominent (208). It has been associated with the death of Socrates (209).

The mechanisms of action of this piperidine alkaloid neurotoxin are not completely understood. There is evidence to show that at least part of the toxin acts as a curare mimetic, blocking the postsynaptic function of the NMJ (210).

III. OCCUPATIONAL NEUROTOXINS

A. Heavy Metals

Numerous polyvalent cations affect neuromuscular transmission, but these effects are seen in physiology and pharmacology laboratories where they have been used as tools to study the basic mechanisms of synaptic transmission. Nearly all of these intoxicants have multiple effects on synaptic transmission. They predominantly block the release of ACh from the presynaptic nerve terminal. All of them also facilitate the spontaneous quantal release of neurotransmitter. These include barium, erbium, cadmium, cobalt, gadolinium, lanthium, manganese, nickel, praseodymium, triethyltin, and zinc (211–223). The mechanisms by which they exert their effects include their ability to block the flux of Ca^{2+} through voltage-gated calcium channels and to disrupt intracellular stores of Ca^{2+} (224).

Heavy-metal intoxication is a rare cause of clinical NMJ toxicity. Interest in this topic arose from the 1971 contamination of grain with a methylmercury fungicide. Despite appropriate warnings, the grain was fed to animals, ground for flour, and used for making bread (225). Symptoms began within a month of consumption ultimately affecting more than 6500 people and killing nearly 8% of them (226). Patients experienced ataxia, fatigue, generalized muscle weakness, and occasionally optic atrophy. While one of the expected abnormalities following mercurial poisoning is a peripheral neuropathy (based on the Minamata experience), extensive electrodiagnostic examinations of the affected Iraqi population did not demonstrate this (227,228). Repetitive nerve stimulation studies demonstrated a decremental response that was partially reversible with cholinesterase inhibitors (229). Similar abnormalities have been demonstrated in experimental animals (230).

There are reports that gadolinium acutely reduced the strength of myasthenic patients (217,231).

B. Organophosphate and Carbamate Poisoning

Organophosphates are a class of compounds that irreversibly inhibit cholinesterases including AChE (232). Exposure to organophosphate compounds occurs in the workplace, in food, drinking water, and in the environment. They are widely used in the agricultural, manufacturing, and pharmaceutical industries and as weapons of mass destruction (233,234). The earliest use of a cholinesterase inhibitor as a neurotoxin is probably attributed to tribesmen in

Africa who used the Calabar bean in a right of passage or as an "ordeal poison" (235). Organophosphate intoxication is uncommon in the United States since organophosphate-containing insecticides are not readily available. However, they are commonly used in many other countries, including those in Europe, where intoxication most commonly results from attempted suicide by ingestion of insecticides, as well as by indiscriminate handling and storage by poorly educated workers (236–239).

The physiochemical properties of these compounds vary. They may be solid, liquid, or gaseous and soluble in various media. Some are highly corrosive, others are not; some are highly volatile whereas others are not. They may be absorbed through dermal contact, respiratory inhalation, and gastrointestinal absorption. These various physiochemical properties lend themselves to the various applications noted above as well as to the inherent dangers of their use (240).

Four neuromuscular toxicologic syndromes occur from organophosphate poisoning: an acute cholinergic crisis (type 1 and 2), an intermediate syndrome, a myopathy, and a delayed neuropathy (241). Only the type 2 cholinergic crisis and the intermediate syndrome are the result of NMJ toxicity. Organophosphate compounds exert their NMJ toxicity by the irreversible inhibition of AChE. This results in the excessive accumulation of ACh at the NMJ as well as at other cholinergic synapses of the central, peripheral, and autonomic nervous systems (242). The excessive accumulation of ACh produces a depolarizing neuromuscular block at the NMJ that is followed by desensitization of the AChR (243–245). Electrodiagnostic studies demonstrate normal nerve conduction studies, reduced CMAP amplitudes, a decremental response to repetitive nerve stimulation, and CMAP after-discharges to a single nerve stimulus (238,246).

Carbamate salts and esters are synthetic analogues of the alkaloid physostigmine (eserine). They are used primarily as pesticides. They may directly or indirectly affect the NMJ. Like the organophosphate compounds, carbamates also inhibit the action of AChE at cholinergic synapses. They are easily absorbed into the CNS because of their lipid solubility characteristics. Unlike organophosphate compounds, the effects of carbamate agents are reversible. However, the symptoms of carbamate poisoning are indistinguishable from those organophosphate poisoning.

Neurotoxicity occurs rapidly following significant exposure to both classes of compounds. Death is usually the result of respiratory paralysis, occurring in 40% of poisoned victims, and carries with it a very high mortality rate (247).

1. Pesticides

Organophosphorus chemistry had its origin around 1820 when Lassainge synthesized triethyl phosphate, but it was not until the turn of the century that these compounds were recognized for their insecticidal properties. The organophosphate insecticides are all derivatives of phosphoric acid. There are many subclasses within this group of compounds, and their various moieties (e.g., sulfur, amides) confer variation in their overall toxicity. Despite recognition of their toxicity, their use is continuing to rise, particularly in developing countries where the demand was predicted to more than double in the last decade (248). Most fatal intoxications occur as the result of suicidal ingestion (236–239,249–252).

Documented cases of carbamate NMJ toxicity are few (253). The largest episode of carbamate poisoning occurred in 1985 when aldicarb was illegally used as an insecticide on watermelons (254). Seventy-seven percent of 1376 exposed individuals were poisoned, with each exhibiting a dose-related spectrum of nicotinic and muscarinic cholinergic receptor toxicity. Fatalities are rare and only occur at very high levels of exposure (255–258). Symptoms appear rapidly, often within an hour, peaking in 2–3 h and recovering fully within 72 h (259).

2. Agents of War and Terrorism

The highly dangerous toxicity of organophosphate compounds was recognized in 1932 leading to the discovery of GB (sarin) and GA (tabun) in 1937, GD (soman) in 1944 and VX (venom X) in 1952 (260). Little is known about a Russian agent, coded VR-55 (261). Great Britain ceased nerve gas weapons research in 1959 and the United States transiently discontinued their efforts between 1969 and 1981 (262). Other countries have continued to develop their weapons programs through the present. Recent examples of the use of nerve gas as an offensive weapon exist. It is speculated that GA was used in the 1980s during the Iraq–Iran conflict causing innumerable deaths (261). Terrorist attacks in Japan resulted in the exposure of civilians to GB and VX (263–267).

The effects of nerve agents depend upon route of exposure (Table 7.5). Symptoms of inhalation exposure to a nerve agent vapor begin within seconds

Table 7.5 Comparative LCt_{50} and LD_{50} to Nerve Agents in Human Exposure

Nerve agent	Inhalation (LCt_{50})	Cutaneous (LD_{50})
VX vapor	10 mg min/m^3	6–10 mg
Soman vapor	50 mg min/m^3	350 mg
Sarin vapor	100 mg min/m^3	1700 mg
Tabun vapor	400 mg min/m^3	1000 mg

LCt_{50} dose of vapor necessary to cause death in 50% of the exposed population where C is concentration and t is time; LD_{50} dose of cutaneous exposure necessary to cause death in 50% of the exposed population.

to minutes depending on the concentration of vapor. Maximal effects occur within a few minutes. The effects of dermal exposure are delayed compared to inhalation exposure. The effects are dependent on dose, body site of exposure, temperature, and humidity. Local effects (sweating, mucosal irritation) occur within seconds to minutes, and in severe exposure paralysis and apnea may occur so quickly that the individual does not recognize what is happening. In some instances the individual may be asymptomatic for up to 18 h only to be followed by the precipitant development of symptoms (268).

C. Treatment

Treatment is directed to the prevention of chemical exposure by appropriate clothing and the decontamination of exposed victims (269). Aggressive cardiopulmonary support is necessary. Atropine is an effective antidote to block the excessive cholinergic activity at muscarinic receptors in both organophosphate and carbamate intoxications. The use of AChE reactivators [oximes such as praoidoxime (2-PAM)] and anticholinergics are often helpful for acute organophosphorus intoxications but appear to have little effect in reversing the weakness caused by the intermediate syndrome. Oximes dissociate the toxic phosphate moiety from the esteratic site on AChE, thus reactivating esterase and restoring the mechanisms of normal neuromuscular transmission (270). Soman is the least responsive of the nerve agents to oxime therapy because the agent–enzyme complex rapidly undergoes "aging," the process whereby the compound undergoes a time-dependent conformational change that is no longer responsive to reactivators (271). In contrast to organophosphate intoxications, oxime reactivators are contraindicated in carbamate poisoning as these compounds enhance the effects of the carbamate and promote further junctional toxicity (272). In cases where the offending compound is not known, it is possible to assay the reactivation of AChE activity in vivo and possibly differentiate between organophosphate and carbamate poisonings (273). Neuromuscular blockade with curariform drugs will block the repetitive discharges, although it is not clear whether there is any clinical benefit to their use (274).

Because nerve agents can cause severe and potentially lethal effects within minutes of exposure, treatment with a postexposure antidote is severely limited. In the face of a chemical exposure, even well-trained personnel will not be uniformly successful in performing self-injection tasks of nerve agent antidotes and the "aging" phenomenon of organophosphate-AChE interaction make oxime therapy much less effective (275). For this reason, the carbamate pyridostigmine was used as a "pretreatment" for organophosphate poisoning during Operation Desert Storm in 1991. It was the first use of prophylactic treatment for organophosphate exposure in a wartime situation. It was believed that a previously administered AChE compound would protect the enzyme from the subsequent exposure to some nerve agents and provide partial protection for 6–8 h. Their use remains controversial. While studies have shown that a 40% inhibition in AChE activity by physostigmine protected experimental animals from the acute cholinergic toxicity following exposure to the nerve agent soman, such findings have not been conclusively demonstrated for pyridostigmine (276). The use of pyridostigmine was complicated by higher than expected gastrointestinal side effects with nearly 50% of 41,650 military personnel developing excessive flatus, loose stools, and abdominal cramps (277). Lesser but significant numbers experienced urinary urgency and frequency. Future efforts are being directed to the development of macromolecules and high-affinity monoclonal antibodies that will inactivate specific nerve agents (278–282).

REFERENCES

1. Montecucco C, Schiavo G. Molecular Microbiology 1994; 13:1–8.
2. Kerner JAC. Neue Beobachtungen uber die in Wurttemberg so haufig vorfallenden todlichen Vergiftungen durch den Genuss geraucherter Wurste. Tubingen: Osiander, 1820.
3. Van Ermengen E. Zeitschrift fur Hygeine und Infektionskrankheiten 1897; 26: 1–56.
4. Durban EE, Durban M, Grecz N. Can J Microbiol 1974; 20:353–358.
5. Hofer JW, Davis J. Tex Med 2002; 68:80–81.
6. Hawrylewicz E, Gowdy B, Ehrlich R. Nature 2002; 193:497.
7. Sakaguchi G, Sakaguchi S, Karashimada T. Characterization of *Clostridium botulinum* type E toxin in "izuchi." In: Toxic Microorganisms. Washington, DC: U.S. Dept. of Interior, 1970.
8. Smith LDS, Sugiyama H. Botulism: The Organism, Its Toxins, The Disease. 2nd ed. Springfield: Charles C Thomas, 1988:1–184.
9. Gimenez D, Ciccarelli A. Boletin de la Oficina Sanitaria Panamericana 1970; 69:505–510.
10. Burgen ASV, Dickens F, Zatman LJ. J Physiol (London) 1949; 109:10–24.
11. Black JD, Dolly JO. JCell Biol 1986; 103:535–544.
12. Pellizzari R, Rossetto O, Washbourne P, Tonello F, Nicotera PL, Montecucco C. Toxicol Lett 1998; 103:191–197.
13. Cherington M, Smith RH, Montecucco C. In: de Wolff FA, ed. Intoxications of the Nervous System. Amsterdam: Elsevier, 1995:209–215.
14. Schiavo G, Benfenati F, Poulain B, Rossetto O, Polverino DL, Dasgupta BR, Montecucco C. Nature Oct. 28, 1992; 359:832–835.
15. Simpson LL. Ann Intern Med Oct. 1, 1996; 125:616–617.
16. Uncini A, Lugaresi A. Muscle Nerve 1999; 22:640–644.
17. Woodruff BA, Griffin PM, McCroskey LM, Smart JF, Wainwright RB, Bryant RG, Hutwagner LC, Hatheway CL. J Infect Dis 1992; 166:1281–1286.

18. McCroskey LM, Hatheway CL, Woodruff BA, Greenberg JA, Jurgenson P. J Clin Microbiol 1991; 29:2618–2620.
19. Hughes JM. In: Scheid WM, Whitley RJ, Durack DT, eds. Infections of the Central Nervous System. New York: Raven Press, 1991:150–153.
20. Jenzer G, Mumenthaler M, Ludin HP, Robert F. Neurology 1975; 25:150–153.
21. Pickett J, Berg B, Chaplin E, Brunstetter-Shafer M. N Engl J Med 1976; 295:770–792.
22. Arnon SS, Midura TF, Damus K, Thompson B, Wood RM, Chin J. J Pediatr 1979; 94:331–336.
23. Schmidt RD, Schmidt TW. J Emerg Med 1992; 10:713–718.
24. Spika JS, Shaffer N, Hargrett-Bean N, Collin S, MacDonald KL, Blake PA. Am J Dis Child 1989; 143:828–832.
25. Cherington M, Ginsburg S. Arch Surg. 1975; 110:436–438.
26. MMWR Morb Mortal Wkly Rep 44: 889-892, Dec. 8, 1995.
27. Jensen T, Jacobsen D, von der LE, Heier MS, Selseth B. Tidsskr Nor Laegeforen Nov. 12, 1998; 118:4363–4365.
28. MacDonald KL, Rutherford SM, Friedman SM, Dieter JA, Kaye BR, McKinley GF, Tenney JH, Cohen ML. Ann Intern Med 1985; 102:616–618.
29. Passaro DJ, Werner SB, McGee J, Mac K, Vugia DJ. JAMA March 18, 1998; 279:859–863.
30. Weber JT, Goodpasture HC, Alexander H, Werner SB, Hatheway CL, Tauxe RV. Clin Infect Dis 1993; 16:635–639.
31. Romanello R, De Santis F, Caione R, Fenicia L, Aureli P. Eur J Clin Microbiol Infect Dis 1998; 17:295–296.
32. Chia JK, Clark JB, Ryan CA, Pollack M. N.Engl J Med 315: 239-241.
33. Dowell VR Jr, McCroskey LM, Hatheway CL, Lombard GL, Hughes JM, Merson MH. JAMA Oct 24, 1977; 238:1829–1832.
34. Griffin PM, Hatheway CL, Rosenbaum RB, Sokolow R. J Infect Dis 1997; 175:633–637.
35. Olney RK, Aminoff MJ, Gelb DJ, Lowenstein DH. Neurology 1988; 38:1780–1783.
36. Sanders DB, Massey EW, Buckley EG. Neurology 1986; 36:545–547.
37. Ansved T, Odergren T, Borg K. Neurology 1997; 48:1440–1442.
38. Kessler KR, Skutta M, Benecke R. J Neurol 1999; 246:265–274.
39. Erbguth F, Claus D, Engelhardt A, Dressler D. J Neurol Neurosurg Psychiatry 1993; 56:1235–1236.
40. Borodic G. Lancet Dec. 5, 1998; 352:1832.
41. Cole LA. Sci Am 1996; 275:60–65.
42. Kadlec RP, Zelicoff AP, Vrtis AM. JAMA Aug. 6, 1997; 278:351–356.
43. Bermudez JS. The Armed Forces of North Korea. London: I.B. Tauris, 2001:1–375.
44. Smithson AE. Toxic Archipelago: Preventing Proliferation from the Former Soviet Chemical and Biological Weapons Complexes. Washington, DC: Henry L. Stimson Center, 1999:1 101.

45. Franz DR. In: Sidell FR, Takafuji ET, Franz DR, eds. Medical Aspects of Chemical and Biological Warfare. Washington: Borden Institute, Walter Reed Army Medical Center, 1997:603–620.

46. Smart JK. In: Sidell FR, Takafuji ET, Franz DR, eds. Textbook of Military Medicine: Medical Aspects of Chemical and Biological Warfare. Washington, DC: Office of the Surgeon General 1997:9–86.

47. Hill EV. Botulism. In: Summary Report on B. W. Investigations. Memorandum to Alden C. Waitt, Chief Chemical Corps, U.S. Army, Dec 12, 1947; tab D. Archived at the U.S. Library of Congress.

48. Bryden J. Deadly Allies: Canada's Secret War, 1937-1947. Toronto: McClelland & Stewart, 1989: 1–316.

49. Carus WS. In: Lederberg J, ed. Biological Weapons: Limiting the Threat. Cambridge: MIT Press, 1999:211–230.

50. Zilinskas RA. JAMA Aug. 6, 1997; 278:418–424.

51. Ekeus R. Memorandum to the Biological Weapons Convention Fourth Review Conference. New York: United Nations Special Commission (UNSCOM). Nov 20, 1996.

52. Kadlec RP, Zelicoff AP, Vrtis AM. In: Lederberg J, ed. Biological Weapons: Limiting the Threat. Cambridge: MIT Press, 1999:95–112.

53. Patocka J, Splino M. ASA Newslett 2002; 02-1:14–23.

54. Thompson JA, Glasgow LA, Warpinski JR, Olson C. Pediatrics 1980; 66:936–942.

55. Cherington M. In: Katirji B, Kaminski HJ, Preston DC, Ruff RL, Shapiro BE, eds. Neuromuscular Disorders in Clinical Practice. Boston: Butterworth Heinemann, 2002:942–952.

56. Cherington M. Muscle Nerve 1982; 5:S28–S29.

57. Gutmann L, Bodensteiner J, Gutierrez A. J Pediatr 1992; 121:835.

58. Cornblath DR, Sladky JT, Summer AJ. Muscle Nerve 1983, 448–452.

59. Girlanda P, Dattola R, Messina C. Acta Neurol Scand 1983; 67:118–123.

60. Schiller HH, Stålberg EV. Arch Neurol 1978; 35:346–349.

61. Mandler RN, Maselli RA. Muscle Nerve 1996; 19:1171–1173.

62. Duchen LW, Strich SJ. QJ Exp Physiol Cogn Med Sci 1968; 53:84–89.

63. Black RE, Gunn RA. Am J Med 2002; 69:567–570.

64. Critchley EM. Postgrad Med J 1991; 67:401.

65. Franz DR, Pitt LM, Clayton MA, Hanes MA, Rose KJ. In: Das Gupta B. ed. Botulinum and Tetanus Neurotoxins and Biomedical Aspects. New York: Plenum Press, 1993:473–476.

66. Middlebrook JL. In: Das Gupta B. ed. Botulinum and Tetanus Neurotoxins and Biomedical Aspects. New York: Plenum Press, 1993:515–519.

67. Ball AP, Hopkinson RB, Farrell ID, Hutchison JG, Paul R, Watson RD, Page AJ, Parker RG, Edwards CW, Snow M, Scott DK, Leone-Ganado A, Hastings A, Ghosh AC, Gilbert RJ. QJ Med 1979; 48:473–491.

68. Cherington M. Arch Neurol 1974; 30:432–437.

69. Cherington M, Greenberg H, Soyer A. Clin Toxicol 1973; 6:83–89.

70. Cherington M. Rocky Mt Med J 1972; 69:55–58.

71. Scaer RC, Tooker J, Cherington M. Neurology 1969; 19:1107.
72. Benz HG, Lunn JN, Foldes FF. Br J Med 1961; 2:241–242.
73. Neal KR, Dunbar EM. Lancet May 26, 1990; 335:1286–1287.
74. Oh SJ, Halsey JH Jr, Briggs DD Jr. Arch Intern Med 1975; 135:726–728.
75. Howard JF, Weiss AS, Donovan MK, Cheshire WP, Braun TG. Muscle Nerve 1992; 15:1202–1203.
76. Siegel LS, Price JI. Toxicon 1987; 25:1015–1018.
77. Siegel LS, Johnson-Winegar AD, Sellin LC. Toxicol App Pharmacol June 30, 1986; 84:255–263.
78. Sanders DB, Kim YI, Howard JF Jr, Goetsch CA. J Neurol Neurosurg Psychiatry 1980; 43:978–985.
79. Ball AP, Snow M, Paul R. Adv Biosci 1982; 35:297–318.
80. Cherington M. Neurology 1976; 26:944–946.
81. Major RH. Classic Descriptions of Disease. Springfield IL: Charles C Thomas, 1965: 134–135.
82. Cook TM, Protheroe RT, Handel JM. Br J Anaesth 2001; 87:477–487.
83. Oladiran I, Meier DE, Ojelade AA, OlaOlorun DA, Adeniran A, Tarpley JL. World J Surg 2002; 26:1282–1285.
84. MMWR Morbid Mortal Weekly Rep Nov. 6, 1988;47: 928-930.
85. MMWR Morbid Mortal Weekly Rep Dec. 9, 1994;43: 885-887.
86. Izurieta HS, Sutter RW, Strebel PM, Bardeneier B, Prevots DR, Wharton M, Hadler SC. MMWR CDC Surveill Summ Feb. 21, 1997; 46:15–25.
87. MMWR - Morbid Mortal Weekly Rep March 6, 1998;47: 149-151
88. Cherubin CE, Sapira JD. Ann Intern Med Nov. 15, 1993; 119:1017–1028.
89. Rossetto O, Deloye F, Poulain B, Pellizzari R, Schiavo G, Montecucco C. J Physiol Paris 1995; 89:43–50.
90. Choe S, Bennett MJ, Fujii G, Curmi PM, Kantardjieff KA, Collier RJ, Eisenberg D. Nature May 21, 1992; 357:216–222.
91. Mellanby J, Green J. Neuroscience 1981; 6:281–300.
92. Brown H. JAMA 1968; 204:614–616.
93. Millard AH. Lancet 1954; 2:844–846.
94. Bagratuni L. Br Med J 1952; 1:461–463.
95. Carrillo AM. Associacion Dental Mexicana 1966; 23:267–268.
96. Clark DC. J Oral Surg 1970; 28:424–431.
97. de Boer MP, Raghoebar GM, Stegenga B, Schoen PJ, Boering G. Quintessence Int 1995; 26:779–784.
98. Epperly TD, Wood TC. Am Fam Physician 1990; 42:102–112.
99. Friedman NR, Mitchell RB, Pereira KD, Younis RT, Lazar RH. Arch Otolaryngol Head Neck Surg. 1997; 123:630–632.
100. Kanesada K, Mogi G. Auris Nasus Larynx 1981; 8:35–39.
101. Szuhay G, Tewfik TL. J Otolaryngol 1998; 27:206–212.
102. van Loosen J, van der DF. Ned Tijdschr Geneeskd April 18, 1987; 131:683.
103. Sandyk R, Brennan MJ. J Neurol Neurosurg Psychiatry 1982; 45:1070.
104. Tokuoka K, Hamano H, Ohta T, Tamura Y, Shinohara Y. Rinsho Shinkeigaku 1997; 37:417–419.

105. Vic-Dupont V, Emile J, Bazin C, Poisson M, Milhaud M, Christol D. Presse Med Jan. 25, 1969; 77:155–158.
106. Moersch FP, Woltman HW. Mayo Clin Proc 1956; 31:421–427.
107. Meinck HM, Ricker K, Hulser PJ, Solimena M. J Neurol 1995; 242:134–142.
108. Thompson PD. J Neurol Neurosurg Psychiatry 1993; 56:121–124.
109. Shimoni Z, Dobrousin A, Cohen J, Pitlik S. Br Med J Oct. 16, 1999; 319.
110. Warren JD, Kimber TE, Thompson PD. Muscle Nerve 1999; 22, 1590–1592.
111. Steinegger T, Wiederkehr M, Ludin HP, Roth F. Schweiz Med Wochenschr March 9, 1996; 126:379–385.
112. Fernandez JM, Ferrandiz M, Larrea L, Ramio R, Boada M. J Neurol Neurosurg Psychiatry 1983; 46:862–866.
113. Poncelet AN. Muscle Nerve 2000; 23:1435–1438.
114. Saady A, Torda TA. Anaesth Intensi Care 1973; 1:226–231.
115. Trujillo MJ, Castillo A, Espana JV, Guevara P, Eganez H. Crit Care Med 1980; 8:419–423.
116. Olsen KM, Hiller FC. Clin Pharmacol 1987; 6:570–574.
117. Udwadia FE, Lall A, Udwadia ZF, Sekhar M, Vora A. Epidemiol Infect 1987; 99:675–684.
118. Ernst ME, Klepser ME, Fouts M, Marangos MN. Ann Pharmacother 1997; 31:1507–1513.
119. Engrand N, Benhamou D. Anaesth Intensi Care 2001; 29:306–307.
120. Reddy VG. Middle East J Anesthesiol 2002; 16:419–442.
121. Boots RJ, Lipman J, O'Callaghan J, Scott P, Fraser J. Anaesth Intens Care 2000; 28:438–442.
122. Corbett JL, Kerr JH, Prys-Roberts C, Smith AC, Spalding JM. Anaesthesia 1969; 24:198–212.
123. Tsueda K, Jean-Francois J, Richter RW. Int Surg 1973; 58:599–603.
124. Corbett JL, Spalding JM, Harris PJ. Br Med J Aug. 25, 1973; 3:423–428.
125. Bhagwanjee S, Bosenberg AT, Muckart DJ. Crit Care Med 1999; 27:1721–1725.
126. Wesley AG, Hariparsad D, Pather M, Rocke DA. Anaesthesia 1983; 38:243–249.
127. Maretic Z. In: Bettini S, ed. Arthropod Venoms. Berlin: Springer-Verlag, 1978: 185–212.
128. Rose I. Can Med Assoc J 1954; 70:175–176.
129. Temple IU. Med Sentinel 1912; 20:507–514.
130. Rosenthal L. Pharmacol Ther 1989; 42:115–134.
131. Hurlbut WP, Iezzi N, Fesce R, Ceccarelli B. J Physiol 1990; 424:501–526.
132. Henkel AW, Sankaranarayanan S. Cess Tissue Res 1999; 296:229–233.
133. Ushkaryov YA, Petrenko AG, Geppert M, Sudhof TC. Science 1992; 257:50–56.
134. Longenecker HE, Hurlbut WP, Mauro A, Clark AW. Nature 1970; 225:701–703.
135. Clark AW, Hurlbut WP, Mauro A. J Cell Biol 1972; 52:1–14.
136. Clark AW, Mauro A, Longenecker HE, Hurlbut WP. Nature 1970; 225:703–705.
137. Ceccarelli B, Grohovaz F, Hurlbut WP. J Cell Biol 1979; 81:163–177.

138. Pumplin DW, Reese TS. J.Physiol. 1977; 273:443–457.
139. Gorio A, Rubin LL, Mauro A. J Neurocytol 1978; 7:193–202.
140. Howard BD. Annu Rev Pharmacol Toxicol 1980; 20:307–336.
141. Gilbert WW, Stewart CM. Am J Med Sci 1935; 189:532–536.
142. Miller TA. Am Fam Physician 1992; 45:181–187.
143. D'Amour EF, Becker FE, Van Riper W. Q Rev Biol 1936; 11:123–160.
144. Todd JL. Can Med Assoc J 1912; 2:1118–1119.
145. Cleland JB. Australas Med Gaz 1912; 32:295–299.
146. Gregson JD. Tick Paralysis: An Appraisal of Natural and Experimental Data. Ottawa: Canada Department of Agriculture, 1978:1–109.
147. Anonymous. JAMA May 15, 1996; 275:1470.
148. Gothe R, Kunze K, Hoogstraal H. J Med Entomol Nov. 23, 1979; 16:357–369.
149. Weingart JL. Minn Med 1967; 50:383–386.
150. Brown AF, Hamilton DL. J Acc Emerg Med 1998; 15:111–113.
151. Felz MW, Smith CD, Swift TR. N Engl J Med Jan 13, 2000; 342:90–94.
152. Cherington M, Synder RD. N Engl J Med Jan 11, 1968; 278:95–97.
153. Swift TR, Ignacio OJ. Neurology 1975; 25:1130–1133.
154. Grattan-Smith PJ, Morris JG, Johnston HM, Yiannikas C, Malik R, Russell R, Ouvrier RA. Brain 1997; 120:1975–1987.
155. Donat JR, Donat JF. Arch Neurol 1981; 38:59–61.
156. Lagos JC, Thies RE. Arch Neurol 1969; 21:471–474.
157. Dworkin MS, Shoemaker PC, Anderson DE. Clin Infect Dis 1999; 29:1435–1439.
158. Jones HR Jr. Curr Opin Pediat 1995; 7:663–668.
159. Stanbury JB, Huyck JH. Medicine 1945; 24:219–242.
160. Crause JC, van Wyngaardt S, Gothe R, Neitz AW. Exp Appl Acarol 1994; 18:51–59.
161. Stone BF, Aylward JH. Toxicon 1992; 30:552–553.
162. Rose I, Gregson JD. Nature 1959; 178:95–96.
163. Gothe R, Neitz AWH. Adv Dis Vector Res 1991; 8:177–204.
164. Stone BF. Adv Dis Vector Res 1988; 5:61–85.
165. Esplin DW, Phillip CB, Hughes LE. Science 1960; 132:958–959.
166. DeBusk FL, O'Connor S. Pediatrics 1972; 50:328–329.
167. Haller JS, Fabara JA. Am J Dis Child 1972; 124:915–917.
168. Warnick JE, Albuquerque EX, Diniz CR. J Pharmacol Exp Ther 1976; 198:155–167.
169. Belghith M, Boussarsar M, Haguiga H, Besbes L, Elatrous S, Touzi N, Boujdaria R, Bchir A, Nouira S, Bouchoucha S, Abroug F. J Toxicol Clin Toxicol 1999; 37:51–57.
170. Sofer S, Shahak E, Gueron M. Pediatrics 1994; 124:973–978.
171. Campbell CH. Contemp Neurol Series 1975; 12:259–293.
172. Vital-Brazil O. In: Cheymol J, ed. Neuromuscular Blocking and Stimulating Agents. New York: Permagon Press, 1972:145–167.
173. Lee CY. Clin Toxicol 1970; 3:457–472.
174. Karlsson E, Arnberg H, Eaker D. Eur J Biochem 1971; 21:1–16.

175. Lee CY, Chang SL, Kau ST, Luh SH. J Chromatogr 1972; 72:71–82.
176. Tu AT, Tu T. In: Halstead BW, ed. Poisonous and Venomous Marine Animals of the World. Washington, DC: US Government Printing Office, 1972:885–903.
177. Barme M. In: Keegan HL, MacFarlane W, eds. Venomous and Poisonous Animals and Noxious Plants of the Pacific Region. Oxford: Pergamon Press 1963:373–378.
178. Karlsson E. In: Lee CY, ed. Snake Venoms. New York: Springer-Verlag, 1979:159–212.
179. Chang CC, Su MJ. Toxicon 1980; 18:641–648.
180. Rowlands JB, Mastaglia FL, Kakulas BA, Hainsworth D. Med J Aust 1969; 1:226–230.
181. Kellaway CH. Aust J Exp Biol Med Sci 1932; 10:181–194.
182. Bouquier JJ, Guibert J, Dupont C, Umdenstock R. Arch Francaises de Pediatrie 1974; 31:285–296.
183. Mitrakul C, Dhamkrong-At A, Futrakul P, Thisyakorn C, Vongsrisart K, Varavithya C, Phancharoen S. Am J Trop Med Hyg 1984; 33:1258–1266.
184. Reid HA. Br Med J 1964; 2:540–545.
185. Warrell DA, Barnes HJ, Piburn MF. Trans R Soc Trop Med Hyg 1976; 70:78–79.
186. Kerrigan KR. Am J Trop Med Hyg 1991; 44:93–99.
187. Ouyang C, Teng C-M, Huang T-F. Toxicon 1992; 30:945–966.
188. Reid HA. Lancet 1975; 1:622–623.
189. Theakston RDG, Phillips RE, Warrell DA, Galagedera Y, Abeysekera DTDJ, Dissanayaka P, De Silva A, Aloysius DJ. Trans R Soc Trop Med Hyg 1990; 84:301–308.
190. Kumar S, Usgaonkar RS. J Ind Med Assoc 1968; 50:428–429.
191. Pettigrew LC, Glass JP. Neurology 1985; 35:589–592.
192. Southcott RV. In: Hornabrook RW, ed. Topics on Tropical Neurology. Philadelphia: F.A. Davis,1975:165–258.
193. Steidinger KA, Steinfield HJ. In: Spector DL, ed. Dinoflagellates. New York: Academic Press, 1984:201–206.
194. Olivera BM, Gray WR, Zeikus R, McIntosh JM, Varga J, Rivier J, de Santos V, Cruz LJ. Science 1985; 230:1338–1343.
195. Kohn AJ. In: Keegan HC, McFarlane WV, eds. Venomous and Poisonous Animals and Noxious Plants of the Pacific Region. Oxford: Permagon Press, 1963:1–456.
196. Kohn AJ. Hawaii Med J 1958; 17:528–532.
197. Cruz LJ, In: White J, Meier J, White J, eds. CRC Handbook on Clinical Toxicology of Animal Venoms and Poisons. Boca Raton: CRC Press, 1995:117–128.
198. Gray WR, Luque A, Olivera BM, Barrett J, Cruz LJ. J Biol Chem 1981; 256:4734–4740.
199. Hopkins C, Grilley M, Miller C, Shon KJ, Cruz LJ, Gray WR, Dykert J, Rivier J, Yoshikami D, Olivera BM. J Biol Chem 1995; 270:22361–22367.
200. McIntosh M, Cruz LJ, Hunkapiller MW, Gray WR, Olivera BM. Arch Biochem Biophys 1982; 218:329–334.

201. McCleskey EW, Fox AP, Feldman D, Cruz LJ, Olivera BM, Tsien RW, Yoshikami D. Proc Nat Acad Sci USA 1987; 84:4327–4331.

202. Adams DJ, Alewood PF, Craik DJ, Drinkwater RD, Lewis RJ. Drug Dev Res 1999; 46:219–234.

203. De Aizpurua HJ, Lambert EH, Griesmann GE, Olivera M, Lennon VA. Cancer Res 1988; 48:4719–4724.

204. Yoshiba S. Jap J Hyg 1984; 39:565–572.

205. Halstead BW. Poisonous and Venomous Marine Animals of the World. Washington, DC: US Government Printing Office, 1970:1–1006.

206. Gwee MC, Gopalakrishnakone P, Yuen R, Khoo HE, Low KS. Pharmacol Ther 1994; 64:509–528.

207. Kreger AS, Molgo J, Comella JX, Hansson B, Thesleff S. Toxicon 1993; 31:307–317.

208. Hardin JW, Arena JW. Human Poisoning from Native and Cultivated Plants. Durham, NC: Duke University Press, 1974:1–174.

209. Davies MI, Davies TA. Med Sci Law 1994; 34:331–333.

210. Panter KE, Keeler RF. In: Cheeke P, ed. Toxicants of Plant Origin. Vol 1. Alkaloids. Boca Raton: CRC Press, 1989:109–130.

211. Silinsky EM. J Physiol (London) 1978; 274:157–171.

212. Silinsky EM. Br J Pharmacol 1977; 59:215–217.

213. Metral S, Bonneton C, Hort-Legrand C, Reynes J. Nature 1978; 271:773–775.

214. Cooper GP, Manalis RS. Eur J Pharmacol 1984; 99:251–256.

215. Forshaw PJ. Eur J Pharmacol 1977; 42:371–377.

216. Weakly JN. J Physiol (London) 1973; 234:597–612.

217. Molgo J, del Pozo E, Banos JE, Angaut-Petit D. Br J Pharmacol 1991; 104:133–138.

218. Kajimoto N, Kirpekar SM. Nature 1972; 235:29–30.

219. Balnave RJ, Gage PW. Br J Pharmacol 1973; 47:339–352.

220. Kita H, Van der Kloot W. Nature 1973; 245:52–53.

221. Alnaes E, Rahaminoff R. Nature 1975; 247:478–479.

222. Allen JE, Gage PW, Leaver DD, Leow ACT. Chem Biol Interact 1980; 31:227–231.

223. Benoit PR, Mambrini J. J Physiol (London) 1970; 210:681–695.

224. Cooper GP, Manalis RS. Neurotoxicology 2001; 4:69–84.

225. Rustam H, Hamdi T. Brain 1974; 97:499–510.

226. Bakir F, Damluji SF, Amin-Saki L, Murthada M, Khalida A, Al-Rawi NY, Tikriti S, Dhahir HJ, Clarkson T, Smith JC, Doherty RA. Science 1973; 181:230–241.

227. Igata A. In: Tsubaki T, Takahashi H, eds. Recent Advances in Minamata Disease Studies. Tokyo: Kodansha, 1986:41–57.

228. LeQuense P, Damluji SF, Berlin M. J Neurol Neurosurg Psychiatry 1974; 37:333–339.

229. Rustam H, von Burg R, Amin-Saki L, Elhassani S. Arch Environ Health 1975; 30:190–195.

230. Atchinson WD, Narahashi T. Neurotoxicology 1982; 3:37–50.

231. Nordenbo AM, Somnier FE. Lancet 1992; 340:1168.
232. Taylor P. In: Gilman AG, Goodman LS, Rall TW, Murad F, eds. The Pharmacological Basis of Therapeutics. New York: Macmillan, 1985:110–129.
233. Edmundson RS. Dictionary of Organphosphorous Compounds [electronic resource]. London: Chapman and Hall, 1988.
234. Gunderson CH, Lehmann CR, Sidell FR, Jabari B. Neurology 1992; 42:946–950.
235. Moore B, Safani M, Keesey J. Lancet 1988; 1:882.
236. Fernando R. Pesticides in Sri Lanka. Colombo: Friedrich-Ebert-Stiftung, 1989: ix–255.
237. Besser R, Gutmann L, Dilimann U, Weilemann LS, Hopf HC. Neurology 1989; 39:561–567.
238. Gutmann L, Besser R. Semin Neurol 1990; 10:46–51.
239. Jeyaratnam J. World Health Stat Q 1990; 43:139–145.
240. Aldridge WN, Reiner E. Enzyme Inhibitors as Substrates. Amsterdam: North-Holland, 1972:1–328.
241. Marrs TC. Pharmacol Thera 1993; 58:51–66.
242. Namba T, Nolte CT, Jackrel J, Grob D. Am J Med 2001; 50:475–492.
243. Karalliedde L, Senanayake N. B J Anaesth 1989; 63:736–750.
244. De Wilde V, Vogblaers D, Colarddyn F, Vanderstraeten G, Van Den Neucker K, DeBleecker J, De Reuck J, Van den Neede M. Klin Wochenschrift 1991; 69:177–183.
245. Good JL, Khurana RK, Mayer RF, Cintra WM, Albuquerque EX. J Neurol Neurosurg Psychiatry 1993; 56:290–294.
246. Maselli RA, Soliven BC. Muscle Nerve 1991; 14:1182–1188.
247. Tsao TC, Juang Y, Lan R, Shieh W, Lee C. Chest 1990; 98:631–636.
248. WHO/UNEP1-128, 1990.
249. Haddad LM. J Toxicol Clin Toxicol 1992; 30:331–332.
250. De Bleecker J, Willems J, Van Den Neucker K, De Reuck J, Vogelaers D. Clin Toxicol 1992; 30:333–345.
251. Güler K, Tascioglu C, Özbey N. Isr J Med Sci 1996; 32:791–792.
252. Chaudhry R, Lall SB, Mishra B, Dhawan B. B Med J 7-25-1998; 317:268–269.
253. Cranmer MF. Neurotoxicology 1986; 7:247–328.
254. Goldman LR, Smith DF, Neutra RR, Saunders LD, Pond EM, Stratton J, Waller K, Jackson J, Kizer KW. Arch Environ Health 1990; 45:229–236.
255. Freslew KE, Hagardorn AN, McCormick WF. J Foren Sci 1992; 37:337–344.
256. Jenis EH, Payne RJ, Goldbaum LR. JAMA 1969; 207:361–362.
257. Klys M, Kosún J, Pach J, Kamenczak A. J Forens Sci 1989; 34:1413–1416.
258. Maddock RK, Bloomer HA. JAMA 1967; 201:123–127.
259. Ecobichon DJ. In: Spencer PS, Schaumburg HH, eds. Experimental and Clinical Neurotoxicology. New York: Oxford University Press, 2000:289–298.
260. Maynard RL. In: Ballantyne B, Marrs T, Turner T, eds. General and Applied Toxicology. New York: Stockton Press, 1993:1253.
261. Spencer PS, Wilson BW, Albuquerque EX. In: Spencer PS, Schaumburg HH, eds. Experimental and Clinical Neurotoxicology. New York: Oxford University Press, 2000:1073–1093.

262. Meselson M, Perry Robinson J. Sci Am 1980; 242:38–47.
263. Nozaki H, Aikawa N, Fujishima S, Suzuki M, Shinozawa Y, Hori S, Nogawa S Lancet 1995; 346:698–699.
264. Nozaki H, Aikawa N, Shinozawa Y, Hori S, Fujishima S, Takuma K, Sagoh M Lancet 1995; 345:980–981.
265. Morita H, Yanagisawa N, Nakajima T, Shimizu M, Hirabayashi H, Okudera H, Nohara M, Midorikawa Y, Mimura S. Lancet 1995; 346:290–293.
266. Nakajima T, Saro S, Morita H, Yanagisawa N. Occ Environ Med 1997; 54:697–701.
267. Woodall J. Lancet 1997; 350:296.
268. Sidell FR. In: Sidell FR, Takafuji ET, Franz DR, eds. Textbook of Military Medicine: Medical Aspects of Chemical and Biological Warfare. Washington, DC: Office of the Surgeon General, 2002:129–179.
269. Holstege CP, Kirk M, Sidell FR. Crit Care Med 1997; 13:923–942.
270. Dawson RM. J App Toxicol 1994; 14:317–331.
271. Becker G, Kawan A, Szinicz L. Arch Toxicol 1997; 71:714–718.
272. Ecobichon DJ. In: Ecobichon DJ, Joy RM, eds. Pesticides and Neurological Disease. Boca Raton: CRC Press, 1994:251–289.
273. Rotenberg M, Shefi M, Dany S, Dore I, Tirosh M, Almog S. Clin Chim Acta 1995; 234:11–21.
274. Besser R, Vogt T, Gutmann L. Muscle Nerve 1991; 14:1197–1201.
275. Michel HO, Hackley BE Jr, Berkowitz L, List G, Hackley EB, Gillilan W, Pankau M. Arch Biochem Biophys 1967; 121:29–34.
276. Miller SA, Blick DW, Kerenyi SZ, Murphy MR. Pharmacology Biochem Behav 1993; 44:343–347.
277. keeler JR, Hurst CG, Dunn MA. JAMA Aug. 7, 1991; 266:693–695.
278. Lenz DE, Yourick JJ, Dawson JS, Scott J. Immunol Lett 1992; 31:131–135.
279. Lenz DE, Brimfield AA, Hunter KW Jr, Benschop HP, de Jong LP, Van Dijk C, Clow TR, Fund Appl Toxicol 1984; 4:S156–S164.
280. Doctor BP, Blick DW, Caranto G, Castro CA, Gentry MK, Larrison R, Maxwell DM, Murphy MR, Schutz M, Waibel K. Chem Biol Interact 1993; 87:285–293.
281. Doctor BP, Raveh L, Wolfe AD, Maxwell DM, Ashani Y. Neurosci.Biobehav.Rev 1991; 15:123–128.
282. Maxwell DM, Castro CA, De La Hoz DM, Gentry MK, Gold MB, Solana RP, Wolfe AD, Doctor BP. Toxicol Appl Pharmacol 1992; 115:44–49.

8

Pharmacologic Neurotoxicology of Neuromuscular Transmission

I. INTRODUCTION

The previous chapter discussed the unique sensitivity of the neuromuscular junction (NMJ) to a variety of neurotoxins including biological, environmental, and chemical substances. Of more concern to the clinical neurologist are those situations that result from the direct effects of various pharmacologic agents routinely used in the practice of medicine that produce significant aberrations of neuromuscular transmission in susceptible individuals (e.g., those with disorders of neuromuscular transmission). Such deleterious events may be encountered in the outpatient arena as well as in the hospital setting. In some instances, the use of such drugs may seemingly precipitate a neuromuscular syndrome in a patient in whom the disorder was subclinical or in whom the disease was not previously recognized.

II. PHARMACOLOGIC BLOCKADE OF NEUROMUSCULAR TRANSMISSION

Categorically, four clinical situations are encountered in which these drugs produce a worsening of neuromuscular function (Table 8.1). First, there is the direct and augmented deleterious effects of the drug on synaptic transmission in an otherwise apparently normal individual; second, there are those related to a drug-induced disturbance of the immune system that results in the development of myasthenia gravis (MG); third, there is the unmasking of subclinical MG or the worsening of muscle strength in patients with disorders of neuromuscular transmission [MG, Lambert-Eaton syndrome (LES), botulism]; and fourth, there are those with delayed recovery of strength, particularly respiratory function, following general anesthesia during which neuromuscular blocking agents may or may not have been used.

Preexisting circumstances, such as altered drug clearance due to renal or hepatic disease, concomitant drug administration, electrolyte disturbances, or direct toxicity, may predispose the patient to neuromuscular weakness in the first situation. Such an example would be the patient with chronic renal failure, undergoing a surgical procedure during which he or she was given a neuromuscular blocking agent and an aminoglycoside antibiotic. The second situation is most commonly encountered in D-penicillamine (D-P)–induced MG and there are a few reports of similar occurrences in patients receiving tiopronine, pyrithioxine, hydantoin drugs, trimethadione, and possibly chloroquine. In the third situation, the failure of the neuromuscular manifestations to resolve following the discontinuation of the drug implies that the disorder was subclinical and brought forth by the use of the pharmalogic agent. This has been seen in otherwise asymptomatic patients given D-P in whom the clinical symptoms and findings did not resolve following discontinuation of the drug.

The adverse effects of drugs on synaptic transmission may be classified in three ways (Table 8.2). They may act presynaptically, with a reduction in acetylcholine (ACh) release secondary to local anesthetic-like activity on the nerve terminal, an alteration or impairment of calcium flux into the nerve terminal, or a hemicholinium effect. They may act postsynaptically, with antibody-like blockade of ACh receptors (AChRs), or have a curare-like effect

Table 8.1 Mechanisms of Pharmacologic Blockade at the Neuromuscular Junction

---

1. Direct deleterious effects on synaptic transmission in an otherwise normal individual
2. Drug-induced disturbance of the immune system with the resulting development of myasthenia gravis
3. Unmasking of subclinical disease or the worsening of muscle strength in patients with disorders of neuromuscular transmission
4. Delayed recovery of strength, particularly respiratory function, following general anesthesia during which neuromuscular blocking agents may or may not have been used

or potentiation of depolarizing or non-depolarizing neuromuscular blocking agents. In some instances the effects may occur with varying degrees of both. Each of these pharmacologic interactions may result in any of the situations described above (Table 8.1). Since the publication of the summaries of Howard, Argov, Swift, and Kaeser describing disorders of neuromuscular transmission occurring as the result of adverse drug reactions, many more reports have surfaced adding to the list of potentially dangerous agents (1–4). Unfortunately, much of the literature is anecdotal, often involving isolated cases of patients experiencing increased weakness in the setting of use of a particular drug, and there are only a few comprehensive in vitro evaluations of selected drugs on the effects of neuromuscular transmission in animal or human nerve–muscle preparations. As such, it is difficult to know with certainty the cause-and-effect relationship between the drug and increasing MG weakness. The potential adverse effects of these medications must be taken into consideration when deciding which drugs to use in managing other diseases in patients who also have disorders of synaptic transmission. For most drugs the actual incidence of adverse effects is unknown because we do not know how many patients with disease of the NMJ have used the same drug without side effects. The problem is further complicated by the fact that some in vitro studies and animal studies may suggest an adverse drug effect, but these observations may not correlate with clinically significant side effects. While it is most desirable to avoid drugs that may adversely affect neuromuscular transmission, in certain instances they must be used for the management of other illness. In such situations a thorough knowledge by the physician of the deleterious side effects can minimize their potential danger. When possible it is wise to use that drug within a class of drugs that has been shown clinically or at least experimentally to have the least effect on neuromuscular transmission.

With the possible exceptions of D-P, botulinum toxin, and perhaps interferon-α, there are no drugs that are absolutely contraindicated in patients with MG and LES. There are, however, numerous drugs that can and will interfere with neuromuscular transmission and will exacerbate the weakness of these patients or prolong the duration of neuromuscular blockade in patients receiving muscle relaxants. Drug-induced disturbances of synaptic

Table 8.2 Mechanisms by Which Drugs Affect Synaptic Transmission

1. Reduced release of ACh from the presynaptic nerve terminal
2. Potentiation of depolarizing or nondepolarizing neuromuscular blocking agents
3. Blockade of postsynaptic AChRs

transmission resemble MG with varying degrees of ptosis, as well as ocular, facial, bulbar, respiratory, and generalized muscle weakness. Treatment includes discontinuation of the offending drug and when necessary reversing the neuromuscular blockade with intravenous infusions of calcium, potassium, or cholinesterase inhibitors.

While these problems are uncommon, the literature suggests that the most common situation encountered is prolonged muscle weakness and respiratory embarrassment postoperatively, although it is this author's experience, dealing with a large neuromuscular population, that the most frequently encountered problems are the effects of antibiotics (aminoglycoside and macroglides) and β-adrenergic blocking agents acutely worsening the strength of patients with MG. This chapter will review the adverse reactions of major classes of drugs on synaptic transmission. An extensive bibliography is provided so that the reader may have access to the anecdotal experiences of others. It is beyond the scope of this chapter to address known anesthetic complications of synaptic transmission.

A. Analgesics

The narcotic analgesics, in therapeutic concentrations, do not appear to directly depress neuromuscular transmission in myasthenic muscle (5,6). We have routinely used morphine sulfate for analgesia in our postthymectomy patients, without difficulty. However, they should be used with extreme care given their potential for respiratory depression. Cholinesterase inhibitors may potentiate the analgesic effects of morphine, hydromorphone, codeine, and opium alkaloids (7). Grob has reported acute death within hours of receiving morphine sulfate (8).

B. Anesthetics: General

There are no controlled studies addressing the advantages or disadvantages of the use of general anesthetics in patients with disorders of neuromuscular transmission. There may be a potentiation of neuromuscular blocking agents in patients with MG (9). The current practice of pretreating the myasthenic patient with, for example, corticosteroids and/or plasma exchange to achieve a state of marked improvement or remission prior to surgery has obviated much of the earlier concern about prolonged postoperative ventilatory failure (10–12). In our experience, the majority of patients receive combinations of ethrane and nitrous oxide without the use of neuromuscular blocking agents. It is the very rare patient who requires postoperative ventilation some the majority of patients are extubated when fully awake in the operating room or the recovery room. The reader is referred to Foldes for an old but comprehensive review of this topic (13).

There is a single case report of the unmasking of a subclinical case of MG in a nurse anesthetist who had routinely administered the inhalation anesthetic methoxyflurane (13,14). Fatigue, weakness, and ptosis occurred repeatedly on exposure to the anesthetic and waned in severity 2–3 h following the cessation of exposure. Similar symptoms produced by a direct challenge to the agent were readily reversed by neostigmine.

Experimental studies have shown that inhalation anesthetics alter the postjunctional sensitivity to ACh, alter ionic conductances, and cause a shortening of channel open time following activation by ACh (15).

C. Anesthetics: Local

Local anesthetics in and of themselves are unlikely to cause neuromuscular weakness in otherwise normal individuals. However, intravenous injections of lidocaine, procaine, and similar local anesthetic agents are capable of potentiating the effects of neuromuscular blocking agents. The mechanisms of action appear varied with both pre- and postsynaptic effects and may be ascribed to an impairment of the propagation of the nerve action potential in the nerve terminal with a reduction in ACh release (16). In addition, others have demonstrated a reduction in the sensitivity of the postjunctional membrane to ACh (17). Procaine has been reported to produce an acute myasthenic crisis although this has been contested by others (18). An acute myasthenic crisis in a young women undergoing a brachial plexus block using large amounts of lidocaine as the anesthetic for shunt placement has been observed (Howard JF, personal observation).

D. Antibiotics

The earliest report of antibiotio-induced neuromuscular blockade in humans was in 1956 although in 1941 it was demonstrated that tyrothricin, one of the first antibiotics, produced respiratory weakness in animals (19,20). Pridgen reported four patients without prior evidence of neuromuscular disease who developed apnea (resulting in death in two) when given intraperitoneal neomycin sulfate. To date there are several hundred case reports of purported neuromuscular weakness resulting from antibiotic effects on the NMJ in otherwise normal patients, those receiving neuromuscular blocking agents, those with MG, those with other diseases that alter the pharmacokinetics of the drug, and in patients receiving other drugs known to be toxic to the NMJ (21–26).

As a group the aminoglycoside antibiotics are well recognized for producing neuromuscular weakness irrespective of the route of administration (24). The weakness is related to dose and the serum levels and is reversible in part by cholinesterase inhibitors, calcium infusion, and the aminopyridines

(27–29). Experimental nerve–muscle preparations have demonstrated that these drugs act pre- and postsynaptically, many with elements of both. For example, tobramycin has predominantly presynaptic effects similar to those reported with high concentrations of magnesium with inhibition of ACh release, and netilmicin is predominantly postsynaptic with blocking of ACh binding to receptor, similar to curare (30–32). Neuromuscular toxicity data exist for several of the antibiotics, including amikacin, gentamicin, kanamycin, neomycin, netilmicin, streptomycin, and tobramycin (33–39). Of the group neomycin is the most toxic; tobramycin the least (30).

Clinically, only gentamicin, kanamycin, neomycin, tobramycin, and streptomycin have been implicated in producing muscle weakness in non-myasthenic patients (4). The weakness of infant botulism is potentiated by these drugs (40,41). The first case reports of myasthenic exacerbation by antibiotics were described in 1964 by Hokkanen citing the acute deterioration of strength in patients receiving a variety of aminoglycoside antibiotics (42). The degree of weakness varied from minimal to ventilatory failure.

Occasionally, myasthenic patients given erythromycin report a mild exacerbation of their weakness though detailed physiologic examinations have not been carried out (Howard JF, personal observations). Erythromycin therapy in normal volunteers demonstrated a facilitatory response with repetitive nerve stimulation studies suggestive of a presynaptic neuromuscular block, though this has not been confirmed with more sensitive techniques to assess synaptic transmission (43). Similarly, myasthenic worsening has also been reported with azithromycin, and telithromycin (44, JF Howard, personal observations).

Neuromuscular blockade is not limited to the aminoglycoside antibiotics. The polypeptide and monobasic amino acid antibiotics, penicillins, sulfonamides, tetracyclines, and fluoroquinolones have been reported to cause transient worsening of myasthenic weakness, to potentiate the weakness of neuromuscular blocking agents, or to have a theoretical basis for blocking synaptic transmission. Lincomycin and clindamycin, monobasic amino acid antibiotics, are slightly different in sturcture from the aminoglycosides but differ considerably in their effects on synaptic transmission (45,46). Both drugs can cause neuromuscular blockade that is not readily reversible with cholinesterase inhibitors. Both have pre-and postjunctional effects causing reductions in miniature endplate potential (MEPP) frequency, evoked transmitter release, and postjunctional ACh sensitivity (47). The neuromuscular blocking effects of lincomycin may be reversed by increasing the calcium concentration or by administering one of the aminopyridines (48). Cholinesterase inhibitors may worsen the effect. Clindamycin appears to block muscle contractility directly, as well as having a local anesthetic action (49).

Vancomycin may potentiate the neuromuscular blockade of succinyl-choline (50).

Polymyxin B, colistimethate, and colistin have also been reported to produce neuromuscular weakness, particularly in patients with renal disease or when used in combination with other antibiotics or neuromuscular blocking agents (51–56). Experimental studies have shown the effects of these drugs to be mixed, with a reduction in ACh release and, to a lesser degree, postjunctional block of the AChR (57–59). Decker reported acute ventilatory failure in a myasthenic patient given a single intramuscular injection of colistimethate (60). Colistin is also reported to acutely exacerbate the strength of myasthenic patients (61).

Tetracycline analogues, oxytetracycline and rolitetracycline, have also been reported to exacerbate MG though the mechanism is unclear (62,63). It has been suggested that the mechanism may be due to the magnesium in the diluent causing a reduction in ACh release from the nerve terminal (63). Others have reported no adverse reactions with tetracycline or alteration of neuromuscular transmission in nerve–muscle preparations (30,42).

More recently, it has been suggested that ampicillin may aggravate the strength of patients with MG or worsen the decrement of repetitive nerve stimulation in rabbits with experimental autoimmune myasthenia gravis (EAMG) (64). Girlanda and coworkers have demonstrated in vivo changes of synaptic transmission in healthy volunteers by single-fiber electromyography (SFEMG), the most sensitive technique to assess synaptic efficacy (65,66). The mechanism of action for the neuromuscular block is not known; bath application of this antibiotic to nerve–muscle preparations has not produced an abnormality of neuromuscular transmission (64).

There are a few case reports suggesting that quinolones may acutely worsen the strength of patients with MG. Ciprofloxacillin, perfloxacin, and norfloxacin have been implicated (67–70). In the author's experience, there are some MG patients who tolerate ciprofloxacillin without difficulty, yet others who experience substantial worsening of their strength. The mechanism of this effect is not known.

E. Anticonvulsants

Diphenylhydantoin (DPH) has been shown to depress both pre- and post-synaptic mechanisms of neuromuscular transmission in experimental systems (71–73). Symptomatic MG has been reported to occur in previously asymptomatic patients receiving a variety of anticonvulsant medications including phenytoin, mephenytoin, trimethadione, and gabapentin (73–78). In some individuals weakness has reversed following discontinuation of the drug, suggesting that there is a direct neuromuscular blocking effect of these drugs. Experimentally phenytoin has been demonstrated to reduce quantal release from the nerve terminal and to simultaneously increase spontaneous neurotransmitter release (MEPPs). This has been explained by a reduction in the amplitude of the nerve action potential or an antagonism of calcium influx into the nerve terminal and its intracellular sequestration. In addition, phenytoin also exerts postsynaptic effects; reducing the amplitude of MEPPs by presumably desensitizing the endplate (72). Osserman has also reported that barbiturates could aggravate myasthenic strength (79). Experimentally it has been shown that barbiturates and ethosuximide will produce a post-synaptic neuromuscular block and carbamazepine exerts most of its effects presynaptically (80,81). Another recent report emphasized the presence of a defect of neuromuscular transmission as demonstrated by a decremental response at high-frequency repetitive stimulation in children who had received an overdose of carbamezapine (82). To date there have been no clinical reports of adverse reactions with ethosuximide.

It has been suggested that trimethadione may induce an autoimmune disorder directed to the NMJ. This is suggested by the development of other autoimmune diseases (systemic lupus erythematosus, nephrotic syndrome) in patients receiving this drug; the demonstration of other autoantibodies against skeletal muscle, nuclear antigens, and thymic tissue; and the prolonged recovery following discontinuation of these agents (76,77,83,84).

In the experience of this author, there has been no acute clinical worsening of strength in those few patients who have required phenytoin therapy for seizures.

F. Cardiovascular Drugs

Many cardiovascular drugs have been implicated in adversely affecting the strength of patients with MG and LES and they, along with the antibiotics, account for the majority of adverse drug reactions in patients with neuromuscular disorders. Certain ones, including quinine, have in the past been used as a diagnostic test for MG (85,86).

1. β-Adrenergic Blocking Agents

β-adrenergic blocking agents, despite their clinical usefulness, may cause serious side effects; in particular, some are implicated in causing symptomatic worsening of strength in patients with MG. Even those drugs instilled topically on the cornea are capable of producing such weakness (see Section K below). The β-blockers oxprenolol, propranolol, practolol, and timolol have been previously reported to potentiate weakness in MG patients (87–91). Weber cites several cases of transient diplopia in patients receiving a variety of β-blockers though extensive evaluation of neuromuscular transmission was not performed (92). In this author's experience, two patients given timolol maleate, one patient given betaxolol for glaucoma, and one patient given pindolol for hypertension experienced abrupt worsening of their strength (Howard JF, personal observation). Furthermore, the onset of myasthenic symptoms coincided with the initiation of drug therapy with the β-blockers propranolol and nadolol in four other patients (Howard JF, personal observations). However, others have disputed this observation (93). To date, much of the previous experimental work has examined the effects of various β-blockers on changes in muscle twitch tension (94–101). There is only one comprehensive study using intracellular electrophysiologic techniques to measure the effects of β-blockers on the pre-and postsynaptic mechanisms of neuromuscular transmission. Atenolol, labetolol, metoprolol, nadolol, propranolol, and timolol cause a dose-dependent reduction in the efficacyof neuromuscular transmission in normal rat skeletal muscle and human myasthenic intercostal muscle biopsies (Howard JF, unpublished observations) (102). Different β-blockers have reproducibly different pre- and postsynaptic effects on neuromuscular transmission at motor endplates. The reduction in MEPP amplitude caused by all of these drugs suggests a postsynaptic site of action. Additional presynaptic effects of these drugs are suggested by the relatively large reductions in endplate potential (EPP) amplitude as compared to MEPP amplitude reduction, drug-induced alterations in MEPP frequency caused by all of the β-blockers other than timolol, and the reduction in quantal content caused by metoprolol and propranolol. Propranolol is the most effective β-blocker for impairing neuromuscular transmission. Compared to propranolol, the other β-blockers had weaker effects on neuromuscular transmission. Atenolol had the least effect of these drugs on neuromuscular transmission.

The molecular mechanisms of β-blocker-induced neuromuscular blockade have yet to be elucidated. One possibility is that these drugs specifically block β-adrenergic receptors whose activation is important for neuromuscular transmission. Another source of natural adrenergic agonists might be the motor nerve terminals themselves. It has been shown that enzymes responsible for the synthesis of catecholamines are present in human and rat nerve terminals (103). β-Receptor stimulation has been implicated in having important functional roles in neuromuscular transmission (104). Adrenaline has been shown to modulate the Na^+, K^+ pump, and this effect can be blocked by propranolol (105). Pump activity is suggested to control endplate depolarization by ACh agonists through its electrogenic effects and to control AChR sensitivity by regulating the phosphorylation state of the receptor (106,107). In addition, β receptors appear to be involved in the modulation of transmitter release from mammalian motor nerve terminals; noradrenaline and isoprenaline enhance neurally evoked transmitter output, and this is blocked by propranolol and atenolol (108). Other alternative mechanisms of action for these drugs other than specific blocking of β-adrenergic receptors could include competitive curare-like actions, channel blockade, reduction of single-channel conductance, and general anesthetic effects (109). The facts that β-blockers had qualitatively different effects on MEPP frequency which were also concentration dependent and that not all drugs had the same qualitative effects on MEPP and EPP time courses suggests that at least some of their effects are not related to β-receptor blockade. Of course, β-blocker-specific and more general effects of these drugs could both contribute to the quantitative and qualitative concentration dependent effects that have been described.

2. Bretylium

Bretylium is a quaternary ammonium compound used previously for refractory ventricular arrhythmias. In high concentrations it is reported to cause significant weakness and to significantly potentiate the neuromuscular block of competitive neuromuscular blocking agents (104,110).

3. Calcium Channel Blockers

The effects of calcium channel blockers on myocardial muscle have been extensively characterized, but their effects on skeletal muscle are less well understood. Studies to date have resulted in conflicting information. Some have demonstrated neuromuscular blockade with postsynaptic curare-like effects, presynaptic inhibition of ACh release, and both pre- and postsynaptic effects (94,111–115). The oral administration of calcium channel blockers to cardiac patients without neuromuscular disease did not produce any evidence of altered neuromuscular transmission by SFEMG (116). There is one reported case of a patient with Duchenne muscular dystrophy who had an acute exacerbation of weakness with respiratory failure following the intravenous administration of verapamil (117). Precise details are not known but it was postulated that the patient had end-stage muscle disease, and even minimal alteration of synaptic efficacy was enough to acutely decompensate the patient. Krendel has reported the temporal association of acute respiratory failure in a patient with LES and small cell carcinoma of the lung who was given oral doses of verapamil (118). One patient with moderately severe, generalized myasthenia developed acute respiratory failure following verapamil initiation (Howard JF, unpublished observations). Elderly myasthenic patients have experienced worsening of their strength after receiving felodipine and nifedipine for arterial hypertension (119). Low doses of verapamil or its timed-release preparation have been used successfully for the management of hypertension in patients with MG receiving cyclosporine (Howard JF, unpublished observations; Phillips JT, personal communication). Others have also reported safe use of these drugs in myasthenic patients (93).

4. Procainamide

Procainamide (Pronestyl) is reported to produce acute worsening of strength in patients with MG (120,121). The rapid onset of neuromuscular blockade and the rapid resolution of symptoms following discontinuation of the drug suggest that the drug has a direct toxic effect on synaptic transmission rather than the induction of an autoimmune response against the NMJ. The postulated mechanism of action is primarily at the presynaptic membrane with impaired formation of ACh and/or its release though it is known to have postsynaptic blocking effects as well.

5. Quinine and Quinidine

The earliest report of quinidine (the stereoisomer of quinine) administration aggravating MG was by Weisman (122). There are several reports of the unmasking of previous unrecognized cases of MG following treatment with quinidine (121,123,124). It has been demonstrated that the neuromuscular block is both presynaptic, impairing either the formation or release of ACh, or, in larger doses, postsynaptic with a curare-like action (125). Sieb et al. studied the effects of quinolone derivatives on neuromuscular transmission using conventional microelectrode and patch-clamp techniques. All three derivatives reduce quantal content of the endplate potential by 37–45% and decrease the amplitude and decay time constant of the MEPP and miniature endplate current (126). At progressively larger concentrations the MEPP becomes undetectable. The effects were not reversed by neostigmine. Single-channel patch-clamp analysis of quinine effects demonstrate a long-lived open-channel and a closed-channel block of the AChR. The literature suggests that the ingestion of small amounts of quinine, in a gin and tonic, will acutely worsen myasthenic symptoms though this can not be substantiated with objective reports (127–129). Quinidine is also capable of potentiating the weakness of non-depolarizing and depolarizing neuromuscular blocking agents (130,131). Quinolone drugs adversely affect both presynaptic and postsynaptic aspects of neuromuscular transmission at concentrations close to those employed in clinical practice. Myasthenic patients receiving standard doses of quinine for management of leg cramps may develop markedly increased weakness within hours to days of starting the medication. Therefore, these drugs should not be used, or should be used only with extreme caution, in disorders having a reduced safety margin of neuromuscular transmission (Pascuzzi, R, personal communication).

6. Trimethaphan

There are isolated case reports that trimethaphan, a ganglionic blocking agent used in hypertensive emergencies, dissecting aortic aneurysms, cerebral aneurysm surgery, and for decreasing cardiac afterload in patients with myocardial infarction, can produce neuromuscular weakness. It has been reported to cause acute respiratory paralysis probably due to curare-like action at the NMJ (132). In addition, it has been reported to potentiate the neuromuscular block in patients receiving both non-depolarizing neuromuscular blocking agents and depolarizing neuromuscular blocking agents (133–135).

G. Hormones

1. Estrogen and Progesterone

Estrogen therapy has been reported to acutely worsen the strength of a patient with MG though the details of this case are subject to question (136). Parenteral progesterone has been reported to aggravate the strength of myasthenic women after a delay of 3–5 days (137). There is an isolated case report of MG occurring in a woman taking birth control pills, but there are no data to suggest that their use increases the incidence of MG or worsens the strength of patients with MG (138). The mechanism of acute worsening in these patients has yet to be elucidated.

2. Thyroid Hormone

The relationship of the thyroid gland to MG is well recognized (139). The older literature states that thyroid hormone and antithyroid medications can aggravate the strength of patients with MG perhaps through a reduction in the release of ACh, although this has not been felt to be a problem of late with newer modes of therapy (140–142).

H. Immune Modulators

Patients treated with interferon-α develop a variety of autoantibodies and autoimmune diseases including MG. The initial reports of interferon-induced MG occurred in 1995 when a 66-year-old man was reported to develop seropositive generalized MG about 6 months after starting interferon-α therapy for leukemia (143). Subsequently, MG has developed in other patients during interferon-α 2b treatment for malignancy (144,145). Patients treated for chronic active hepatitis C with interferon-α have also developed autoimmune MG with onset from 6 to 9 months after starting treatment. In one case MG symptoms persisted for at least 7 months following cessation of drug (146,147). Fulminating myasthenic crisis may occur after interferon-α therapy (148).

Regarding the mechanism of interferon-induced MG, the expression of interferon-γ at motor endplates of transgenic mice results in generalized weakness, abnormal NMJ function, and improvement with cholinesterase inhibitors. Immunoprecipitation analysis indicates that a previously unidentified 87-kD target antigen is recognized by sera from those transgenic mice and also from human MG patients. Such studies suggest that the expression of interferon-γ at motor endplates in these transgenic mice provokes an autoimmune humoral response, similar to that which occurs in human MG (149). While the number of anecdotal case reports has increased to suggest a cause-and-effect relationship between interferon-α and MG, recent reports have also suggested that MG may occur independently in association with hepatitis C (150–153).

I. Magnesium

Hypermagnesemia is an uncommon clinical situation associated with the use of magnesium-containing drugs (154). Magnesium (Mg^{2+}) is contained in some antacids and laxatives. Magnesium sulfate ($MgSO_4$) is used in the management of pre-eclampsia and eclampsia, for hemodynamic control during anesthesia and the early postoperative period, and in patients depleted of Mg^{2+} (such as in chronic alcoholism) (155). Normal serum magnesium runs 1.5–2.5 mEq/L (2–3 mg/dL) which is stabilized through exchange with tissue stores in bone, liver, muscle, and brain; also, serum Mg^{2+} concentration is maintained via renal excretion. Patients having renal failure are predisposed to developing hypermagnesemia, and should avoid magnesium-containing antacids and laxatives for this reason (156,157). Elevated serum magnesium levels due to oral use of magnesium-containing compounds is very uncommon, so long as the patient has normal renal function (158,159). Hypermagnesemia is occasionally seen with use of enemas, but this usually occurs in patients with an underlying gastrointestinal tract disorder (158,160). In the management of preeclampsia, hypermagnesemia occurs commonly due to administration of high doses of parenteral $MgSO_4$, at times resulting in serious side effects in the mother or the newborn (161–163). The clinical features of hypermagnesemia correlate fairly well with the serum magnesium levels (158,164,165). In treating patients with pre-eclampsia, the neuromuscular transmission effects are monitored and used as a limiting factor in dosage. With serum levels above 5 mEq/L, the muscle stretch reflexes become reduced, while levels of 9–10 mEq/L are associated with absent reflexes and clinically significant weakness. In treating patients with pre-eclampsia, muscle stretch reflexes are tested serially, and magnesium administration is stopped if the reflexes disappear (162). Serum levels between 3.5 and 7 mEq/L are usually associated with no significant adverse effects in preeclamptic women, but clinical weakness is common with levels greater than 10 mEq/L and death from respiratory failure can occur (161,162). Serum levels above 14 mEq/L can induce acute cardiac arrhythmia including heart block and arrest. Additional symptoms from autonomic nervous system involvement include dry mouth, pupil delations urinary retention, hypotension, and skin flushing thought to be caused by presynaptic blockade at autonomic ganglia (166). Although patients can develop severe weakness, mental status is usually not directly affected (165). Reduced level of consciousness may occur indirectly as a result of hypoxia, hypercarbia, or hypotension. The muscles of ocular motility tend to be spared.

Magnesium interferes with neuromuscular transmission by inhibiting the release of ACh by competitively blocking calcium entry at the motor nerve terminal (167). There may also be a more mild postsynaptic effect. Clinically, hypermagnesemia resembles LES more so than autoimmune MG (168). In addition, magnesium can potentiate the action of neuromuscular blocking agents, which has been emphasized in women who had cesarean section after treatment with Mg^{2+} for preeclamsia (169,170). Patients with underlying junctional disorders are more sensitive to Mg^{2+}-induced weakness. Patients with MG and LES have been reported to exacerbate in the setting of Mg^{2+} use in spite of normal or only mildly elevated serum levels (171–175). Typically, increased MG symptoms occur with parenteral magnesium administration, but on occasion is seen with oral use (175). Therefore, parenteral Mg^{2+} administration should be avoided and oral Mg^{2+} preparations used with caution in patients with known disorders of synaptic transmission (e.g. MG, LES, botulism, etc.).

The effect of standard parenteral doses of $MgSO_4$ on neuromuscular transmission of preeclamptic or preterm labor patients is significant though largely subclinical. Train-of-four (TOF) recordings obtained from the thenar muscles before and 30 min after $MgSO_4$ infusion shows an increase in tension of the contractile response in the control or baseline recordings, but the postinfusion TOF shows no increase but rather fading of the response (176). These data suggest that in this patient population clinically relevant infusions of $MgSO_4$ produced significant changes in neuromuscular transmission as manifested by loss of the "treppe phenomenon" and diminished TOF response to nerve stimulation. $MgSO_4$ (60 mg/kg) effects on residual neuromuscular block after administration of vecuronium is also significant (155). Patients given Mg^{2+} immediately upon recovery from vecuronium block or 1 h later demonstrate rapid and profound recurarization as measured by EMG and TOF studies.

Treatment of the hypermagnesemic patient depend on the severity of clinical symptoms. Discontinuation of magnesium is the first step; if the patient is significantly weak, administration of intravenous calcium gluconate, 1 g over 3 min, can produce rapid but temporary improvement (so long as the patient has normal renal function typical for a patient being treated for pre-eclampsia). If hypermagnesemia is more severe or if there are life-threatening side effects such as cardiac arrhythmia or renal failure, hemodialysis is indicated (177). If patients have MG or LES, they will respond poorly to calcium. Such patients may respond better to cholinesterase inhibitors (172).

J. Neuromuscular Blocking Drugs

It is common to categorize the muscle relaxants as depolarizing agents or non-depolarizing agents depending on their effects on the muscle membrane potential. The actions of these neuromuscular blocking agents are modified by a number of factors, including the degree of neuromuscular blockade, associated disease states, acid–base status, and electrolyte imbalance (178). Competitive, non-depolarizing neuromuscular blocking agents can be many times more sensitive in their effects in myasthenic and presumably LES patients than in those individuals without these diseases. As such, small amounts of these drugs may produce a greater degree of and a more prolonged period of neuromuscular blockade. Depolarizing agents such as succinylcholine also must be used with caution; the inhibition of hydrolysis by cholinesterase inhibitors prolongs its duration of action (13). In addition, patients with MG are less sensitive to this drug, being lulled into a sense of false security and thus ending up with prolonged blockade because of the larger amount of drug used. The occasional unmasking of MG in patients given these drugs is recognized by those seeing large numbers of myasthenic patients and has been reported (Howard JF, personal observations; 14). In addition to the effects of disease, the pharmacologic effects of these neuromuscular blocking agents are potentiated by a number of different drugs (see above), including antibiotics, general anesthetics, local anesthetics, and antiarrhythmics. While the newer neuromuscular blocking agents are of much shorter duration, the same concerns and guidelines would apply when used in patients with MG or LES. Prolonged muscle weakness has been reported in myasthenic patients receiving these drugs. Benzing reports a myasthenic child who developed severe, generalized muscle weakness that persisted for 6 weeks after receiving muscle relaxants for 1 week while requiring ventilator support (179).

Prolonged apnea and muscle weakness in patients given depolarizing neuromuscular blocking agents may also occur in situations where plasma cholinesterase levels are reduced, either by plasma exchange or in patients with genetic abnormalities of plasma cholinesterase (180,181).

K. Ophthalmic Drugs

The β-adrenergic blocking eye drops Timoptic (timolol maleate) and Betopic (betaxolol hydrochloride) (Howard JF, unpublished observations) have been reported to be associated with the temporal exacerbation of MG (89–91). Their mechanism of neuromuscular blockade is as described above (see Section F above). Ecothiophate, a long-acting cholinesterase inhibitor used in the management of open-angle glaucoma, is reported to produce muscle weakness and fatigue that resolved following the discontinuation of the drug (182). While the mechanism of weakness was not determined it is possible that the use of a long-acting cholinesterase inhibitor could produce additive effects, i.e., cholinergic weakness, in patients with MG currently receiving cholinesterase inhibitors or potentiate the weakness induced by depolarizing neuromuscular blocking agents (183).

L. Psychotropic Drugs

1. Phenothiazines

Chlorpromazine was first reported to produce an acute exacerbation of muscle weakness following the administration of this drug in a myasthenic schizophrenic patient by McQuillen and colleagues (184). This finding confirmed previous pharmacologic studies on nerve-muscle preparations that chlorpromazine produces a postsynaptic block with a reduction in MEPP and EPP amplitudes without alteration in quantal content or MEPP frequency, although others have suggested that there are presynaptic effects as well (185). Phenothiazines (chlorpromazine and promazine) can antagonize applied ACh and may prolong the effects of succinylcholine. Anecdotal reports exist of prolonged neuromuscular blockade in patients given depolarizing neuromuscular blocking drugs while receiving promazine and phenelzine (186,187).

2. Lithium

Long-term lithium carbonate administration has been reported to produce varying degrees of muscle weakness, although in the majority of instances the mechanism for such occurences are not known. The experimental literature is conflicting; some investigators have postulated a progressive accumulation of lithium inside the presynaptic nerve terminal where it functions as a competitive cation for calcium resulting in an inhibition of ACh synthesis and a reduction in quantal release (188,189). Others have demonstrated a reduction in the number of ACh receptors in denervated muscle preparations, suggesting that lithium selectively increases the rate of receptor degradation without altering their synthesis (190). Several anecdotal reports of prolonged neuromuscular blockade in patients receiving long-term lithium therapy and neuromuscular blocking agents have appeared (191–193). Neil describes the best account of the development of fatigable weakness responsive to cholinesterase inhibitors and electrophysiologic abnormalities consistent with the diagnosis of MG (194). Granacher reports the development of ptosis and weakness within 48 h of receiving lithium, although that patient did not respond to cholinesterase inhibitors and decremental responses were not seen with repetitive nerve stimulation (195). Acute worsening of the decremental response to repetitive nerve stimulation has been observed in a patient recovering from the hidden form of botulism who was given lithium for her bipolar disorder (Howard, JF, unpublished observations).

3. Others

Argov and Mastaglia have also implicated amitriptyline, amphetamines, droperidol, haloperidol, imipramine, paraldehyde, and trichloroethanol as all being capable of interfering with synaptic transmission under experimental systems (2).

M. Rheumatologic Drugs

1. Chloroquine

Chloroquine is used primarily as an antimalarial but in higher doses is also used in the management of several collagen vascular disorders including rheumatoid arthritis, discoid lupus erythematosus, and porphyria cutanea. It may produce a number of neurologic side effects among which are myopathies and disorders of neuromuscular transmission. The reported mechanisms of action for the latter have been both presynaptic, with a reduction in EPP amplitude resulting from a decrease in the amplitude of nerve action potentials and ACh release, and postsynaptic, with competitive postjunctional blockade (196,197). In addition, it is reported that chloroquine will directly suppress the excitability of the muscle membrane.

There is some evidence to suggest that chloroquine may alter immune regulation and produce a clinical syndrome of MG similar to that reported with D-P. Two cases are reported, one with rheumatoid arthritis and the other with systemic lupus erythematosus. In both cases, following prolonged treatment with chloroquine the patient developed the typical clinical, physiologic, and pharmacologic signs of MG. Antibodies to the AChR were present and subsequently slowly disappeared, as did the clinical and electrophysiologic abnormalities, with discontinuation of the drug (198,199).

De Bleeker reports a case of persistent MG following the intermittent use of antimalarial (200). Robberecht and colleagues report the transient development of a postjunctional disorder of neuromuscular transmission following a week of chloroquine therapy (201). In this case, AChR antibodies were not demonstrated, and the rapid resolution of symptoms suggested that this syndrome was related to a direct toxic effect at the NMJ rather than a derangement of immune function as mentioned above. That this drug could have both effects of neuromuscular transmission is not unheard of; the hydantoin drugs exert their effects similarly.

2. D-Penicillamine

D-Penicillamine is used in the management of rheumatoid arthritis (RA), Wilson's disease, and cystinuria. A number of autoimmune diseases occur in patients receiving D-P, including immune complex nephritis, pemphigus, polymyositis, systemic lupus erythematosus and, most frequently, MG (202–210). The myasthenia induced by D-P is usually mild and may be restricted to the ocular muscles. In many patients the symptoms are not recognized and it may be difficult to demonstrate mild weakness of the limbs in the presence of severe arthritis. The diagnosis can be confirmed by the response to cholinesterase inhibitors, EMG abnormalities and elevated serum AChR antibodies (211–213). In our experience, repetitive stimulation studies are abnormal less often than is SFEMG, reflecting the relatively mild degree of neuromuscular abnormality present in most of these patients. Intercostal muscle biopsy studies have shown reduced MEPP amplitude as seen in acquired MG (212).

In normal rats, D-P given in doses equivalent to the human therapeutic dose produces no neuromuscular abnormality (214). In guinea pigs, chronic administration of doses more than 10 times the therapeutic level produced a mild degree of neuromuscular blockade (215). These studies provide no evidence that D-P produces a direct, clinically significant effect on neuromuscular transmission. It is unlikely that D-P has a direct effect on neuromuscular transmission. MG begins after prolonged D-P therapy in most patients and has a relatively low incidence in patients receiving D-P for Wilson's disease compared to those receiving it for RA. D-P has been reported to produce a variety of other autoimmune disorders (210,211). It is more likely that D-P induces MG by stimulating or enhancing an immunologic reaction against the NMJ.

Similarly, tiopronine and pyrithioxine have been reported to induce MG after prolonged administration of the drug (216,217). In each, antibodies to the AChR were demonstrated and the time course of resolution was prolonged. This suggests that the effects of these drugs are not due to direct toxicity to the NMJ but rather that an alteration of immune function occurs, as is the case with D-P.

It is not rare to see MG and RA in the same patient. When myasthenia begins while the patient is receiving D-P, it remits in 70% of patients within a year after the drug is discontinued (218). As the myasthenia improves, the AChR antibody titer falls and the electromyographic abnormalities improve or disappear altogether (212,213,218; Sanders DB, Howard JF, unpublished observations). In a few patients the MG persists after D-P is discontinued, implying that a subclinical myasthenic state existed prior to the initiation of D-P (Howard JF, personal observations).

N. Miscellaneous

D,L-Carnitine, but not L-carnitine, has been reported to acutely worsen the strength of patients with MG undergoing dialysis (219). The precise mechanism of neuromuscular blockade is not known but postulated to be a presynaptic block similar to that produced by hemicholinium or a postsynaptic block by the accumulation of acylcarnitine esters (220).

Diuretics have been suggested to aggravate the strength of patients with MG, probably by potassium wasting (221). It has been long recognized that myasthenic patients are uniquely sensitive to hypokalemia or even low-normal levels of serum potassium.

Emetine, originally used as an amebicide and the principal ingredient of ipecac syrup, has been reported to produce acute neuromuscular weakness in nonmyasthenic patients receiving the drug as an amebicide (222,222). One of the postulated mechanisms of action in experimental preparations is to inhibit indirectly elicited action potentials that are not reversed with cholinesterase inhibitors (223).

Hutchinson has reported acute crisis in MG patients given enemas preparatory to radiographic procedures. This has not been confirmed by others (224), but it could be postulated that the abrupt removal of cholinesterase inhibitors from the gastrointestinal tract could precipitate acute myasthenic worsening in the brittle patient or a large magnesium load could reduce ACh release from the nerve terminal.

The intravenous infusion of iodinated contrast agents has been reported to acutely worsen the strength of patients with MG or precipitate a myasthenic crisis (225,226). Others have not found such problems in a retrospective study of their patient population though the recommendation for caution was made (227). The mechanism of these adverse reactions in MG patients is not known. There is one report of a single patient with LES who developed transient, severe respiratory insufficiency following the intravenous infusion of iodinated contrast material (228). The postulated mechanism of action is an acute hypocalcemia due to direct binding by the contrast agent resulting in further presynaptic blockade with a reduction in ACh release.

The intravenous infusion of sodium lactate is reported to worsen the strength, including respiratory function, in patients with MG (127). The mechanism for this is not known but is postulated to be related to transient hypocalcemia resulting in impaired neurotransmitter release from the nerve terminal.

There is a single case report of myasthenic weakness following administration of tetanus antitoxin (229).

Trasylol, a proteolytic enzyme inhibitor that is no longer available, is reported to potentiate the action of suxamethonium and tubocurarine (230).

Trihexiphenidyl (Artane) is reported to unmask and worsen the strength of a single patient with MG. In this case report it is stated that the concentration of AChR antibody paralleled the degree of weakness when challenged with this drug (231).

Botulinum neurotoxin, when used therapeutically for treatment of focal dystonias, has unmasked subclinical LES (232). Myasthenic crisis or worsening of muscle strength has been reported following injections of botulism toxin (233,234). The use of botulinum toxin is considered to be a relative contraindication in patients with a known defect of neuromuscular transmission.

Numerous drugs have been demonstrated to produce or exacerbate a neuromuscular block in experimental situations. To date there are no known reports of clinical adverse reactions with these drugs in patients with neuromuscular disorders or the precipitation of muscle weakness in otherwise normal patients. Amantadine appears to reduce the postjunctional sensitivity to inotophoretically applied ACh by interacting with the ionic channel of the AChR (235). Ironically, azathioprine, often used as treatment for MG, has been shown to potentiate the neuromuscular block of succinylcholine in cat nerve–muscle preparations but to antagonize the neuromuscular block of curare (236). Like theophylline, it has been found to inhibit the action of phosphodiesterase, the enzyme that hydrolyzes cyclic AMP. The increased concentration of cyclic AMP produces increased neurotransmitter release. It has been postulated that such an effect occurs because of the inhibition of phosphodiesterase in the motor nerve terminal. In this author's experience, there have been no untoward neuromuscular blocking effects in myasthenic patients receiving this drug as part of their treatment. Diphenhydramine has been shown to potentiate the neuromuscular block of barbiturates and neuromuscular blocking agents, and to reduce the amount of neurotransmitter released from the NMJ (237).

REFERENCES

1. Howard JF. Semin Neurol 1990; 10:89–102.
2. Argov Z, Mastaglia FL. N Eng Jo Med 1979; 301:409–413.
3. Swift TR. Muscle Nerve 1981; 4:334–353.
4. Kaeser HE. Acta Neurol Scand 1984; 70:39–37.
5. Kim YI, Howard JF, Sanders DB. Soc Neurosci Abstr 1979; 5:482–482.
6. Sanders DB, Kim YI, Howard JF, Johns TR, Muller WH. Ann NY Acad Sci 1981; 377:544–566.
7. Slaughter D. Arch Int Pharmacodyn 1950; 83:143–148.
8. Grob D. J Chronic Dis 1958; 8:536–566.
9. Baraka A, Afifi A, Muallem M, Kachachi T, Frayha F. Bri J Anaesth 1971; 43:91–95.
10. Howard JF. Semin Neurol 1982; 2:273–279.
11. Howard JF, Sanders DB. In: Albuquerque EX, Eldefrawi AT, eds. Myasthenia Gravis. London: Chapman and Hall, 1983:457–489.
12. Sanders DB, Howard JF. In: Bradley WG, Daroff RB, Fenichel GM, Marsden CD, eds. Neurology in Clinical Practice. Boston: Butterworth, 1991:1819–1842.
13. Foldes FF, McNall PG. Anesthesiology 1962; 23:837–872.
14. Elder BF, Beal H, DeWald W, Cobb S. Anesth Analg 1971; 50:383–387.
15. Gage PW, Hamill OP. Br J Pharmacol 1976; 57:263–272.
16. Matthews EK, Quilliam JP. Br J Pharmacol 2000; 22:415–440.
17. Hirst GDS, Wood DR. Br J Pharmacol 1971; 41:94–104.
18. Katz RL, Gissen AJ. Acta Anaesthesiol Scand 1969; 36:103–113.
19. Pridgen JE. Surgery 1956; 40:571–574.
20. Robinson J, Molitor H. Surgery 1956; 40:571–574.
21. Benz HG, Lunn JN, Foldes FF. Br J Med 1961; 2:241–242.
22. Bodley PO, Brett JE. Anaesthesia 1962; 17:438–443.
23. McQuillen MP, et al. Arch Neurol 1968; 18:402–402.
24. Pittinger CB, Eryasa Y, Adamson R. Anesth Analg 1970; 49:487–487.
25. Albiero L. Arch Int Pharmacodyn Ther 1978; 233:343–343.
26. Burkett L, et al. Anesth Analg 1979; 58:107–115.
27. Singh YN, Harvey AL, Marshall IG. Anesthesiology 1978; 48:418–424.
28. Singh YN, Marshall IG, Harvey AL. J Pharm Pharmacol 1978; 30:249–250.
29. Maeno T, Enomoto K. Proc Jpn Acad 1980; 56(7):486–491.
30. Caputy AJ, Kim YI, Sanders DB. J Pharmacol Exp Therap 1981; 217:369–378.
31. Waterman PM, Smith RB. Anesth Analg 1977; 56:587–588.
32. Dretchen KL, Gergis SD, Sokoll MD, et al. Eur J Pharmacol 1972; 18:201–203.
33. Singh YN, Marshall IG, Harvey AL. B J Anaesth 1978; 50:109–109.
34. Torda T. Br Jo Anaesth 1980; 52:325–325.
35. Paradelis AG, Triantaphyllidis C, Giala MM. Metha Find Expt Clin Pharmacol 1980; 2(1):45–51.
36. Elmqvist D, Josefsson JO. Acta Physiol Scand 1962; 54:105–110.
37. Albiero L. Eur J Pharmacol 1978; 50:1–7.
38. Dretchen KL, Sokoll MD, Gergis SD. Eur J Pharmacol 1973; 22:10–16.

39. De Rosayro M, Healy TEJ. Br J Anaesth 1978; 50:251–251.

40. L'Hommedieu C, Stough R, Brown L, Kettrick R, Polin R. J Pediatrics 1979; 95:1065–1070.

41. Santos JI, Swenson P, Glasgow LA. Pediatrics 1981; 68:50–54.

42. Hokkanen E. Acta Neurol Scand 1964; 40:346–352.

43. Herishanu Y, Taustein I. Confinia Neurol 1971; 33:41–45.

44. Cadisch R, Streit E, Hartmann K. Schweizerische Med Wochenschr J Suisse Med Feb 24, 1996; 126:308–310.

45. Samuelson RJ, Giesecke AH Jr, Kallus FT, Stanley VF. Anesth Analg 1975; 54:103–105.

46. Fogdall RP, Miller RD. Anesthesiology 1974; 41:407–408.

47. Rubbo JT, Gergis SD, Sokoll MD. Anesth Analg 1977; 56:329–332.

48. Booij LHD, Miller RD, Crul JF. Anesth Analg 1978; 57:316–321.

49. Wright JM, Collier B. Cana J Physiol Pharmacol 1976; 54:926–936.

50. Albrecht RF, Lanier WL. Anesth Analg 1993; 77:1300–1302.

51. Pittinger C, Adamson R. Annu Rev Pharmacol 1972; 12:109–184.

52. McQuillen MP, Engbaek L. Arch Neurol 1975; 32:235–238.

53. Parisi AF, Kaplan MH. JAMA 1965; 194:298–299.

54. Pohlmann G. JAMA 1966; 196:181–183.

55. Gold GN, Richardson AP. Am J Med 1966; 41:316–321.

56. Lindesmith LA, Baines RD, Bigelow DB, Petty TL. Ann Intern Med 1968; 68:318–327.

57. Durant NN, Lambert JJ. Br J Pharmacol 1981; 72:41–47.

58. Viswanath DV, Jenkins HJ. J Pharm Sci 1978; 67(9):1275–1275.

59. Wright JM, Collier B. Can J Physiol Pharm 1976; 54:937–944.

60. Decker DA, Fincham RW. Arch Neurol 1971; 25:141–144.

61. Herishanu Y. Confinia Neurol 1969; 31:370–373.

62. Gibbels E. Dtsch Med Wochenschr 1967; 92:1153–1154.

63. Wullen F, Kast G, Bruck A. Dtsch Med Wochenschr 1967; 92:667–669.

64. Argov Z, Brenner T, Abramsky O. Arch Neurol 1986; 43:255–256.

65. Girlanda P, Venuto C, Mangiapane R. Eur Neurol 1989; 29:36–38.

66. Sanders DB, Howard JF. Muscle Nerve 1986; 9:809–819.

67. Moore B, Safani M, Keesey J. Lancet 1988; 1:882–882.

68. Roquer J, Cano A, Seoane JL, Pou SA. Acta Neurol Scand 1996; 94:419–420.

69. Vial T, Chauplannaz G, Brunel P, Leriche B, Evreux JC. Rev Neurol (Paris) 1995; 151:286–287.

70. Rauser EH, Ariano RE, Anderson BA. Drug Intell Clin Pharm 1990; 24:207–208.

71. Yaari Y, et al. Ann Neurol 1977; 1:334–338.

72. Yaari Y, Pincus JH, Argov Z. Brain Res 1979; 160:479–487.

73. Norris F, Colella J, McFarlin D. Neurology (Minneapolis) 1964; 14:869–876.

74. Brumlik J, Jacobs RS. Can J Neurol Sci 1974; 1:127–129.

75. Regli F, Guggenheim P. Nervenarzt 1965; 36:315–318.

76. Peterson H. N Engl J Med 1966; 274:506–507.

77. Booker HE, Chun RWM, Sanguino M. JAMA 1970; 212:2262–2263.

78. Boneva N, Brenner T, Argov Z. Muscle Nerve 2000; 23:1204–1208.
79. Osserman KE, Genkins G. Mt Sinai J Med 1971; 38:497–537.
80. Alderdice MT, Trommer BA. J Pharmacol Exp Thera 1980; 215:92–96.
81. Thesleff S. Acta Physiol Scand 1956; 37:335–349.
82. Zaidat OO, Kaminski HJ, Berenson F, Katirji B. Muscle Nerve 1999; 22:1293–1296.
83. Rallison ML, Carlisle JW, Less RE, Vernier RL, Good RA. Am J Dis Child 1961; 101:725–738.
84. Talamo RC, Crawford JD. N Engl J Med 1963; 269:15–18.
85. Eaton LM. Proc Staff Meet Mayo Clin 1943; 18:230–236.
86. Harvey AM, Whitehill MR. Bull Johns Hopkins Hosp 1937; 61:216–217.
87. Hughes RO, Zacharias FJ. Br Med J 1976; 1:460–461.
88. Herishanu Y, Rosenberg P. Ann Intern Med 1975; 83:834–835.
89. Coppeto JR. Am J Ophthalmol 1984; 98:244–245.
90. Shaivitz SA. JAMA 1979; 242:1611–1612.
91. Verkijk A. Ann Neurol 1985; 17:211–212.
92. Weber JCP. Lancet 1982; 2:826–827.
93. Jonkers I, Swerup C, Pirskanen R, Bjelak S, Matell G. Muscle Nerve 1996; 19:959–965.
94. Chiarandini DJ. Br J Pharmacol 1980; 69:13–19.
95. Turker K, Kiran B. Arch Int Pharmacodyn 1965; 155(2):356–364.
96. Wislicki L, Rosenblum I. Br J Anaeth 1967; 39:939–942.
97. Usubiaga J. Anesthesiology 1968; 29:484–492.
98. Davis WG. J Pharm Pharmacol 1970; 22:284–290.
99. Patel VK, Jindal MN, Kelkar VV. Ind J Physiol Pharmacol 1974; 18(2):126–128.
100. Harry JD, Linden RJ, Snow HM. Br J Pharmacol 1975; 52:275–281.
101. Lilleheil G, Roed A. Arch Int Pharmacodyn 1971; 194:129–140.
102. Howard JF, Johnson BR, Quint SR. Soc Neurosci Abstr 1987; 13:147–147.
103. Chan-Palay V, Engel AG, Wu JY, Palay SL. Proc Natl Acad Sci USA 1982; 79:7027–7030.
104. Bowman WC. In: Szekeres L, ed. Handbook of Experimental Pharmacology. Berlin: Springer-Verlag, 1981:47–128.
105. K Kaibara, T Akasu, T Tokimasa, K Koketsu, Pflugers Arch, 405: 24–28, 1111
106. Creese R, Head SD, Jenkinson DF. J Physiology 1987; 384:377–403.
107. Ayrapetyan SN, Arvaov VL, Maginyan SB, Azatyan KV. Cell Mol Neurobiol 1985; 5:231–243.
108. Wessler I, Anschutz S. Br J Pharmacol 1988; 94:669–674.
109. Colquhoun D. In: Kharkevich DA, ed. New Neuromuscular Blocking Agents: Handbook of Experimental Pharmacology. Berlin: Springer-Verlag, 1986:59–113.
110. Campbell EDR, Montuschi E. Lancet 1960; 2:789–789.
111. Chiarandini DJ, Bentley PJ. J Pharmacol Exp Ther 1978; 205:49–57.
112. Bikhazi GB, Leung I, Foldes FF. Anesthesiology 1982; 57:A268–A268.
113. Bikhazi GB, Leung I, Foldes FF. Anesthesiology 1983; 59:A269–A269.
114. Van der Kloot W, Kita H. Com Biochem Physiol 1975; 50C:121–125.

115. Ribera AB, Nastuk WL. Com Biochem Physiol C: Compar Pharmacol Toxicol 1989; 93C:137–141.
116. Adams RJ, Rivner MH, Salazar J, Swift TR. Neurology 1984; 34:132–133.
117. Zalman F, Perloff JK, Durant NN, Campion DS. Am Heart J 1983; 105:510–511.
118. Krendel DA, Hopkins LC. Muscle Nerve 1986; 9:519–522.
119. Pina Latorre MA, Cobeta JC, Rodilla F, Navarro N, Zabala S. J Clin Pharm Ther 1998; 23:399–401.
120. Drachman DA, Skom JH. Arch Neurol 1965; 13:316–320.
121. Kornfeld P, Horowitz SH, Genkins G, Papatestas AE. Mt Sinai J Med 1976; 43:10–14.
122. Weisman SJ. JAMA 1949; 141:917–918.
123. Stoffer SS, Chandler JH. Arch Intern Med 1980; 140:283–284.
124. Shy ME, Lange DJ, Howard JF, Gold AP, Lovelace RE, Penn AS. Ann Neurol 1985; 18:120–120.
125. Miller RD, Way WL, Katzung BG. Proc Soc Exp Biol Med 1968; 129:215–218.
126. Sieb JP, Milone M, Engel AG. Brain Res 1996; 712:179–189.
127. Engel WK, Festoff BW, Patten BM, Swerdlow ML, Newball HH, Thompson MD. Ann Intern Med 1974; 81:225–246.
128. Patten BM. Muscle Nerve 1978; 1:190–205.
129. Donaldson JO. Neurology of Pregnancy. Philadelphia: WB Saunders, 1978:58.
130. Grogono AW. Lancet 1963; 2:1039–1040.
131. Way WL, Katzung BG, Larson CP. JAMA 1967; 200:153–154.
132. Dale RC, Schroeder ET. Arch Intern Med 1976; 136:816–818.
133. Wilson SL, Miller RN, Wright C, Hasse D. Anesth Analg Curr Res 1976; 35:1202–1207.
134. Nakamura K, Koide M, Imanaga T, Ogasawara H, Takahashi M, Yoshikawa M. Anaesthesia 1980; 35:1202–1207.
135. Poulton TJ, James FM, Lockridge O. Anesthesiology 1979; 50:54–56.
136. Vacca JB, Knight WA. Mo Med 1957; 54:337–340.
137. Frenkel M, Ehrlich EN. Ann Intern Med 1964; 60:971–981.
138. Bickerstaff ER. Neurological Complication of Oral Contraceptives. London: Oxford University Press, 1975:1–107.
139. Drachman DB. N Engl J Med 1962; 266:330–333.
140. MacLean B, Wilson JAC. Lancet 1954; 2:950–953.
141. Thorner MW. Arch Intern Med 1939; 64:330–335.
142. McEachern D, Parnell JL. J Clin Endocrinol 1948; 8:842–850.
143. Perez A, Perella M, Pastor E, Cano M, Escudero J. Am J Hematol 1995; 49:365–366.
144. Batocchi AP, Evoli A, Servidei S, Palmisani MT, Apollo F, Tonali P. Neurology 1995; 45:382–383.
145. Lensch E, Faust J, Nix WA, Wandel E. Muscle Nerve 1996; 19:927–928.
146. Piccolo G, Franciotta D, Versino M, Alfonsi E, Lombardi M, Poma G. J Neurol Neurosur Psychiatry 1996; 60:348.

147. Mase G, Zorzon M, Biasutti E, Vitrani B, Cazzato G, Urban F, Frezza M. J Neurol Neurosurg Psychiatry 1996; 60:348–349.
148. Konishi T. Rinsho Shinkeigaku Clin Neurol 1996; 36:980–985.
149. Gu D, Wogensen L, Calcutt N, Zhu S, Merlie JP, Fox HS, Lindstrom JM, Powell HC, Sarvetnick N. J Exp Med 1995; 18:547–557.
150. Bora I, Karli N, Bakar M, Zarifoglu M, Turan F, Ogul E. Eur Neurol 1997; 38:68.
151. Uyama E, Fujiki N, Uchino M. J Neurol Sci 1996; 144:221–222.
152. Gurtubay IG, Morales G, Arechaga O, Gallego J. Electromyogr Clin Neurophysiol 1999; 39:75–78.
153. Eddy S, Wim R, Peter VE, Tanja R, Jan T, Werner VS. Dig Dis Sci 1999; 44:186–189.
154. Krendel DA. Semin Neurol 1990; 10:42–45.
155. Fuchs-Buder T, Tassonyi E. B J Anaesth 1996; 76:565–566.
156. Castlebaum AR, Donofrio PD, Walker FO, Troost BT. Neurology 1989; 39:746–747.
157. Randall RE, Cohen MD, Spray CC, Rossmeise EC. Ann Intern Med 1964; 61:73–88.
158. Mordes JP, Wacker WEC. Pharmacol Rev 1978; 29:273–300.
159. Lemcke B, Fucks C. Contrib Nephrol 1984; 38:185–194.
160. Collins EN, Russell PW. Cleveland Clin Q 2002; 16:162–166.
161. Flowers CJ. Am Jo Obstet Gynecol 1965; 91:763–776.
162. Pritchard JA. J Reprod Med 1979; 23:107–114.
163. Lipsitz PJ. Pediatrics 1971; 47:501–509.
164. Fishman RA. Arch Neurol 1965; 12:562–596.
165. Somjen G, Hilmy M, Stephen CR. J Pharmacol Exp Ther 1966; 154:652–659.
166. Hutter OF, Kostial K. J Physiol 1954; 124:234–241.
167. Del Castillo J, Engback L. J Physiol 1954; 124:370–384.
168. Swift TR. Muscle Nerve 1979; 2:295–298.
169. De Silva AJC. Br J Anaesth 1973; 45:1228–1229.
170. Ghoneim MM, Long JP. Anesthesiology 1970; 32:23–27.
171. Bashuk RG, Krendell DA. Muscle Nerve 1987; 10:666–666.
172. Cohen BA, London RS, Goldstein PJ. Obstet Gynecol 1976; 48:35S–37S.
173. George WK, Han CL. Lancet 1962; 2:561–561.
174. Gutmann L, Takamori M. Neurology 1973; 23:977–980.
175. Strieb EW. Ann Neurol 1973; 2:175–176.
176. Ross RM, Baker T. J Clin Anesth 1996; 8:202–204.
177. Alfrey AC, Terman DS, Brettschneider L, Simpson KM, Ogden DA. Ann Intern Med 1970; 73:367–371.
178. Miller RD. Can J Anaesth 1979; 26(2):83–83.
179. Benzing G III, Iannaccone ST, Bove KE, Keebler PJ, Shockley LL. Pediatr Neurol 1990; 6:190–196.
180. Evans RT, MacDonald R, Robinson A. Anaesthesia 1980; 35:198–201.
181. Viby-Mogensen J. Anesthesiology 1981; 55:429–434.
182. Alexander WD. Br Med J 1981; 282.1359–1359.

183. Gesztes T. Br Jo Anaesth 1966; 38:408–409.

184. McQuillen MP, Gross M, Johns RJ. Arch Neurol 1963; 8:402–415.

185. Argov Z, Yaari Y. Brain Res 1979; 164:227–236.

186. Regan AG, Aldrete JA. Anesth Analg 1967; 46:315–318.

187. Bodley PO, Halwax K, Potts L. Br Med J 1969; 3:510–512.

188. Havdala HS, Borison RL, Diamond BI. Anesthesiology 1979; 50:534–537.

189. Vizi ES, Illes P, Ronai A, Knoll J. Neuropharmacology 1972; 11:521–530.

190. Pestronk A, Drachman DB. Science 1980; 210:342–343.

191. Hill GE, Wong KC, Hodges MR. Anesthesiology 1976; 44(5):439–442.

192. Borden H, Clark MT, Katz H. Can Anaesth Soc J 1974; 21:79–82.

193. Eaton LM. Proc Mayo Clin 1947; 22:4–7.

194. Neil JF, Himmelhoch JM, Licata SM. Arch Gen Psychiatry 1976; 33:1090–1092.

195. Granacher RP Jr Am J Psychiatry 1977; 134:702–702.

196. Vartanian GA, Chinyanga HM. Can J Physiol Pharmacol 1972; 50:1099–1103.

197. Jui-Yen T. Jpn J Anesth 1971; 50:491–503.

198. Schumm F, Wietholter H, Fateh-Moghadam A. Dtsch Med Wochenschri 1981; 25:1745–1747.

199. Sghirlanzoni A, Mantegazza R, Mora M, Pareyson D, Cornelio F. Muscle Nerve 1988; 11:114–119.

200. De Bleecker J, De Reuck J, Quatacker J, Meire F. Acta Clin Belg 1991; 46:401–406.

201. Robberecht W, Bednarik J, Bourgeois P, Van Hees J, Carton H. Arch Neurol 1989; 46:464–468.

202. Balint G, Szobor A, Temesvari P, Zahumenszky Z, Bozsoky S. Scand J Rheumatol 1975; 12–21.

203. Dische FE, Swinson DR, Hamilton EBRPV. J Rheumatol 1976; 3:145–154.

204. Hewit J, Benveniste M, Lessana-Leibowitch M. Br Med J 1975; 3:371–371.

205. Cucher BG, Goldman AL. Ann Intern Med 1976; 85:615–616.

206. Schraeder PL. Arch Neurol 1972; 27:456–457.

207. Petersen J, Halberg P, Hojgaard K, Lyon BB, Ullman S. Scand J Rheumatol 1978; 7:113–117.

208. Ansell BM. Postgrad Med J 1974; 50:78–80.

209. Bucknall RC, et al. Br Med J 1975; 1:600–602.

210. Czlonkowska A. Br Med J 1975.

211. Masters CL, et al. Am J Med 1977; 63:689–694.

212. Vincent A, Newsom-Davis J, Martin V. Lancet 1978; 1:1254–1254.

213. Russell AS, Lindstrom JM. Neurology 1978; 28:847–849.

214. Aldrich MS, Kim YI, Sanders DB. Muscle Nerve 1979; 2:180–185.

215. Burres SA, et al. Muscle Nerve 1979; 2:186–190.

216. Menkes CJ, Job-Deslandre C, Bauer-Vinassac D, Rouillon A, Rousseau R. Presse Med 1988; 17:1156–1157.

217. Kirjner M, Lebourges J, Camus JP. La Nouvelle Presse Med 1980; 9:3098.

218. Albers JW, Hodach RJ, Kimmel DW, Treacy WL. Neurology (Minneapolis) 1980; 30:1246–1250.

219. Bazzato G, Coli U, Landini S, Mezzina C, Ciman M. Lancet 1981; 1:1209–1209.
220. De Grandis D, Mezzina C, Fiaschi A, et al. J Neurol Sci 1980; 46:365–371.
221. Jenkins RB, Witorsch P, Smythe NPD. South Med J 1970; 46:365–371.
222. Brown PW. JAMA 1935; 105:1319–1325.
223. Ng KKF. Br J Pharmacol Chemother 1966; 28:228–237.
224. Russell JGB. Br J Radiol 1984; 57:655–655.
225. Canal N, Franceschi M. Lancet 1983; 1:1288.
226. Chagnac Y, Hadanin M, Goldhammer Y. Neurology 1985; 35:1219–1220.
227. Frank JH, Cooper GW, Black WC, Phillips LH. Neurology 1987; 37:1400–1402.
228. Van den Bergh P, Kelly JJ, Carter B, Munsat TL. Ann Neurol 1986; 19:206–207.
229. Ionescu-Drinea M, Vioculescu V, Serbanescu G, Nicolau C. Rev Roum Neurol 1973; 10:239–243.
230. Chasapakis G, Dimas C. Br J Anaesth 1966; 38:838–839.
231. Ueno S, Takahashi M, Kajiyama K, Okahisa N, Hazama T, Yorifuji S, Tarui S. Neurology 1987; 37:832–833.
232. Erbguth F, Claus D, Engelhardt A, Dressler D. J Neurol Neurosurg Psychiatry 1993; 56:1235–1236.
233. Borodic G. Lancet Dec 5, 1998; 352:1832.
234. J Emmerson, Mov Disord 9:367–1994
235. Tsai MC, Mansour NA, Eldefrawi AT, Eldefrawi ME, Albuquerque EX. Mol Pharmacol 1978; 14:787–803.
236. Dretchen KL, Morgenroth VH. Anesthesiology 1976; 45:604–609.
237. Abdel-Aziz A, Bakry N. Eur J Pharmacol 1973; 22:169–174.

Index

Acetyl coenzyme A (acetyl-CoA),
23–24
Acetylcholine (ACh)
binding, 25–26
hydrolysis, 25
release (*see* Synaptic vesicles)
in synaptic vesicles, 5
synthesis of, 23–24, 192
Acetylcholine receptor (AchR),
9–13
adult
in extraocular muscles, 9–10
vs. fetal, 9–10, 26
agrin and aggregation of, 13
binding sites, 10–11, 12*f*
clustering, 13
deficiency, 217–220
fetal, 9–10, 193
half-life of, 107
ion passage, 25–26
main immunogenic region, 11
rapsyn and aggregation of, 13, 193
structure of, 9–11
subunits, 9–11, 193–195

[Acetylcholine receptor (AchR)]
genes encoding, 195*t*
as target autoantigen in MG,
104–105
turnover, 13
Acetylcholine receptor antibodies,
90–91
binding, 90–91, 114
blocking, 92, 114
false positive, 91
modulating, 92, 114
Acetylcholinesterase (AChE)
location at the endplate, 8–9, 9*f*
role in neuromuscular transmission,
25
Acetylcholinesterase inhibitors
ambenonium chloride (Mytelase),
118, 119*t*
edrophonium, 114–115
equivalent doses, 118–119, 119*t*
in Lambert-Eaton syndrome, 180
in myasthenia gravis, 117–119
in neonatal myasthenia gravis,
143

about the authors...

MATTHEW N. MERIGGIOLI is Director of the Neuromuscular Disorders Section, the Electromyography Laboratory, and the Myasthenia Gravis Clinic, as well as Assistant Clinical Professor, Rush-Presbyterian-St. Luke's Medical Center, Chicago, Illinois. The author or coauthor of numerous professional publications, he is a member of the American Academy of Neurology, the American Association of Electrodiagnostic Medicine, and serves on the scientific advisory board of the Myasthenia Gravis Foundation of America, among other organizations. He received the B.S. degree (1982) in biology and mathematics from Loyola University of Chicago, Illinois, and the M.D. degree (1990) from the University of Health Sciences/The Chicago Medical School, North Chicago, Illinois. Dr. Meriggioli completed his residency (1994) in neurology at the Loyola University of Chicago, Illinois, and his fellowship in neuromuscular disease (1996) at Duke University, Durham, North Carolina.

JAMES F. HOWARD, JR. is Chief of the Neuromuscular Disorders Section, Director of the EMG Laboratory, Department of Neurology, and Professor of Neurology and Medicine, University of North Carolina at Chapel Hill. He is also Codirector of the Muscular Dystrophy Association Clinic. The author or coauthor of numerous professional publications, he serves on the Board of Directors for the American Association of Electrodiagnostic Medicine and is Chair of the National Medical and Scientific Advisory Board of the Myasthenia Gravis Foundation of America. He is a member of the Medical Advisory Committee of the Muscular Dystrophy Association and founding associate editor of the *Journal of Clinical Neuromuscular Diseases*. He received the B.S. degree (1970) from the University of Vermont, Burlington, and the M.D. degree (1974) from the University of Vermont School of Medicine, Burlington.

C. MICHEL HARPER, JR. is Director of the Electromyography Lab and Codirector of the Neuromuscular Clinic, Department of Neurology Mayo Clinic, Vice Chair of the Department of Neurology; and Associate Professor of Neurology, Mayo Clinic Foundation, Rochester, Minnesota. The author or coauthor of numerous professional publications, he is a member of the American Board of Electrodiagnostic Medicine, the American Board of Psychiatry and Neurology, and the Myasthenia Gravis Foundation of America, among other organizations. He received the M.S. degree (1978) from the University of Nebraska Medical Center, Omaha, and the M.D. degree (1981) from the University of Nebraska College of Medicine, Omaha.

ISBN 0-8247-4079-3